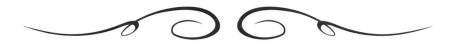

Clinical Perspectives on Multiple Personality Disorder

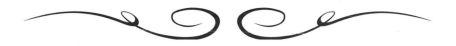

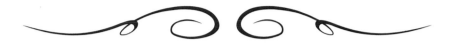

Clinical Perspectives on Multiple Personality Disorder

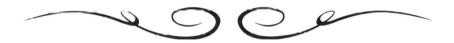

Edited by

Richard P. Kluft, M.D.
Director, Dissociative Disorders Program
The Institute of Pennsylvania Hospital
Clinical Professor of Psychiatry
Temple University School of Medicine
Philadelphia, Pennsylvania

Catherine G. Fine, Ph.D.
Program Coordinator, Dissociative
  Disorders Program
The Institute of Pennsylvania Hospital
Clinical Assistant Professor of Psychiatry
Temple University School of Medicine
Philadelphia, Pennsylvania

Washington, DC
London, England

Copyright © 1993 American Psychiatric Press
ALL RIGHTS RESERVED
Manufactured in the United States of America on acid-free paper
96 95 94 93   4 3 2
First Edition

American Psychiatric Press, Inc.
1400 K Street, N.W., Washington, DC 20005

Library of Congress Cataloging-in-Publication Data
Clinical perspectives on multiple personality disorder / edited by
  Richard P. Kluft, Catherine G. Fine. — 1st ed.
      p. cm.
    Includes bibliographical references and index.
    ISBN 0-88048-365-2 (alk. paper)
    1. Multiple personality.   I. Kluft, Richard P., 1943–   .
  II. Fine, Catherine G., 1950–   .
      [DNLM: 1. Multiple-Personality Disorder—therapy. WM 173.6 C641]
    RC569.5.M8C55 1993
    616.85'236—dc20
    DNLM/DLC   92-48949
    for Library of Congress   CIP

British Library Cataloguing in Publication Data
A CIP record is available from the British Library.

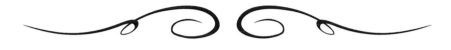

To Connie

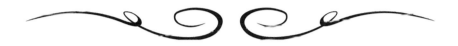

In memory of
Cornelia B. Wilbur, M.D.,
who passed away
April 10, 1992

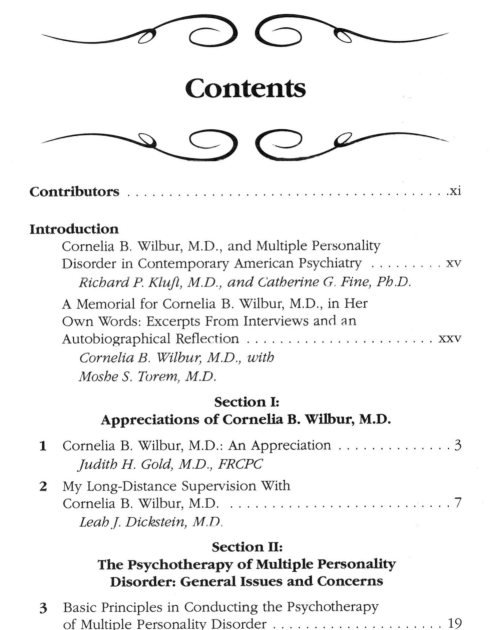

Contents

Section IV:
Contemporary Issues and Concerns in the
Study of Multiple Personality Disorder

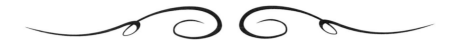

Contributors

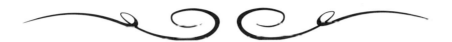

Andy Andrei
Supportive Counselor, Bangor Mental Health Institute, Bangor, Maine

Reina Attias, Ph.D.
Psychotherapist in Private Practice, Albuquerque and Santa Fe, New Mexico

Bennett G. Braun, M.D.
Director, Section on Psychiatric Trauma, Rush-Presbyterian-St. Luke's Medical Center, Chicago, Illinois; Medical Director, Dissociative Disorders Program, Rush-North Shore Medical Center, Skokie, Illinois

Philip M. Coons, M.D.
Associate Professor of Psychiatry, Indiana University School of Medicine, and Staff Psychiatrist, Larue D. Carter Memorial Hospital, Indianapolis, Indiana

Robert A. deVito, M.D.
Professor and Chairman, Department of Psychiatry, Stritch School of Medicine, Loyola University, and Chief, Psychiatry Service, Loyola University Medical Center, Chicago, Illinois

Leah J. Dickstein, M.D.
Professor, Department of Psychiatry and Behavioral Sciences, and Associate Dean for Faculty and Student Advocacy, University of Louisville School of Medicine, Louisville, Kentucky

Joen Fagan, Ph.D.
Regents Professor Emeritus, Department of Psychology,
Georgia State University, and Psychologist in Private Practice,
Atlanta, Georgia

Catherine G. Fine, Ph.D.
Program Coordinator, Dissociative Disorders Program, The
Institute of Pennsylvania Hospital, and Clinical Assistant
Professor of Psychiatry, Temple University School of Medicine,
Philadelphia, Pennsylvania

David L. Fink, M.D.
Associate Director, Dissociative Disorders Program,
The Institute of Pennsylvania Hospital,
Philadelphia, Pennsylvania

Judith H. Gold, M.D., FRCPC
Psychiatrist in Private Practice, Halifax, Nova Scotia

Jean M. Goodwin, M.D., M.P.H.
Professor of Psychiatry, Department of Psychiatry and
Behavioral Sciences, University of Texas Medical Branch,
Galveston, Texas

George B. Greaves, Ph.D.
Clinical and Forensic Psychologist in Private Practice,
Atlanta, Georgia

Richard P. Kluft, M.D.
Director, Dissociative Disorders Program, The Institute of
Pennsylvania Hospital, and Clinical Professor of Psychiatry,
Temple University School of Medicine,
Philadelphia, Pennsylvania

Richard J. Loewenstein, M.D.
Director, Dissociative Disorders Program, Sheppard and
Enoch Pratt Hospital, and Assistant Clinical Professor of
Psychiatry, University of Maryland School of Medicine,
Baltimore, Maryland

Polly Paul McMahon, Ph.D.
Psychologist in Private Practice, Macon, Georgia

Frank W. Putnam, Jr., M.D.
Chief, Unit on Dissociative Disorders, Laboratory of
Developmental Psychology, National Institute of Mental Health,
Bethesda, Maryland

Lucy G. Quimby, Ph.D.
Psychologist in Private Practice, Bangor, Maine

Roberta G. Sachs, Ph.D.
Senior Clinical Consultant, Dissociative Disorders Program,
Rush-North Shore Medical Center, Skokie, Illinois

David Spiegel, M.D.
Professor, Department of Psychiatry and Behavioral Science,
Stanford University Medical Center, Stanford, California

Moshe S. Torem, M.D.
Professor and Chairman, Department of Psychiatry,
Northeastern Ohio Universities College of Medicine, Rootstown,
Ohio; Chairman, Department of Psychiatry, Akron General
Medical Center, Akron, Ohio

Helen H. Watkins, M.A.
Formerly Staff Therapist, University of Montana Counseling
Center, Missoula, Montana; Psychologist in Private Practice,
Missoula, Montana

John G. Watkins, Ph.D.
Professor Emeritus, Department of Psychology, University of
Montana, Missoula, Montana

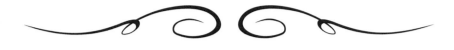

Introduction

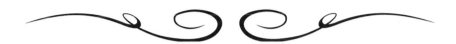

Cornelia B. Wilbur, M.D., and
Multiple Personality Disorder in
Contemporary American Psychiatry

The advent of the current renaissance of interest in multiple personality disorder (MPD) is inextricably intertwined with the career and the landmark contributions of Cornelia B. Wilbur, M.D. Although her publications were few and most contemporary authors in the field make minimal reference to her name and work, the articles we read today are nonetheless suffused with her thought, bear the mark of her influence, and attest to the lasting impact of her presence. Cornelia B. Wilbur, M.D., known to her colleagues and friends as Connie, provided the role model and inspiration for the generation of clinicians, scholars, and scientific investigators whose efforts, observations, and explorations followed, developed, and mapped the trails that she had blazed—all too often in solitude and isolation. Her death on April 10, 1992, leaves us saddened and bereft of a friend and leader. She passed away while *Clinical Perspectives on Multiple Personality Disorder* was in production, but she was well aware of the project and had enjoyed many of the articles in draft form before her final illness.

There is a tired and well-worn jest: "You can always tell who the pioneers are: they're the ones with the most arrows in their backs."

Connie wore the dubious decorations of the pioneer with grace and forbearance. She endured more than her fair share of adversity—she was a woman at a time when medicine was preeminently a man's field. Moreover, she was a strong woman with ambition and keen insights who would not graciously "stay in her place." Her courage, compassion, and creativity brought her to the fore. Her most striking contributions were made in an area still fraught with controversy, but that, in her day, was treated with condescension, lack of interest, and arrogant disdain. Those few who became associated with the study of MPD literally were taking their careers and their reputations in their hands. It is discouraging to reflect that many of the most useful insights into the treatment of MPD that have been published in the last decade by other authors might have been available a quarter of a century earlier had the scientific literature of her day not rejected the still unpublished clinical papers of Connie Wilbur. It is painfully ironic that Connie's first scientific publications on the treatment of MPD occurred virtually on the eve of her retirement from clinical practice.

However, it is a blessing that Connie was able to influence as many mental health professionals as she did. Whether they came to know her from Flora Rheta Schreiber's *Sybil* (1973) or in the movie of the same name, heard her lecture, received instruction in workshops, or sought her out for consultation or supervision, they came away inspired, enriched, enlightened, and often amazed. Connie was a gifted teacher and clinician whose trademarks were generosity, honesty, integrity, courage, compassion, and directness. Nonetheless, she was both gentle and tolerant, eager to help others develop to their fullest potential in their own way, and quick to warn the overidealizing neophyte against slavish imitation.

It may well be that just because Connie was so generous in helping others to grow in their own way and so disinclined to be lionized that there are hardly any dramatic or striking Connie Wilbur stories that get passed along among those who were so influenced by her. When Connie comes up in conversation among those in the dissociative disorders field, there are no intriguing tales to tell—only unsensational but sensitive accounts that acknowledge her consistent courage, her generous helpfulness, and the importance of her example and her advice. A few illustrations of the nature of her quiet but powerful impact may serve to explain to those who have never met her the high esteem in which she was and always will be held.

In the mid-1970s one of us (Richard P. Kluft), barely out of training, sought out Connie after one of her lectures and told her he had seen a few patients with MPD and was encountering rather negative reactions from colleagues. The interchange was brief, and a most striking aspect of the conversation was the total absence of any dramatic utterances or striking pronouncements. Connie was not inclined to show off her capacities or to try to make an impression. She listened attentively and reacted with seriousness and respect in a way that erased the differential of years and experience that might have created a barrier between them. She made a sensitive acknowledgment of the difficulties described to her and offered a few words of encouragement. The conversation could go no further, because there were many others present who wanted to speak to Connie, but it had a striking impact because of the quality of respect Connie was able to convey in just a few words—a respect that magnified the impact of whatever she had to say. With Connie, one always knew one had been listened to and heard. Over the years there were several other brief encounters, and finally a friendship, but the tenor of the relationship was always the same—interest, respect, encouragement.

One of us (Catherine G. Fine) entered the dissociative disorders field just as Connie was reducing her clinical and teaching obligations. Her actual contact with Connie was minimal. However, in that contact it was impossible not to be touched and influenced by the role model Connie provided. At an age when she was entitled to do little but accept acknowledgments and compliments, Connie continued as a frontline teacher, although she taught less frequently than before. With a stature that entitled her to the most special considerations, she requested none and would accept none. She was a team player who worked well in workshop settings with those she once had taught and encouraged. With a fame that might justify her restricting her availability, Connie spent hours at conferences surrounded by those who wanted her advice or who simply wanted to meet the woman who had done so much for the advancement of our understanding of MPD. It is easy to recall dozens of images of

Connie, listening and responding to colleague after colleague, always with an easy grace and genuine friendliness. Connie's example has been widely emulated throughout the field, making the annual International Conferences on Multiple Personality/Dissociation warm and welcoming events, where the accessibility of the major workers in the field to those who attend is the rule rather than the exception.

What has become of MPD since Connie Wilbur began her groundbreaking work and her encouragement of those who took an interest in the plight of patients with MPD? Few if any mental disorders have entered the clinical mainstream with such rapidity and in such an atypical manner. In the 1970s and up to the early 1980s, MPD was regarded as a rarity. The scientific literature was minimal up to 1980—alone among major mental disorders, MPD was depicted more commonly in the media and the lay literature than in scientific publications. With its often striking phenomena and the complex and intricate lives often led by those afflicted by it, MPD seemed to be a subject fit more for soap opera than for science. The drama and fascination that surrounded MPD contributed to the skepticism of the mental health professions and the disdain for work in this area.

In the intervening years a burgeoning literature has demonstrated that MPD is a rather commonplace dissociative variant of the adaptive responses of children overwhelmed by exogenous trauma. A preoccupation with the arresting phenomena of the personalities has given way to a grim realization that MPD is no more than the attempt of a beleaguered youngster, unable to escape or defend against external adversity, to flee inwardly and create alternative selves and alternative constructs of reality that allow the possibility of psychological survival. The belief that MPD could be treated only by a handful of specially gifted clinicians has yielded to an appreciation that the conscientious mental health professional who makes a serious attempt to master the challenges involved in working with such patients can move from a position of feeling exasperated and deskilled to a stance of competence and expertise. Those who once worked in isolation can now network, collaborate, and meet with colleagues struggling with similar clinical concerns. Study groups have sprung up in most areas of the United States. A wealth of courses, conferences, and workshops are available to the clinician who wants to acquire or refine the clinical skills necessary for work with MPD patients. In 1993, MPD is a clinical commonplace in many parts of the country and is recognized with increasing frequency abroad.

An intriguing aspect of this rapid advance is that the vast majority of significant contributions in the MPD field have not been made by scientific investigators and clinicians who were senior, established, and well-recognized contributors to the literature. In the main, the study of MPD has been a bottom-up rather than a top-down phenomenon. A mere handful of grants have been awarded for the study of the dissociative disorders. Most published papers have emerged from work undertaken, sustained, and supported at the initiative and expense of the authors. Many of them have been primarily clinicians, attempting to organize the observations they have made in the course of their clinical work. As a result, the spread of knowledge about the dissociative disorders often has been from the clinician to the researcher and from those outside of academe to those within. Fortunately, the efforts of the early contributors has been sufficient to establish the field and generate an interest in MPD and dissociative phenomena within research and academic circles. The last few years have witnessed an escalation of such involvement.

As more mental health professionals have taken an interest in MPD and have begun to contend with the clinical challenge of treating MPD patients, the need to make clinically relevant information more readily available has become apparent. To a certain extent this is addressed by books by Braun (1986), Putnam (1989), and Ross (1989) and by the journal *Dissociation*. However, the field remains so new that many basic clinical issues have yet to be addressed, and it has progressed so fast that its recent history has yet to be recorded.

Clinical Perspectives on Multiple Personality Disorder began as a Festschrift in honor of Connie Wilbur. It was expanded in scope because it seemed a truer testimony to Connie to address a wide variety of topics that are of relevance to those who work with MPD patients but that, for the most part, have not yet been explored in depth in the available literature. The first section of *Clinical Perspectives* is made up of appreciations of Connie Wilbur and follows a vivid interview portrait of Connie. The second section consists of a series of articles that outline some overarching concerns in the psychotherapy of MPD that have not been explored in depth elsewhere; the third continues to demonstrate, in case-oriented illustrations, aspects of the treatment of MPD that are of considerable importance, but are largely absent from the literature to date. *Clinical Perspectives* concludes with a section that presents a discussion of a number of issues that concern contemporary clinicians, and with a review of the recent history of MPD.

The first section of this book is preceded by a memorial to Connie Wilbur in her own words. We are indebted to Moshe S. Torem, M.D., for his kindness in allowing the reprinting of portions of one of the few recorded interviews with Connie, and excerpts of an autobiographical piece of Connie's that he edited to her approval. Chapters 1 and 2 are by Judith H. Gold and Leah J. Dickstein, both of whom knew Connie well. Their personal accounts testify to the contributions Connie made simply in the course of being herself and by making herself available to her colleagues.

The next group of six chapters concerns general issues in the treatment of MPD. In Chapter 3, Richard P. Kluft discusses basic principles in the psychotherapy of MPD, condensing findings from experience in treating patients with MPD and consulting to hundreds of other therapists. He attempts to outline those stances that seem, pragmatically, to be associated with successful treatments, and discusses the problems associated with their alteration or omission. Next, in Chapter 4, Richard J. Loewenstein offers thoughtful insights into the impact of traumatic experiences and dissociative phenomena on transference and countertransference in the treatment of MPD, sharing new and helpful insights into some of the most difficult and frequently disconcerting aspects of work with such patients. This is followed by the observations of David Spiegel in Chapter 5 on the treatment of MPD as a posttraumatic condition. He perceives MPD as a series of posttraumatic adjustments that can be approached with primary attention to trauma and the restructuring of dissociative phenomena.

Then, Richard P. Kluft offers a general overview in Chapter 6 of the process of integration, a central aspect of the treatment of patients with MPD that he believes can be illustrated far more easily than it can be understood. Attempts to articulate cohesive overall treatment strategies in MPD are rare. In Chapter 7, Catherine G. Fine discusses pacing and formulates the perspective of the tactical integrationalist approach, in which integration is achieved by the accomplishment of a series of intermediate graded therapeutic objectives. The simplicity of her recommendations and approaches makes them readily accessible models. Concluding this section, Bennett G. Braun offers in Chapter 8 a rich series of experience-based perspectives on the hospital treatment of MPD, drawing on his familiarity with the treatment of such patients in a number of inpatient settings. His recommendations and caveats are useful guidelines.

The third section consists of case studies that illustrate the application of techniques, approaches, and insights that are considered important, but are difficult to learn because they have not been documented in detail in the literature. In Chapter 9, Frank W. Putnam, Jr., demolishes the usual stereotype of the MPD patient (the intelligent, articulate, and creative woman) by his sensitive and often wrenching account of the treatment of an aggressive, difficult, and often uncommunicative inner-city African American adolescent male with MPD. His ability to modify techniques and approaches in the face of his patient's unique circumstances is enlightening. Lucy G. Quimby, Andy Andrei, and Frank W. Putnam, Jr., in Chapter 10 study the dilemma of the MPD patient who has long been institutionalized under erroneous diagnoses. They offer a model for resocializing the chronic patient that respects and works within the limitations of resources and personnel encountered in the state hospital system.

The use of Amytal-facilitated interviews in the treatment of MPD is often alluded to, yet rarely depicted. In Chapter 11, Robert A. deVito makes it possible to follow a patient from diagnosis through integration with a focus on the role of this modality, and describes the procedure and some interviews in helpful detail. One of the ongoing problems in bringing together the rich literature of psychoanalysis with the clinical phenomena encountered in MPD is the difficulty many authors have had in remaining true to both areas of knowledge without distorting the one to fit the findings or theories of the other. In Chapter 12, David L. Fink demonstrates the usefulness of Winnicott's observations on transitional objects and transitional phenomena in understanding a number of rarely discussed but frequently encountered MPD behaviors.

There is increasing interest in the recognition and treatment of children with dissociative disorders, but no extensive case studies of such therapies has been available. Polly Paul McMahon and Joen Fagan remedy this deficit in Chapter 13 with their description of the play therapy of such a child. Ego-state therapy is often discussed in connection with the dissociative disorders. In Chapter 14, Helen H. Watkins and John G. Watkins offer a detailed description of the application of this technique with a patient with a mild ego-state disorder that has the underlying structure of MPD. Those in the MPD field are eager to learn and employ any new approach that will facilitate the treatment of such patients. This section ends with an innovative discussion in Chapter 15 from Roberta G. Sachs of the application of sand tray methods to their treatment.

The final section of *Clinical Perspectives* touches on some contemporary concerns in the field and on the recent history of the study of MPD, the context in which the contributions of Connie Wilbur and others must be understood and appreciated. In Chapter 16, Philip M. Coons describes his experiences in setting up a clinic for the assessment of suspected MPD patients and illustrates some of the typical types of concerns that are encountered in offering consultation to a wide variety of colleagues. The coexistence of eating disorders and MPD is a frequent clinical phenomenon, and the appreciation and treatment of the coexisting pathologies can prove to be a challenge. In separate chapters (17 and 18), Jean M. Goodwin and Reina Attias as well as Moshe S. Torem offer important contributions to the study of these phenomena. *Clinical Perspectives* concludes with fascinating perspectives on the history of MPD from George B. Greaves and his attempt to reformulate the condition in view of that history and in consideration of certain vexing clinical phenomena. Chapter 19 is thus the first contemporary effort to document the events of the last several years in the MPD field and is written by a participant observer who himself is unquestionably among the pioneers.

Richard P. Kluft, M.D.
Catherine G. Fine, Ph.D.

References

Braun BG (ed): Treatment of Multiple Personality Disorder. Washington, DC, American Psychiatric Press, 1986

Putnam FW: The Diagnosis and Treatment of Multiple Personality Disorder. New York, Guilford, 1989

Ross CA: Multiple Personality Disorder: Diagnosis, Clinical Features, and Treatment. New York, Wiley, 1989

Schreiber FR: Sybil. Chicago, IL, Regnery, 1973

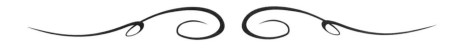

A Memorial for
Cornelia B. Wilbur, M.D.,
in Her Own Words:
Excerpts From Interviews and
an Autobiographical Reflection

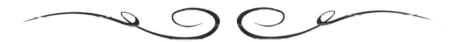

Cornelia B. Wilbur, M.D., with Moshe S. Torem, M.D.

Cornelia B. Wilbur, M.D., died on April 10, 1992, while the final revisions to the text of this book were being made. The young clinicians of today will remember her portrayal in Sybil *(Schreiber 1973) and hear about her from those who knew her. That is, for the most part, they must conjure up a picture of her from her representations in lay sources and from the recollections of others. Fortunately, Moshe S. Torem, M.D., interviewed Connie shortly before she became ill and unable to continue her lecturing and teaching, and he edited her autobiographical remarks to her approval. Both the interview and the autobiographical piece, humorously entitled "Sybil and Me: How I Got That Way," appeared in* Trauma and Recovery *in 1990 and 1991 (Torem 1990; Wilbur 1991). With Dr. Torem's permission and the consent of* Trauma and Recovery, *we present some excerpts that allow Connie to speak for herself. In the interest of readability, we have not indicated omissions from the original text.—The Editors*

I suppose the publication of *Sybil* and the forerunners and aftermath were a function of the times as well as my personality style, my professional background and training. I was the only daughter of a very intelligent couple, and I had two older brothers. My paternal grandfather, my father, and I all had red hair; thus I was identified with them from birth. The identification was rather powerful. My father had a Ph.D. in chemistry. It was anticipated that since I was like my father, I would have my father's brain power. I was expected to have reasonably good grades. If I was puzzled [at school] I could ask all the questions I wanted and get all of the answers at home.

I lived in Montana until age 10, the last 6 years on a ranch. The teacher happened to be my father, who was the only well-educated individual in the area and began the school because there were children there who needed to be taught.

[After living in Cleveland] when I was ready for college it was assumed that I was going into chemistry because it was my father's field. At the end of 2 years it was obvious that the girl's college which I attended did not have sufficient education in chemistry for me to continue. [On my father's advice I transferred to Michigan where] I subsequently got my bachelor's degree with a major in chemistry.

It was the beginning of the Great Depression, 1930, when I graduated with a bachelor's degree. I could find no work, so I arranged to go back to school to get a master's degree in chemistry. I did this, but found that I became very bored with chemistry; and by the end of the last semester of my master's work, I felt that if I had to deal with any more test tubes, I would deal with them by dropping them on the floor and breaking them.

I went to the medical school and told the dean that I would like to go into medicine. Applications had dropped off significantly because of the Great Depression. I entered medical school and developed acute thyroid disease. I was taken out of school, operated on, and told to go home and return, to begin again. I graduated without difficulty in 1939 and was accepted for an internship and residency in psychiatry at the University of Michigan.

In the late winter of my first year of residency, Dr. Waggener [the chairman] informed me that my contract would not be renewed. This was unusual, unless you wished to go, or unless you had done something that created difficulties for you and were asked to leave. Neither of these were true of me, so I was shaken and completely astounded. I finally got the courage to [see Dr. Waggener]. I asked him why my contract was not being renewed. I thought the question was quite plain, but Dr. Waggener replied, "You have a great deal of nerve to question my decision." Since I wasn't questioning his decision, I simply sat there with my mouth open because what I really wanted to know was what I had done which put me in jeopardy with him and with my future. He was very angry and stood up behind his desk, leaned across it toward me and said, "I have some advice for you, young lady; I know that you are deeply in debt, and I would advise you to go to a State Hospital and make enough money to get out of debt, and then, not only get out of psychiatry, but get out of medicine." He dismissed me. I was simply terribly angry and recognized I was being treated unfairly, but did not know why.

I went to Pontiac State Hospital and was more than welcomed. I was treated well and given a great deal of information, education, and opportunity to work with many patients.

By this time, World War II was on, and I found a position with A. E. Bennett at the University of Nebraska that paid much better and also provided neurological training. There I worked on the average 12 hours a day, 7 days a week. I had one of my first experiences with [a patient with] unadulterated hysteria. I learned to administer electroconvulsive treatment without noticeable muscular trauma, since Dr. Bennett was the individual who developed the use of curare with electroshock therapy. I also had an opportunity to do research with Thorazine.

At the end of the war, the physician whose place I had taken came back and I decided to go to New York and get my analytic training. So, I went to New York where I was offered a position as Head of Education for the outpatient services of the Veterans Administration in New York City. Under this program, I had residents from all five medical schools in the area, but after 2 years the Veterans Administration refused to fund it and we were forced to close many clinics. Since this took all the joy out of the efforts we were making, I decided to go into private practice.

Now, I need to return to a time when I was in Omaha. I was asked to see a young lady who seemed to have some difficulties. I diagnosed her as having hysteria. I saw her for several months. She was a school teacher and had told me that she wanted to get her master's degree in the teaching of art at Columbia University. In 1952, she came to New York and began her training. I began to see her on a once-a-week basis. One day, when she was talking to me about something that should have made her angry, she jumped off the couch, went over and stuck her fist through one of the window panes in my office. I jumped out of my chair, ran over, grabbed her wrist and said, "Let me see if you cut yourself." She ducked down, hunched her shoulders, peered up at me and said, "Let me go." I said, "No, I want to see your hand, and if you cut yourself." She looked at me and said, "Am I more important than the window?" I said, "Certainly. A handyman can fix the window, but if you are cut, it would take a doctor to sew you up." She had not cut herself, but she was not talking like her typical self. She looked younger and frightened, so I asked her a spontaneous question, "Who are you?" She said, "I am Peggy." I thought immediately that this must be a dual personality, but I said nothing to the patient about this.

The next time this patient was due in the office, I opened the door, and here was a young woman in high heels, hair piled on top of her head, very elegant looking, who looked at me and said, "I am sorry, Sybil was ill today, so I came—I am Vicky." I said, "Come in," and during this hour "Vicky" apprised me of the fact that, yes there is "Peggy" and herself and "others" as well as Sybil, but I should not tell Sybil this because it would upset her. So, here I was with a Multiple Personality, never having diagnosed one before, never having treated one, and not really knowing what to do. I was, as usual, very excited about this new kind of case.

I went on working with Sybil and wrote papers on dissociation and hysteria, and Multiple Personality. When I sent them for publication, I was told that it was a very unusual condition, so rare that this journal would not be able to use it.

After a number of these rejections, I decided I was going to get published no matter what, so I gave a paper on transference and countertransference in Multiple Personality at the meeting of the

American Academy of Psychoanalysis. Now, the American Academy of Psychoanalysis had a yearly meeting at which a number of papers were presented and all of them were published, so that I expected mine to be published too. Three months after the meeting was held, the individual who was responsible for the publication of the papers called me and said the publisher had space limitations. I got angry and decided that if I could not depend on my colleagues, I could certainly depend on the public. The public would find this very interesting, and they might be able to persuade psychiatrists to look for it, diagnose it, and treat it.

I had the good fortune to have been interviewed by Flora Rheta Schreiber for a piece, and she had written everything absolutely correct.

Therefore, I called her and asked her if she would like to write up this case for popular consumption and she was interested, but she wanted to meet the person first, and then said she would not begin the work until the patient was completely integrated as one individual. This eventually happened, and Flora Schreiber spent a considerable amount of time with me and Sybil and came up with a manuscript for a book.

The agent sold the book to [a company that sold] their book publishing to Henry Regnery Publishing Co. in Chicago. They received the manuscript, but by this time, the Regnery Publishing Company had been turned over to Henry Regnery's son-in-law, who informed us that he did not want the manuscript. However, he did give the manuscript to his wife to read. I was told that she, without doing the dishes or spending any time putting the children to bed, read the entire manuscript, and at 3:00 A.M. dropped it on top of her husband when he was asleep and said, "Publish this." So, the book was published, and of course, became a best-seller. Then, it was picked up to be produced as a television movie by Lorimar Productions. It is interesting that *Sybil's* success tended to rescue contemporary books from something of adult doldrums, and it put Lorimar Productions on the map.

However, I was not treated as kindly as either the publisher or the filmmaker.

The book was reviewed by Dominique A. Barbara, M.D., [who

wrote] "Flora Schreiber has given us a brilliant and powerful portrayal of a Multiple Personality, This book is destined to stand as a significant landmark in both psychiatry and literature." [However] in the *American Journal of Psychiatry*, 132:2, February 1975, a letter appeared from Dr. George Victor, a psychologist from Livingston, New Jersey, who stated: "The proper diagnosis is folie à deux." [Dr. Victor went on to accuse me of talking Sybil into believing in her personalities. Dr. Barbara wrote a reply in my defense, emphasizing the legitimacy of the diagnosis.]

I have had individuals stand at meetings where I am present and say that Multiple Personality Disorder is fakery, is produced by the psychiatrist, therapist, and so forth.

I have never seen a formal thought disorder in a Multiple Personality. Mentation is not disordered in MPD. Many patients with MPD have been diagnosed with Borderline Personality Disorder simply because they read people and tend to use what they know to defend themselves. This is considered manipulative. Because they have had to cope with abusive parents, relatives, neighbors, and so forth from infancy on, they become quite adept at influencing people in order to protect themselves. This is not true of borderline patients, who are manipulative for other reasons. MPD is clearly a defense disorder against overwhelming emotional and physical trauma and is more closely related to [post]traumatic stress disorder than anything else. The diagnosis of MPD, from my standpoint, is obtained like any other scientific fact, and is sustained by observation. Therefore, I tend to consider the individuals who do not make the diagnosis of MPD, from time to time, as very poor observers, or simply ignorant. MPD cannot be treated by any medication, except for occasional medication for overriding symptoms. These patients can be treated by any individual who has a clear view of how to treat [post]traumatic stress disorder or severe character disorders.

I think that Sybil and I have contributed to the recovery of a good many MPD patients and to fascinating and ongoing research.

Amen to that, Connie!—The Editors

References

Schreiber FR: Sybil. New York, Regnery, 1973

Torem MS: A dialogue with Dr. Cornelia Wilbur. Trauma and Recovery 3(1):8–12, 1990

Wilbur CB: Sybil and me: how I got this way. Trauma and Recovery 4(2):4–7, 1991

Section I

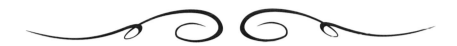

Appreciations
of
Cornelia B. Wilbur, M.D.

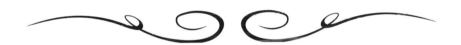

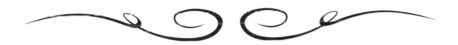

Chapter 1

Cornelia B. Wilbur, M.D.:
An Appreciation

Judith H. Gold, M.D., FRCPC

About 12 years ago, at a psychiatric meeting in Texas, a woman with orange-blonde hair, big blue eyes, and long eyelashes came up to me and said "I'm Connie Wilbur. Where did you get that gold chain?" After that initial meeting, I met her at many such conferences and had the pleasure of spending many enjoyable and educational hours with one of America's most famous psychotherapists.

Connie endeared herself to generations of psychotherapists by her interest in them as people and by her willingness to listen to their clinical problems and assist them. Always available to give advice and supervision, she answered telephone requests and spent time at meetings with colleagues. Interspersed with this was her ability to share herself and her own experiences with others, while never hesitating to join a party or to address an audience.

It is this happy combination of qualities that made her an outspoken and effective advocate for the equality of women, especially in their professional lives, while rebutting all challenges to the existence of the clinical entity of multiple personality disorder (MPD). In the book *Women Physicians in Leadership Roles* (Dickstein and Nadelson 1985), Connie described her early years in psychiatry. Her words made clear her personal familiarity with the struggles women still encounter today in progressing in our profession.

Connie usually said very little about the lack of recognition of her work by the general psychiatric world. Being a trailblazer was never easy. She chose a path that still is not accepted unequivocally but that has gained considerable acceptance, due in large part to her own efforts and the work of those she influenced. As biological psychiatry grew more and more prominent, Connie continued to write and speak about conditions that required hundreds of hours of psycho-therapeutic time, therapeutic skills, and empathy—not a popular treatment form in our age of impatience and quick solutions. Never-theless, she persisted and brought forth a wealth of clinical data that could not be ignored. Now the diagnosis is recognized in DSM-III-R (American Psychiatric Association 1987), and articles on MPD are accepted by learned journals that refused earlier, similar submissions. Connie herself became a member of the Editorial Board of *Dissocia-tion: Progress in the Dissociative Disorders* and continued her active involvement with the field until her death in 1992.

Connie linked MPD with sexual, physical, and psychological child abuse. This etiological understanding has gained more and more importance today as our profession's awareness of such abuse grows. It gave a comprehensibility to the development of the disor-der that was as logical as it was compelling. She showed how this condition emerges as a defense against overwhelming stress. Finally, she trained dozens of men and women in the intricacies of treating these patients, while never ignoring the growing body of knowledge of the organic and neurological.

Many of us instantly connect Connie with the book *Sybil* (Schrei-ber 1973) as well as the movie, both of which certainly popularized the condition of MPD and its treatment. Others will always recall her as the empathic teacher, the woman who was a pioneer in psychia-try, the woman who never hesitated to speak her opinion publicly and forcibly. To me, in addition, she will forever be linked by a gold coin on a chain.

References

American Psychiatric Association: Diagnostic and Statistical Manual of Mental Disorders, 3rd Edition, Revised. Washington, DC, American Psychiatric Association, 1987

Dickstein L, Nadelson C: Women Physicians in Leadership Roles. Washington, DC, American Psychiatric Press, 1985

Schreiber FR: Sybil. Chicago, IL, Regnery, 1973

Chapter 2

My Long-Distance Supervision With Cornelia B. Wilbur, M.D.

Leah J. Dickstein, M.D.

" To Joan with best wishes . . . Dr. Cornelia B. Wilbur." This 1978 inscription, on the frontispiece of a paperback copy of *Sybil* (Schreiber 1973) that belonged to my first patient with multiple personality disorder (MPD), represents an important and unique aspect of my long-distance and long-term intermittent "prn" supervision by Connie Wilbur: her extraordinary empathy and respect for all who sought her assistance.

As a psychiatry resident at the University of Louisville, I, like many others in psychiatry and the other mental health specialties, became extremely interested in MPD with the publication of *Sybil* in 1973. I suspect my interest may have been somewhat heightened because Dr. Wilbur lived in Lexington, Kentucky, only 75 miles southeast of Louisville. I had already met her several times at our Kentucky Psychiatric Association district branch annual and interim meetings. Ever on the lookout for mentors and role models, I was immediately captivated by Connie's warm, direct comments about anything and everything related to psychiatry and patient care. With the publication of *Sybil,* I borrowed a second-year resident's copy and read it immediately. I would ply Connie with questions about the etiology and treatment of MPD every time we met.

In September 1977, the Student Health Service secretary, Jean Tucker, asked me if I could see a student "for only a moment." The student was complaining of gastrointestinal symptoms and test anxiety. She admitted that she was under the care of another psychiatrist. Because this request sounded appropriate, I consented and saw the student at once.

She, Joan, or Joanie (a pseudonym), was a 27-year-old white divorced female in her first semester at the University of Louisville. She had graduated with honors from our local community college. She indeed seemed anxious. I took a short history and asked about her current symptoms of "diarrhea and nervousness" about a forthcoming exam. Our brief session ended after I offered empathic reassurance about how understandable it was to experience a period of "adjustment" to a large university.

However, Joan continued to return almost daily "just to say hey." Sometimes she looked more relaxed and a bit friendlier, and at other times she seemed as anxious as she had been the first time she came. I did not want to interfere with her ongoing psychiatric treatment, so I kept these contacts superficial and short.

Finally, not wanting to give the appearance of rejecting her, I asked Joan if she would like to join a group, if her psychiatrist thought it would be all right. She returned to say he assented. I then called him to confirm that I was only offering her a group experience that would not interfere with her individual therapy, but that might help her adjust to the demands of her new life at the university. He agreed.

At the end of our first 3 weeks of contacts, which had consisted of individual "cameo" appearances at the group session in which she appeared extremely anxious and left in the middle, I sensed something more was amiss. Putting these behaviors together with some additional observations, I asked the fateful question, "Do you lose time?" The answer was an immediate and honest "yes." Thus began an incredible 4-year safari into the unknown for me and Joanie and the 25 "others."

Not completely trusting my psychiatric acumen, and with Joanie's and her initial psychiatrist's consent, I called Connie Wilbur and asked if she would be willing to see my patient in consultation. Her immediate, firm, and generous answer was "Yes, of course." Connie's unhesitating, affirmative, and patient responses to my ongoing requests continues to influence my reactions to others to this day and, I hope, will continue to do so throughout all the years I have contact with and attempt to help patients.

The trip to Lexington for consultation in January 1978 was uneventful, but I was "prepared" just in case a calamity occurred. A student health nurse, Carol, equipped with a syringe filled with diazepam, agreed to accompany us to Connie's office. I had shared my suspicions about Joanie's diagnosis with the student health staff. From the outset, Carol, a minister's wife, a mother, and a warm and caring professional, had been supportive and reassuring, although I suspect she was somewhat skeptical about the diagnosis at times (as I was myself). She and Joanie sat in the back seat, and I chauffeured. As I drove, I talked primarily to Joanie in an effort to reassure her that everything would be all right. The sound of my voice was also reassuring to me. I was apprehensive and silently wished that Joanie or one of the other alters would not bolt out of the car door while we were in motion.

Connie was waiting for us and ushered Joanie and me into her office. She asked Joanie to tell her what she had been feeling and experiencing, and for how long her problems had been going on. Connie sat in a comfortable armchair with her feet on a hassock and Joanie sat on a sofa. I sat nearby, silent and watchful. Connie was calmly reassuring. She evidenced complete understanding and acceptance of what Joanie told her. She asked about alters, when they came and why, how the original personality handled the time and memory losses, and how much she (the original personality) knew of the alters. Connie used no hypnosis. She told me afterward that it simply wasn't necessary with Joanie, because Joanie was able to share their history.

The 1-hour session was exhilarating to me, especially when Connie matter-of-factly told me, "Of course you're right—she is a multiple." When I asked Connie why "they" told me, their sixteenth therapist, about themselves and the loss of time, Connie said, "They trust you—it's common that MPD patients will finally tell one therapist that they lose time and that there are other parts of themselves who take over time."

Before we left her office, Connie had spontaneously told me, "You're doing fine in therapy with her. Just continue as you have been, get to know the other alters and help them get to know each other. Call me when you need to."

Connie's confirmation of my neophyte's diagnostic impression increased my personal estimation of my psychiatric prowess. Needless to say, the return ride home was more relaxing to all of us. Carol talked more, expressing optimism to Joanie about her recovery. Jean, another alter, talked about how "skeered" she had been but that Dr. Wilbur "was so nice, not like Momma." As for me, I stopped imaging "the great escape," a car accident, or an hysterical outbreak.

In addition to my exhilaration with having diagnosed Joanie's illness correctly, I was enthralled with the possibility of ongoing supervisory contacts with Connie. And there were many.

I recall one of the most dramatic consultations quite vividly. Joanie called from where she was standing, which was on the ledge of her third-floor apartment window. I continued to talk to her calmly, encouraging her and the alters to not be angry with each other, but rather to come inside carefully. Different alters continued to argue, blame, berate, cry, and sob. Expressions of anguish were broken by unsettling spells of silence. During these times, I would try to think, "What would Connie do?" Those words reverberated in my thoughts throughout the next 3½ years. I did call Connie after the window ledge episode. As usual, she seemed neither shocked nor critical, but instead supported my instinctive patience and encouragement to Joanie and the other alters. Our patients continue to remind us that they repeat our words when they are alone in difficult situations. In a parallel fashion, any efforts to think of what might have been Connie's words appeared to aid me in my inexperienced yet concerted efforts to remain steadfast in my determination to conduct the psychotherapy of Joanie, a patient with a challenging mental illness that in 1977 was allegedly rare and generally misdiagnosed.

At our twice-yearly meetings of the Kentucky Psychiatric Association and at district branch board meetings, when Connie was the chair of our first Committee on Women and I was District Branch Secretary or Treasurer, I always attempted to spend some time with her, asking what must have appeared to be endless questions: "How do you handle this situation?" or "How do you respond to that situation?" Connie not only responded with direction and recommendations, but she always made time for me. It was obvious that she took time from her myriad other activities and interests to recount relevant disguised case examples from her own extensive clinical practice in which the same or similar issues were important, and to discuss stepwise recommendations I might follow.

These informal supervisory sessions were all the more generous and appreciated because during this time—the decade following the publication of *Sybil*—Connie was deluged with calls for both consultation and advice from psychiatrists nationwide and from around the world. Beyond these expected professional requests, oftentimes patients in treatment with other professionals, and patient's families (particularly if patients were minors), contacted her from all over. To all of these letters and calls Connie responded with referrals and thoughtful, careful recommendations. Without identifying locations and names, Connie shared these fascinating educational vignettes with me. It was really like being part of a group supervision seminar on a controversial psychiatric disorder that had not yet gained credence and acceptance by the majority of psychiatrists and other mental health professionals.

Connie often shared with me her pioneering attempts not only to develop a therapeutic protocol to treat this disorder, but also her persistent struggles to share with her colleagues what she had independently and (in my words) "perceptively and brilliantly formulated." She had been able to describe MPD comprehensively and to link its origin to overwhelming childhood circumstances.

Connie was personally strong and independent enough to tell me that although she submitted numerous papers detailing her work to professional journals, their editors continually and consistently offered excuses and rejections. These articles never were published before 1984! Early in her investigations Connie also offered to share her findings at professional meetings. The audience feedback she received might have shaken the professional souls of less indomitable colleagues, but it did not deter her. Her poignant experience and determined resolve helped me persist as a young unpublished professional, as I collected my own array of rejections.

In response to my request for information about her experiences, I received the following from Connie, dated March 1990:

Dear Leah,

There was a meeting of the Southern Psychiatric Association where the association gave a resident award to a resident for a paper on the history of MPD. After the resident read the paper and the prizes were bestowed, Dr. Phillips, who was the Chairman, asked if anyone had any comments. A middle-aged man in a grey suit got up from the back of the audience and went to the podium. I did not know him then, nor do I know him or his name now. But he started on a tirade (not a discussion) about MPD being a fake disease, being a hoax, and being presented either by a fool or someone excessively naive who really produced the disease themselves, without knowing it, or deliberately for self-aggrandizement. He also said, "I do not believe in Multiple Personality Disorder." He really raved, and the audience as astonished.

When the man sat down, Dr. Phillips asked if there was anyone else who wanted to say anything, and there was dead silence. I happened to be sitting in the front row and Dr. Phillips leaned over to me and said, "Wouldn't you like to say something?"

I started to reply that I didn't want to say anything, but I got an inspiration so I said, "Yes, I think I would like to say something." I then told the audience that I did not believe in MPD either, which produced gasps because I had been a member for a number of years and most of the audience knew me.

I went on to say that it was not a matter of a belief system, that I had been raised in a family of pure scientists. My father had a Ph.D. in chemistry; my brother had a degree in chemical engineering; I myself had a master's degree in chemistry before I went to medical school.

I went on to say that when I came across Sybil, whose symptoms were quite different, I decided to use the scientific method to deal with this case. I began to collect data: symptomatic information detailed by the history, answers to certain questions (such as, did she have blackouts? did time seem to pass when she didn't know what happened to it?), and any other questions I could think of that suggested episodes of amnesia.

I stated that when I had succeeded in detailing between 60 and 80 findings, I carefully reviewed them and tried to subsume to this listing a diagnosis that would cover most of the findings, if not all. I discovered, among other things, that there were other personalities functioning during amnesic periods, and I told the audience that they could call it whatever they wanted to, abracadabra, if necessary. But since there were several quite distinct and separate personalities functioning in one physical body, calling it Multiple Personality Disorder seemed reasonable to me.

I concluded with the remark that I felt that people who did not make the diagnosis of MPD at any time were poor observers.

Dr. Phillips' request for any other discussant was met with silence.

Connie served as a professional mentor for many young women and men psychiatrists in Lexington and Louisville and beyond Kentucky. Wherever she was invited to speak, Connie gave unstintingly of her knowledge and support to interested yet inexperienced therapists. At the early American Psychiatric Association courses on MPD, Connie and other pioneers in the field gave their maximum efforts to teach in 1½ days what they had learned in years of creative trial-and-error attempts to recognize and treat those apparent "treatment failures" and often misdiagnosed patients—those who have MPD.

Like other women leaders in European and American psychiatry, Connie served as an outstanding role model for women. As a woman who excelled as a psychoanalyst, psychiatrist, researcher, clinician, and teacher, she was an inspiration to me and to countless others. As a founding member of the American College of Psychiatrists, Connie once more legitimized women's place, responsibility, and acceptance in psychiatric leadership. The strengths she modeled for us are many. She continuously strove to be the best psychiatrist and psychoanalyst she could be. Her standards were from within rather than from without. She made time for her family, friends, and students, and (what is so important for many of us to emulate today in our complicated lives) she also made time for herself. Repeatedly, she recounted to me the choices she faced throughout her career, from her premedical days through internship, residency, and beyond. She appeared to harbor few grudges toward those who truly had impeded her professional life, though she could regale me with tales of professional frustration and temporary impediments and stalemates. To Connie, surmounting obstacles was simply an accepted aspect of one's career.

From part of my informal supervision with Connie, I observed clearly that she used humor constructively, both for personal pleasure and for effective professional and personal communication. People incontrovertibly got the point, and Connie got to guffaw. She also talked about her commitment to her health. Swimming was her important daily exercise; she regarded it as so important that she had an all-season bubble cover made for her backyard pool.

Connie was a role model for me in other important ways as well. She always considered it important to teach nonpsychiatric mental health professionals, lay groups, and government and legal agency workers what she knew about child abuse and its long-term effects and possible repercussions. Her "big picture" approach to informing others was probably unusual for one trained to be a superspecialist.

My experience in long-distance "prn" psychotherapy supervision with Connie resulted in my being better able to care for my patients with MPD, their families, and their significant others. Whether this supervision took place during the day, in the evening, or even on weekends, Connie always responded to my telephone calls and messages with patience, tact, and practical answers. Her advice was unswervingly in the correct, detailed service of patients and their significant others, but was never frustrating or offered critically. Rather, she seemed to appreciate my enthusiasm and my desire to do the best I could and to learn as much as possible. Beyond my own trial-and-error experience and my reading, clearly my best supervision emanated from Connie.

Although many others in fact gladly pay for supervisory sessions, Connie never broached such a topic. Instead, she took me to dinners at meetings, came to my home for dinner, and unswervingly and adamantly responded to my requests humanely, patiently, and expertly.

When I asked this woman—role model to thousands and mentor

to dozens—to yet again make time to allow me to interview her for a chapter in a book on women physicians in leadership roles, with Carol Nadelson as my coeditor, she once again consented. Several years before this request, I had interviewed her for a chapter about her, for my as-yet-unpublished book on the history of women physicians of Kentucky. Furthermore, when Connie received audiotapes of a conference she did on MPD, she surprised me with a gift of the tapes!

Perhaps what one must learn and emulate most from a supervisor-mentor is that, first and last, "to thine own self be true." Clearly and unquestionably, Cornelia B. Wilbur, M.D., evidenced these priceless qualities for me, first as a long-distance role model and supervisor, and in later years as colleague and cherished friend. Since *Sybil* has in fact been translated into 15 languages, I know many professionals throughout the world have recognized through the pages of this book the qualities I saw in Connie. On behalf of all the colleagues in many mental health disciplines and the patients with MPD that were helped by her example and advice, I want to say a final word of thanks. Thank you, Connie Wilbur, for your brilliant professional sensitivity, astuteness, insights, independence, doggedness, creativity, love, empathy, and successes. Thank you also for sharing them with all of us in the service of those who already have MPD and those who, unfortunately, will have it in the future. While we work toward the prevention of child abuse of all types and degrees, we have your knowledge and guidance to help many of its survivors toward integration and health.

References

Schreiber FR: Sybil. Chicago, IL, Regnery, 1973

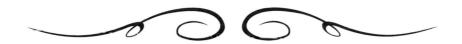

The Psychotherapy of Multiple Personality Disorder: General Issues and Concerns

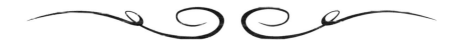

Chapter 3

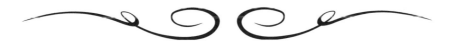

Basic Principles in Conducting the Psychotherapy of Multiple Personality Disorder

Richard P. Kluft, M.D.

Two decades ago, when the publication of *Sybil* (Schreiber 1973) created a renewed interest in multiple personality disorder (MPD), the report of a single case of this allegedly rare condition was considered noteworthy; treating one such patient could establish a therapist as a veritable expert in the field. Today MPD is no longer considered a rarity (American Psychiatric Association 1987). It is understood to be a not uncommon sequela of overwhelming childhood experiences. Several large series of 50 to more than 300 MPD patients have been reported (e.g., Coons et al. 1988; Putnam et al. 1986; Ross et al. 1989; Schultz et al. 1989). Many psychotherapists have worked with large numbers of such patients (e.g., Kluft 1984a, 1986). Contemporary authorities warn against attempting to generalize from findings in single case studies or drawing firm conclusions from small series of MPD patients. The mental health professions are gradually assimilating information about the diagnosis and treatment of this condition and beginning to function with a higher level of awareness that MPD patients, whose clinical presentations can overlap with those of patients with a wide variety of other mental disorders, may be encountered in virtually any clinical setting.

Acquiring the skill to recognize the signs of MPD can be difficult, but a useful literature is available to guide the clinician's efforts (e.g., Bernstein and Putnam 1986; Coons 1980, 1984; Franklin 1988, 1990; Kluft 1985a, 1987a, 1987b, 1987c, 1991a, 1991b; Loewenstein 1991; Putnam 1989; Ross 1989; Solomon and Solomon 1982; Steinberg et al. 1990). With patience, persistence, and occasional consultation, the sensitized clinician is in a position to approach and resolve most diagnostic dilemmas.

With regard to treatment, there are many useful general resources (e.g., Braun 1984, 1986; Kluft 1984a, 1985b, 1991b; Putnam 1989; Ross 1989) and scores of helpful and more specialized articles, but considerable confusion remains about basic ground rules for conducting the therapy. It is my experience as a consultant to more than 1,000 MPD psychotherapies in progress (Kluft 1988a, 1988b) that clinicians often emerge from their study of the literature with valuable insights, but with residual uncertainty about fundamental concerns. Although it is possible to learn to treat MPD by trial and error (the inevitable route followed by the pioneers in the field), this is a prolonged and difficult process. When one "flies by the seat of one's pants," months or years may pass before one realizes that a particular effort or stance is proving counterproductive; additional time may be lost in trying to salvage or redirect the treatment. Extended or intransigent stalemates may occur; at times it may even be necessary to discontinue the treatment and/or to transfer the patient.

Notwithstanding many advances and significant achievements, the dissociative disorders field is quite new. Research on the treatment of MPD is just beginning. It has been demonstrated that MPD can be treated successfully (Kluft 1984a, 1986), but there are no controlled studies that demonstrate the superiority of one approach or point of view over another. Major figures in the field express a diversity of opinion with respect to the theoretical orientations, recommended goals, and technical approaches that they advocate. Differences of opinion can be found on major issues; a unifying paradigm has not emerged. Furthermore, therapists beginning to work with MPD come from a variety of backgrounds and practice innumerable models of therapy. It is very possible for a well-trained and intelligent clinician to emerge from an encounter with the contemporary MPD literature confused and uncertain. He or she may remain perplexed about how to apply new insights within the structure and model of therapy in which he or she was trained.

Contemporary Approaches to the Treatment of MPD

It is a curiosity in the field that although certain approaches have been demonstrated to be effective in the hands of experienced clinicians (Kluft 1984a, 1986), many psychotherapists have elected neither to utilize these methods nor to endorse the perspectives that they embody. Several treatment philosophies and therapeutic stratagems have emerged.

Elsewhere (Kluft 1988c), I attempted to describe several contemporary approaches to the treatment of MPD. I observed many therapists conducting chaotic therapies characterized by frenetic attempts to find "something that works" (desperate eclecticism). This is most commonly encountered among neophytes who have yet to educate themselves about the clinical realities of MPD. In addition, some therapists attempt to force MPD patients to conform to their preferred theories and practices (Procrustean rigidity). This is not infrequent among therapists whose theoretical orientation is also a belief system and constitutes a major portion of their personal as well as professional identities. Furthermore, some therapists attempt to minimize attention to the MPD phenomena, in the hope that a failure to "reinforce" them will lead to their subsiding (minimization). This view is widely held, especially among senior individuals who believe that they, in their long and distinguished careers, have had little or no contact with MPD, and maintain that most if not all contemporary cases are iatrogenic. These three approaches have yet to demonstrate their efficacy. Many MPD patients who are transferred to therapists who are more experienced with MPD have had treatments in which one or more of these approaches were attempted.

Still another approach to therapy is widely practiced (especially by relatively naive therapists) and might be called a reparenting approach. It implicitly if not explicitly accords the alters face validity as people and attempts to nurture them into health by means of a variety of corrective emotional experiences, some of which may become quite tangible in form. The assumption that the personalities are real people (e.g., a child alter is a real child that needs to be helped to mature in a more benign and caring environment) is without foundation, despite the fact that such beliefs may be experienced by the patient as compelling subjective realities. When therapists subscribe to such beliefs, their use of themselves as the curative agent becomes central. Conventional therapeutic boundaries are often violated and the violations rationalized. Unfortunately, such approaches often prove so gratifying to patient and therapist alike that one or both may have difficulties in acknowledging that the treatment is not succeeding, and they may be reluctant to extricate themselves from the endeavor. Although occasional dramatic successes have been achieved in this manner, "forever therapies" and gross misadventures are not uncommon outcomes. Such approaches cannot be recommended.

Several approaches are acknowledged to have helped considerable numbers of MPD patients. Of these, integrationalism is the most widely advocated. There is a considerable body of experience and some uncontrolled research findings that indicate that it is the most desirable stance for the therapist to adopt (Kluft 1984a, 1985c, 1986). Integrationalism and integration itself is the subject of another chapter in this volume (see Chapter 6). Integrationalism has two forms, both of which aim to integrate the personality in the course of the overall resolution of the patient's symptoms and difficulties in living. In strategic integrationalism, the focus is on rendering the dissociative defenses and structures that sustain the MPD both less necessary and less viable, so that, in essence, the MPD collapses from within. The therapy is understood as an ongoing process of defense analysis and conflict resolution, consistent with the psychoanalytic tradition. Techniques and interventions are valued less for themselves than for their contributions to long-term goals. This approach has its origins in the work of Cornelia B. Wilbur, M.D.

Tactical integrationalism (see Chapter 7) is characterized by a greater focus on the tactics and techniques by which a series of therapeutic objectives can be attained. The deliberateness and planfulness of the treatment is quite conspicuous. It is more consistent with the tenor of eclectic hypnotherapy, cognitive therapy, behavior therapy, and short-term psychodynamic psychotherapy. Although it has its roots in the landmark contributions of Despine and Janet, the first authors who expressed tactical integrationalist views in the modern literature were pragmatic hypnotherapists: Margaretta K. Bowers and her colleagues (1971) and Ralph Allison (1974). Although some major theoretical differences underlie the assumptions of these two integrationalist views, in actual practice, many therapies are characterized by periods in which strategic and tactical considerations alternate, but integration is always the goal. This was certainly the case in the successful treatments I reported (Kluft 1984a, 1986).

Personality-focused approaches emerge largely from the work of John and Helen Watkins (1979) and John Beahrs (1982) and those who have been influenced by them. Clinicians influenced by this paradigm take the stance that dividedness in and of itself is a human norm, and not problematic as long as the alters function smoothly together (Beahrs 1982; Torem 1986; H. H. Watkins 1984; J. G. Watkins 1978; J. G. Watkins and H. H. Watkins 1981). Such therapies take the form of a problem-solving inner diplomacy or group or family therapy among a number of selves, all of which are encouraged to collaborate more smoothly and harmoniously without necessarily ceding their separateness or autonomy. Integration is not devalued and may be pursued if the patient so desires, but a more facile and functional arrangement among the elements of the mind is the major objective. Such an objective is an inevitable aspect of the middle phases of integrationalist treatments but, from that perspective, is seen as an intermediate goal rather than a desirable end point.

Another approach might be termed adaptationalism. Such therapists describe themselves as pragmatists; they prioritize helping their

MPD patients manage their lives more smoothly and function more effectively. They acknowledge integration as a desirable goal, but they indicate that integration may require more therapeutic resources and motivation and ego strength on the part of the patient than can be brought to bear. This is a legitimate and useful stance with patients motivated primarily for symptomatic relief whose resources and/or life circumstances preclude a more intense treatment, and those who absolutely refuse to work toward either integration or the processing of past traumata. Because the treatment of most MPD patients involves many such periods, an adaptationalist orientation dominates certain phases of the majority of MPD treatments.

Any of the approaches discussed here may dominate certain phases of a given therapy, but one or the other generally informs the therapist's overall strategy. For example, in the course of an 8-year treatment that resulted in total integration, the early phases of a woman's treatment were governed by strategic integrationalist concerns, with the slow and gradual analysis of defense and gentle uncovering. When the alters were accessible and quite active, a personality-oriented phase occurred, followed by a tactical integrationalist period in which hypnotic techniques were used in a structured manner to work on painful material. When the patient abruptly was left by her husband, a switch was made to an adaptationalist stance. This crisis weathered, for a while the therapy was dominated again by tactical integrationalism. The prolonged process of working-through and the last few integrations marked a return to strategic integrationalism.

Principles of the Successful Psychotherapy of MPD

Therapists who practice very different forms of treatment, perceive themselves to be affiliated with a wide variety of theoretical orientations, and use a bewildering panoply of techniques may nonetheless endorse similar general stances toward the MPD patient and achieve similarly excellent results. In the late 1970s and early 1980s, Bennett

G. Braun, M.D., studied videotapes of the work of many therapists who were expert in the treatment of MPD. He observed that despite these therapists' avowed differences in their orientations and the diversity of their techniques, many of their interventions were identical in substance. Braun concluded that the clinical realities of MPD were a more powerful determinant of the actions of the expert MPD therapists than the rationales that they consciously avowed to be their guides (Braun, quoted in Kluft 1984a). Braun's original observations have held up well. In my experience at literally hundreds of workshops, it remains a commonplace for expert MPD therapists of different avowed orientations to find themselves in substantial agreement as to what type of intervention needs to be made in a given case at a given juncture. They are far less likely to agree with the recommendations of less expert and experienced therapists with whom they share a common theoretical background.

In the spirit of such findings, and in the context of many therapists' expressed confusion as to how to conduct the treatment of the MPD patient, it appears timely to assemble a series of observations and general principles derived from the successful treatment of contemporary MPD patients—general principles that are, for the most part, pragmatic, atheoretical, and amenable to being used by therapists employing a wide variety of treatments and orientations. The principles to be advanced are drawn from my own experience, which includes the successful integration of more than 140 MPD patients and more than 1,000 consultations to colleagues who were working with MPD patients. They are consistent with suggestions advocated in the classic 1971 article by Margaretta K. Bowers and her collaborators (with the exception of their recommendation that group therapy be used to confront the MPD patient about disavowed behavior). These principles assume that the goal of the treatment in question is the integration of the MPD patients. Where they clash with the goals of the personality-oriented and adaptationalist stances, those clashes will be acknowledged.

Once these principles were outlined in 1986 (with the exception of one added more recently), I used them to assess hundreds of consultation situations over the years since. I was impressed that the successful therapies that I reviewed had respected these principles, and that those that were stalemated and/or otherwise problematic inevitably failed to adhere to one or more of them. Therefore, although these principles are not offered as absolutely authoritative, they appear to have been adhered to in every successful MPD therapy known to me, with two exceptions.

It must be acknowledged that there are occasional successes reported by therapists pursuing the reparenting approach, which is problematic and prone to instances of countertransference misadventure and the exploitation of both the patient and the therapist. However, this approach is too problematic to be advocated. Also, there are many cultures that endorse a different approach to the understanding and treatment of MPD and MPD-related phenomena, such as dissociative possession states. In some cultures, exorcistic procedures and other unique methods remain potent healing rituals. Of course it remains possible that there are substantial numbers of MPD patients who have been successfully treated in psychotherapies that violate these principles; but in my 20 years of work with dissociative disorder patients, such patient cohorts have not been called to my attention. The principles explored herein have been discussed elsewhere in summary form (Kluft 1991b).

Pragmatic Principles for the Treatment of MPD

---

1. Maintain a Secure Frame and Firm Boundaries

First, MPD is a condition that was created by broken boundaries. Had the patient not been overwhelmed during childhood, usually by the gross violation of societal mores, a dissociative defense would not have eventuated. *Therefore, a successful treatment will have a secure treatment frame and firm, consistent boundaries.* It is quite common for the therapist to become fascinated by the MPD patient's phenomena and overwhelmed by the MPD patient's material, pain, and (apparent) neediness. This begets a host of countertransferentially-based treatment frame violations that will ultimately complicate and prolong the treatment. The patient needs the therapist to be a consistent, compassionate, and considerate person who safeguards the treatment setting and maintains him- or herself in the role of the therapist. To break the ground rules of therapy is to recapitulate the boundary violations of the patient's childhood and to demonstrate that the therapist is corruptible rather than reliable. An excellent but demanding psychoanalytic discussion of the deleterious impact of altering the treatment frame is found in the work of Langs (1976, 1979).

Case Study 1.   I saw in consultation a therapist who was planning to write a book about the MPD patient he was treating. As the manuscript progressed, the treatment deteriorated. In the consultation, it became clear to me that the therapist was talking more about the book than the patient. To his credit, he rapidly appreciated that the treatment was being sabotaged by his dual relationship with the patient, and thereafter he restricted his efforts to the therapy. The book project was canceled, and the patient healed rapidly.

Case Study 2.   A gifted psychologist saw his work with an MPD patient as an opportunity for interesting research. Gradually the sessions became permeated with nontherapeutic concerns. The therapy failed.

Case Study 3.   A caring therapist became so involved with her MPD patient that she began to perceive her as her friend. They lunched and went to professional meetings together. Although they valued one another, the treatment foundered. The therapist finally withdrew as therapist and remained a friend. Unable to find an equally gratifying relationship with another therapist, and unwilling to tolerate a more standard arrangement, the patient refused to pursue the treatment she needed.

It is a useful caution for the therapist to reflect: "Would I be doing this with a patient with another sort of condition?" If the answer is "no," it is possible that one is involved in a countertransference-mediated violation of the treatment frame. When in doubt, it is best to get consultation and/or supervision.

2. Focus on Achieving Mastery

MPD is a condition of subjective and at times objective dyscontrol. Assaults and unwanted experiences were passively endured by a relatively helpless youngster. Amnestic barriers and the inner battles of alters make the patient feel helpless in the face of his or her symptoms. The MPD patient comes to feel that his or her locus of control is external. *Therefore, there must be a focus on mastery and the patient's active participation in the treatment process.* This speaks to the centrality of the therapeutic alliance, which I will discussed further. Therapy must be done with rather than to the patient.

One of my informal rules is that except in certain crises, I should not be working harder than the patient. Therapy should proceed in a manner that allows the patient to become a meaningful partner in it. It cannot be allowed to become an arcane art form in which the therapist's insights and skills appear so special that they cannot be understood by a mere mortal, and in which the work of the therapy is made to appear beyond the ken of the patient. The therapist who is enamored of sophisticated exposition and Delphic utterances must find other channels for the fulfillment of his or her narcissistic needs and must make efforts to be sure that the treatment is empowering to the patient. Failing this, the patient will not achieve a sufficiently internalized sense of mastery of the therapeutic process, will not form an identification with the therapist that is optimally structure-building, and will have difficulty internalizing his or her gains and gaining a sense of ownership of his or her own progress. The therapy and things therapeutic will be perceived as belonging to the therapist, and dependent on his or her presence and/or good graces.

Case Study 1.   A sensitive therapist was doing a generally excellent treatment of a difficult MPD patient, but he was concerned with the patient's failure to internalize a sense of self-control and her passivity in pursuing difficult material. When we reviewed his process notes, we found that they recorded little more than his elegant interpretations of the patient's dynamics. As he reflected further on this phenomenon, he learned that the patient believed that only the therapist could understand her, and that her own insights were meaningless.

Behind her idealization of him and her self-depreciation was reaction formation and a reenactment of her experience of never feeling that what she thought was valued by her abusive father, who insisted that he was always right. She was enraged at both her father's mistreatment of her and his self-aggrandizement at her expense. The therapist's relatively benign narcissistic investment in his interpretive skill proved to have meshed neatly with a set of past experiences in an inadvertent reenactment that interfered with the treatment. As the therapist took pains to express himself in a more pedestrian manner, the patient became more active. She volunteered that she had experienced his eloquence as demeaning of her, had become angry at him, and was determined not to let him "get to her."

Case Study 2.   An MPD patient in truly deplorable life circumstances was being treated by a therapist who, resonating with her difficulties, took pains to make the treatment and her life as easy as possible. She was so supportive in word and deed that the patient was "spared" much of the work of treatment, and her dealing with reality problems was often cushioned or expedited. When seen in consultation, it became clear that the patient felt both loved and infantilized by the therapist. Fortunately, the therapist was able to explore the situation with the patient and put the treatment on a more constructive course.

If the patient is not undertaking an increasingly active role in the therapeutic process, a close scrutiny of the situation is desirable. I am one of many experienced therapists who, except in emergencies and unusual circumstances, will not begin to work on the uncovering and processing of painful material until I perceive the patient to be an active partner in the work of treatment (Kluft 1992, in press). To do otherwise is to risk having an overwhelmed patient who lacks any sense that he or she has the capacity to resolve rather than be retraumatized by the misfortunes of the past.

---

3. Establish and Maintain a Strong Therapeutic Alliance

MPD is a condition of both genuine and subjectively perceived involuntariness. People with MPD did not elect to be traumatized, and they find their symptoms often are beyond their control. *Therefore, the therapy must be based on a strong therapeutic alliance, and efforts to establish this must be undertaken throughout the entire treatment process.* Again and again, the patient must be educated about and reminded of his or her role and duties in the therapy, and the patient's voluntary efforts must be encouraged. Unless the therapist takes such steps, he or she will find it difficult to confront the MPD patient who is resistant and/or noncompliant. Confrontation will be met with protestations of helplessness and wounded innocence. The concept of the therapeutic alliance is especially difficult for those MPD patients who are nurture-seeking in their orientation and who find in the therapist's warmth and acceptance an implicit endorsement of their wish to be cared for and an absolution of the need to face painful material and share the burdens of the work of the therapy. They rarely are able to appreciate that only their active efforts will secure for them what they hope will be granted magically.

It is especially important to realize that the therapeutic alliance may be very different with each of the several personalities, and subjects that some alters are prepared to discuss may be unacceptable to others. Furthermore, the therapeutic alliance with a given alter may vary with intercurrent stressors, with the influences of the other alters (both the lingering impact of those who have recently had control, and the passive influence of the alters upon one another from "behind the scenes"), and with therapeutically induced and/or spontaneous reconfigurations among the system of alters. It is often worthwhile for the therapist to ask how the patient feels about pursuing a specific subject and inquire as to which alters may be influenced by the subject under discussion. Often it is useful to ask the patient's permission to approach a particular piece of work. It is a common mistake to confuse elements of the real relationship and the transference (especially positive transferences) with the therapeutic alliance. An excellent discussion of these topics can be found in Greenson (1967).

Not uncommonly, the reassessment of the patient who is alleged to have a good therapeutic alliance but is not prospering in treatment reveals that the patient is working to please or appease the therapist, but he or she experiences the therapeutic work as something to be endured in order to obtain the therapist's care rather than as valuable in and of itself. The patient may be highly motivated to achieve symptomatic relief and to be involved in a relationship in which he or she feels accepted and liked, but he or she may have difficulty in accepting that treatment does not consist solely of the use of the therapist as a need-fulfilling object. It is far from rare to find that the patient is essentially without the motivation to do the work of the therapy and will need assistance in appreciating the true nature of the treatment.

Case Study 1.   A patient appeared to be working hard in treatment but was becoming increasingly agitated. The therapist insisted that the transference was positive and the therapeutic alliance was solid. In consultation, it became clear that the patient was experiencing the therapist as a terrifying authority who had to be given all that she wanted and to be told that the patient enjoyed providing it. This proved to be a reenactment of her attempts to please her sadistic father, who insisted that she regale him with accounts of how dearly she cherished his sexual usage of her. The agitation was related to anticipation that soon the therapist would beat her as father had done. The therapist was not pleased to find that the patient's "hard work" had been done in the conscious reenactment of a negative transference, and even less pleased to find that most of the material that had been produced had been made up in an effort to divert the therapist from abusing her.

Case Study 2.   An MPD patient exasperated her therapist by producing little work while protesting how hard she was trying. Exploration revealed that a powerful alter was threatening to punish any alter who revealed any information of substance. Only after months of working with the punitive alter were the other alters able to rejoin the treatment process.

Case Study 3.   An MPD patient seen in emergency consultation appeared to be decompensating. My evaluation revealed that she had developed a strong affectionate tie to her therapist and had mobilized powerful regressive transference phenomena, but that she had virtually no understanding of the therapeutic process in which she was involved. She was so decompensated that hospitalization was necessary. The focus of her hospital-based treatment was her education as to how to go about being in therapy (Kluft 1989). Extensive consultation with the therapist led the therapist to seek ongoing supervision.

Whenever possible, I spend months working on the therapeutic alliance before proceeding to work on affect-laden material. The therapy is very much a shared venture, and I want my partner in the endeavor to understand his or her role across as many alters as possible before proceeding. One would not take a sailboat away from the dock without ascertaining the crew's knowledge of sailing— whether they can swim, whether the appropriate equipment is on board, and so on. In the midst of a difficult situation is not the time to learn that no one on board is able to be of assistance. A psychotherapeutic endeavor requires an analogous degree of preparedness and willingness to collaborate toward a goal that is valued.

---

4. Deal With Buried Traumata and Affect

MPD is a condition of buried traumata and sequestered affect. *Therefore, what has been hidden away must be uncovered, and what feeling has been buried must be abreacted. It is occasionally possible to achieve a salubrious reconfiguration of the alters without dealing with the past and to direct the therapy to the smoother functioning of the alters, but integration cannot be achieved without dealing with the impact of the past.* There is considerable difference of opinion among skilled therapists as to how much of the trauma of the past must be worked with in order to move toward resolution and integration. Some have maintained that virtually all traumatic material must be abreacted, whereas others believe that work on a traumatic incident that is emblematic of many traumata may be effective.

My clinical experience is that if one approaches such patients with the expectation or expresses the attitude that not all of their traumata must be dealt with explicitly, a high percentage of them feel that their suffering and pain is being minimized (i.e., that they are being told to forget it or that their misery is being treated as of little account).

It is astonishing how frequently therapists who are quite empathic with the patient who has experienced a single traumatic event fail to act with similar respect toward each incident that has befallen the repeatedly traumatized patient. It often helps to bear in mind that many alters are created to deal with specific traumata; premature efforts to condense traumata may be perceived as invalidating their reasons for being. However, if a therapist begins to work on traumata one at a time, in the majority of cases he or she finds that work on one trauma may become generalized to the extent that work on other similar incidents takes less time, and/or that alters related to traumata analogous to that being worked with feel their concerns have been addressed and may even integrate along with the alters associated with the traumata that have been processed. It is a rare patient in whom each and every traumatic event requires individual processing, but such patients do exist.

Case Study 1. When she moved, an allegedly integrated MPD patient was referred to another therapist for follow-up care. The therapist rapidly discovered that most of the alters had remained separate. The first therapist had taken the stance that unless an incident could be documented, it would not be worked with in therapy and abreacted. Hence, all of the alters whose issues were not deemed worthy of being addressed ceased to present themselves in the therapy.

Case Study 2. A therapist was keenly aware of the possibility that aggressive exploration of her MPD patient's past might generate confabulations or pseudo-memories, and she declined to work with traumata in depth lest she appear to validate what she could not be sure had occurred. When seen in consultation, the patient was in a frenzy of obsessional doubting. She had flashbacks and traumatic dreams that upset her, but she felt that these were being treated rather casually in the therapy and could neither be validated nor disproven. She felt she had to know the truth in order to get well and that it was wrong to work on material the reality of which she could not prove. I advised the therapist to work with the material despite her reservations, cautioning her that because neither she nor the patient could confirm or disconfirm the material, it might be a more conservative therapeutic stance to help the patient with what appeared to ail her. This proved quite useful. A year later, a sibling was able to confirm several aspects of the incidents in the patient's flashbacks.

Case Study 3.   I took in transfer a patient who was still dealing with material that was alleged to have been abreacted and worked through. It emerged that both the patient and the prior therapist had been rather tentative and apprehensive about such efforts and, as a result, their efforts had been incomplete.

Abreaction without mastery may prove to be little more than retraumatization. It is crucial to help patients process, reframe, and take new meaning from what has befallen them. Many MPD patients believe that they were abused by virtue of their weakness ("I should have been able to stop it") or badness ("I deserved it"). Usually a meticulous exploration of the events under discussion refutes these contentions (e.g., Fine 1988).

---

5. Reduce Separateness and Conflict Among Alters

MPD is a condition of perceived separateness and conflict among the alters. *Therefore, therapy must emphasize their collaboration, co-operation, empathy, and identification with one another so that their separateness becomes redundant and their conflicts muted.* Once alters treat one another with respect and can see one another's perspective, the way is paved for the steps that lead to integration. When the alters protest about one another to me, I am likely to empathize, but to remind the alter doing the protesting, "You are all in this together." I frequently insist that the alters attempt to reason through difficult situations in an internal dialogue instead of turning to me from a stance of helplessness. I encourage their communication and teamwork, all of which is in the service of eroding narcissistic investments in uniqueness and separateness and promoting integration. Efforts on the part of the therapist to take sides in the alters' internal wars reify the condition and prolong the treatment. Advocating rational efforts to seek common objectives or to respect different priorities are often reasonably successful in the long run.

Case Study 1. A very skilled therapist had drawn the inference from Braun (1986) that personalities are more important than less fully articulated entities that Braun calls fragments. As a result, his strategy was to deal exclusively with the personalities. The result was an inner apartheid in which the alters believed to be fragments were treated in a differentially prejudicial manner—a stance the alters designated personalities adopted readily. Braun had never intended his terms to be used in such a manner. He and I (Kluft 1988c) concur that such distinctions have minimal place in the clinical as opposed to the research setting. When I saw this patient in consultation, it became clear that the result of the strategy had been to intensify rather than relieve inner turmoil. I strongly advised that all alters be treated equally (see section on shattered basic assumptions) and engage in dialogue toward collaboration. Shortly thereafter the therapist, who adopted this advice, called to indicate that therapy was proceeding smoothly toward integration, which was achieved within a year.

Case Study 2. Several personalities convinced a therapist that they should have nothing to do with certain other alters because they were "so different." By agreeing, the therapist had accepted the inner myth of the alters as a concrete reality and made progress in therapy impossible. Despite consultation, the therapist was not able to perceive that this stance was counterproductive. On follow-up consultation years later, the situation was unchanged.

Case Study 3. A pastoral counselor saw in MPD an affirmation of his perceptions of the eternal struggle of good versus evil. He coached the alters he perceived as good in his MPD patient to shun those he saw as bad. Therapy went nowhere.

Any action that conveys to the MPD patient that the therapist is validating rather than compassionately exploring the mythic structures of the patient's inner world is likely to prolong if not completely undermine the therapy. The patient (from the integrationalist perspective) must be addressed as both one and many at once, and the many must be discouraged from irresponsible autonomy (Bowers et al. 1971) on the way to integration. From a personality-centered or adaptationalist perspective, the prohibition against irresponsible autonomy is also essential, but this is in the service of smoother functioning toward achieving reasonable goals that are consistent with the patient's overall best interest.

---

6. Work to Achieve Congruence of Perception

MPD patients are highly hypnotizable and have most of the characteristics of highly hypnotizable subjects. One aspect of this is their ability to endorse alternative realities, even rather contradictory ones, without being overly troubled by their discrepancies. They may be said to have a concomitant multiple reality disorder. A common example of this occurs when parts of the mind try to live in a reality that denies troubling perceptions or events (e.g., the MPD patient who in some alters idealizes the father and denies ever having been abused by him despite the fact that the father is incarcerated for incest). *Therefore, the therapist's communications must be clear and straight. There is no room for confusing communications.* There are several implications of this principle. The first is that techniques based on engendering confusion or reconfiguring the patient's perceptions of his or her life are contraindicated. The second is that much confrontation and clarification is essential.

Case Study 1.   Appalled by the stark misery of an MPD patient's circumstances, her therapist tried to use hypnotic techniques to give the patient the impression that she had had a good and nurturing family when this was not the case. This enhanced the patient's strong pressure to deny what had befallen her. When these efforts collapsed, the patient was left not only with her misery, but with the sense that her therapist could not be trusted to tell the truth.

Case Study 2.   An MPD patient was treated by a therapist who valued the confusional techniques practiced within Eriksonian hypnosis. This unwittingly recapitulated her abusers' efforts to cause her to doubt her perceptions and bend to their will. Ultimately, therapy came to a stalemate.

A corollary of this principle is that the language used to address the MPD patient must be clear and the sentences should be crisp. Elegance of expression must yield to the need for unequivocal clarity of communication. The MPD patient must be shown over and over that he or she is entertaining mutually contradictory perceptions and be asked to explore this phenomenon. Patients' pressure to persist in these distortions require the therapist's ongoing attention.

7. Treat All Personalities Evenhandedly and With Consistency

MPD is a condition related to the inconsistency of important others. Most MPD patients were brought up under conditions in which the powerful figures in their environment changed drastically and menacingly, and the patients developed different alters to relate to these different behaviors. *Therefore, the therapist must be evenhanded to all of the alters and must avoid "playing favorites" or dramatically altering his or her own behavior toward the different personalities. The therapist's consistency across all of the different alters is one of the most powerful assaults on the patient's dissociative defenses.* The MPD patient whose therapist changes in response to which alter is in executive control has multiple therapist disorder. Conversely, the therapist who is consistent no matter which alter is out has planted the seed of the destruction of the dissociative barriers. He or she has become the one object representation that is the same no matter which alter is in control. There is no getting away from the therapist by switching, because the therapist is the same in all of the mental data banks. This is the meaning of my clinical axiom that one must be sufficiently unchanging and consistent to "bore the patient into health." I acknowledge the inevitability of the therapist's behaving somewhat differently, especially immediately after the patient switches; but it is important to rebound to one's baseline way of being as soon as possible. Granted, transference will guarantee that one is not perceived consistently despite one's efforts, but considerations of degree are quite important.

It is important to qualify that here I am talking about the therapist's way of being with the patient, not about a uniformity of therapeutic approaches. In a given therapy, some alters may be quite verbal, whereas others only write or draw, or work best with play therapy. Some will sit in one seat in the office, others in another. These issues are superficial in comparison to the therapist's overall deportment.

Case Study 1.   A therapist became very involved with the child alters in her MPD cases and spent many hours in play with them. She rarely talked to other groups of alters, maintaining that they did not want to come to therapy and that when they did, they were difficult to deal with. Although it was mutually gratifying, this therapy failed to help the patient.

Case Study 2.   A therapist worked extensively with several alters that were perceived as cooperative, and he did little with those who caused him problems. Eventually the alters neglected in the treatment took over and left therapy.

Neophyte MPD therapists often feel overwhelmed by encountering more and more alters and focus their efforts on those that are most cooperative and most readily accessed. Experienced MPD therapists take great efforts to involve many of the alters in the therapy at as early a stage as possible, and they focus their efforts on the alters that are among the most challenging and reluctant to enter the treatment. The advantage of the latter stance is that it is made clear from the first that the therapy is directed toward the entire human being, not just those aspects that behave or produce what is wanted on demand. Much of the patient's overall strength may be allocated to alters that are oppositional or identify with aggressors. If a therapist is fortunate enough to convert such alters early in the therapy, the treatment is more likely to proceed with fewer crises. One cannot always do so, but it is always worth the effort to try. Even efforts that fail but convey the message "I accept and am ready to work with every aspect of you as a human being" may lead to more reasonable behaviors from these alters when they are encountered. As a consultant, I am often amazed with how readily this can be done in patients whose therapists assumed it was impossible and had never attempted such interventions.

8. Restore Shattered Basic Assumptions

MPD patients, like other trauma victims, often emerge from their ordeals with shattered basic assumptions: that one is relatively invulnerable, that life is meaningful, and that one can see oneself in a positive light (Janoff-Bulman 1985). *Therefore, the therapy must make positive efforts to restore morale and to inculcate realistic hopes.* Most MPD patients feel very badly about themselves. They are prone to the full spectrum of revictimization behaviors that I have called the "sitting duck syndrome" (Kluft 1990). They experience profound moral masochism. Their reading of their pasts is that they have little grounds on which to hope for a positive outcome. I have found that such patients handle general supportive or encouraging statements quite poorly. They reject the positive statements and feel that the person who has made them is stupid, has been fooled by them, or is setting the stage to exploit them. In some extreme cases, patients are so upset by compliments that they will inflict self-injury as a result.

It is my experience that MPD patients can slowly rebuild their assumptions if the positive feedback they receive is incontrovertible and based on shared experiences within the therapeutic dyad. For example, an MPD patient was sure that facing the next bit of difficult material would destroy her, or at least destabilize her to a point at which she would become convinced that she could never recover. I reminded her of her similar reactions to her diagnosis, the first flashbacks of traumatic material, her terrible memories, her fears of integration as death—and that in each case, despite much pain and difficulty and her dire predictions, we had succeeded in doing what had to be done. "Based on what we have seen and been through together," I said, "I am reasonably confident that you will, despite your fear and in spite of the pain to be faced, come through this all right." The patient admitted, "I guess you're right, but it sure doesn't feel that way," and proceeded.

Case Study 1.   A therapist took great efforts to be supportive to her patient, complimenting her on her strengths and assets, but this appeared to make the patient feel worse. They came together to a consultant, who observed, "When she says those nice things to you, you become convinced that she does not understand you, and you begin to fear that the therapy will be unable to help you." The patient began to weep and admitted that this was the case.

The therapist supports best by accurate, empathic understanding. The MPD patient's masochism and shattered assumptions will be repaired slowly. Countertransference-based urgency to alleviate such entrenched misery often leads therapists to make well-intentioned efforts that in fact fail and may even worsen the situation. The therapist who cannot control the urge to be "nice and supportive" in the general sense must learn to follow up such statements in a way that takes the burden off the patient: "When I see how you say such unrealistically negative things about yourself, I find myself trying to correct your misperceptions. At times like that, I forget for the moment that it is premature to ask you to see things from other perspectives, and that from your own point of view, what I said seems to be implausible and inaccurate."

---

9. Minimize Avoidable Overwhelming Experiences

MPD is a condition stemming from overwhelming experiences. *Therefore, it is essential to pace the therapy.* Many if not most treatment failures occur when the pace of the therapy outstrips the patient's ability to tolerate the material under discussion. I advocate an axiom that has been linked with my name, "Kluft's rule of thirds." If a therapist cannot get into the material he or she had planned to address in the first third of the session, in order to work on it in the remainder of the first and throughout the second third, and to process it and restabilize the patient in the last third, it is best to avoid approaching the material, lest the patient leave the session in an overwhelmed state. This rule applies to sessions in which there is an agreed-upon agenda to explore particular material. There are many sessions in which difficult material emerges near the end, and the patient does not have adequate time to come to grips with it and to leave the session with some semblance of composure. Whenever possible, however, it is best to manage sessions so that the patient leaves in good control. It is the patient who loses confidence in the capacity of therapy to provide a safe venue for work with difficult material who becomes desperate to have access to the therapist by telephone on an ad-lib basis, or who begins to feel that he or she needs the safety of a hospital setting to work on painful material.

It is important to realize that both the patient and the therapist may unwittingly collude in the belief that the "good" sessions are those with blood-and-guts abreactions and the recovery of painful material. This leads to an overemphasis on abreaction and to the devaluing of the working-through process. In my experience, for many patients only two or three out of five sessions should have such a focus; in some cases, each bit of recovered material may require many sessions for its processing. It is true that for very complex patients, many of whose alters are based on discrete traumatic events, there may be many consecutive sessions in which one alter's material is abreacted and processed, and the alter may be integrated. However, in such cases, the alter into which the integration has occurred may need sessions to focus on the impact of such events. The overarching concern is to avoid running the patient into the ground and retraumatizing him or her in the name of therapy. A good rule of thumb is that when in doubt as to whether an MPD patient is ready for or capable of tolerating a particular intervention or bit of information, the therapist should not proceed.

Case Study 1. An eager-to-please MPD patient did intense abreactive work session after session, with little time allocated for restabilization and working-through. Within weeks she was continuously overwhelmed by flashbacks, traumatic nightmares, and dysphoric switching. She became unable to function at work and was hospitalized, ostensibly to do the abreactive work in a safe and structured setting. I was called in consultation, and I recommended that no such work be done beyond the minimum necessary to process material already retrieved and to allow the patient to restabilize. I suggested that the therapist change the emphasis of the treatment. This advice was not heeded. The patient lost her job and underwent a series of hospitalizations.

Case Study 2.   A therapist encouraged an MPD patient to do strenuous abreactive work up to the end of the sessions. The patient would sit in the therapist's waiting room for hours thereafter in an overwhelmed state, and she frequently upset subsequent patients or caused the therapist to delay the other patients' sessions by making further interventions with her. Therapist and patient spent time on the phone every night. Finally, for this patient the therapist set limits on her availability. Distraught and hopeless, the patient attempted suicide.

It is essential to realize that the MPD patient is very vulnerable to destabilization and by virtue of the condition cannot mobilize ego assets in a reliable and uniform manner (Kluft 1984b). Despite this, the verbal facility of most MPD patients and/or the excellent function of a few alters can lead the therapist to grossly overestimate their overall ego strength. In fact, many MPD patients can rise to the occasion frequently enough to camouflage their vulnerability. This frequently leads to an overestimation of their resilience and staying power, with a consequent potential for misadventure. The wise therapist is conservative in his or her assessment of how much the MPD patient can tolerate and is always attuned to "the weakest link."

A corollary of these observations is that the circumspect therapist only communicates to the MPD patient what the patient is able to hear and process, not what the material would allow one to interpret. It is essential that the therapist's zeal and narcissistic investment in communicating his or her understandings be tempered by an appreciation of what the patient is prepared to manage. It is useless to have an apparently productive session with more compensated alters that is followed by a severe suicidal or parasuicidal effort on the part of alters that were unable to tolerate what transpired. Many of my patients tell me that I am less astute and say less of substance than their prior therapists. They marvel that anyone can get well in the hands of such a "boring" person. It is my experience that "the slower you go, the faster you get there"—that is, the fewer messes and complications a therapist has to deal with, the more rapidly the therapy can be concluded.

10. Model, Teach, and Reinforce Responsibility

MPD is a condition that often results from the irresponsibility of others. *Therefore, the therapist must be very responsible and must hold the patient to a high standard of responsibility once the therapist is confident that the patient, across alters, actually understands what reasonable responsibility entails.* Usually MPD patients have been the victims of irrational blame imposed by others who took no responsibility for their actions. They often, in different alters, manifest the signs of both a sadistic conscience directed toward themselves and a callous, self-exonerating disregard of the impact of their actions on other alters and others. The therapist must hold the MPD patient responsible in a supportive, empathic, and educative manner, avoiding a punitive and critical stance. Initially, confrontation should be kind, firm, matter-of-fact, and incorruptible. Once it is clear that the patient understands what is required but behaves inappropriately nonetheless, more forthright confrontation may have a role. This may be especially forceful if the issue concerns cooperation with therapy. What is more important than what the therapist says is what the therapist does—that model will serve for identification.

Case Study 1.   A patient asked her psychiatrist to make her prescriptions out in the name of a friend whose benefits included free medication. He declined. The patient complained, but then associated to therapists who are corruptible and to a therapist who had sexualized their work together. Then she said to the psychiatrist, "I guess you did the right thing, you rigid son of a bitch!"

Case Study 2.   A therapist allowed an MPD patient to leave her bills unpaid. She later learned that the patient was continuing antisocial behaviors. A consultant concluded that the therapist was implicitly encouraging irresponsibility and advised a crackdown in all areas. The patient protested vigorously, but she ultimately curtailed the problematic activities.

Case Study 3.   A therapist allowed an MPD patient to escape without consequences for behaviors the host personality did not remember. When confronted, she showed such exquisite wounded innocence that the therapist could not bring himself to impose any sanctions or controls. A consultant observed that the therapist was treating the personalities as separate people rather than as aspects of one mind, and he was not addressing his comments to the whole mind. The therapist imposed consequences, despite his discomfort. To his astonishment, the patient "shaped up" in short order, despite moaning and complaining of impressive intensity.

Two countertransferential stances are common among those relatively unfamiliar with MPD, and both represent essential misperceptions of the nature of the psychopathology. Some see MPD as essentially malingering and take a punitive law-and-order stance that is without empathy for or interest in correcting the MPD patient's confusing plight. Others, often despite their denial, treat the alters as if they were separate people and are upset if one alter is held accountable for the activities of another. They forget that several alters usually are listening in at any given time, and that one can talk over the host to others and communicate with them in this manner (Kluft 1982). The therapist does the patient little good if he or she either overestimates or underestimates the MPD patient's capacity to comprehend and to conform behavior in a reasonable manner. Although complete communication and compliance is rarely achieved, it is of note that the hospital units that operate on the principles outlined here have an excellent record of interrupting dysfunctional behaviors in MPD patients.

---

11. Take an Active, Warm, and Flexible Therapeutic Stance

MPD is a condition that often results from people who could have protected a child doing nothing. *The therapist can anticipate that passivity, affective blandness, and technical neutrality will be experienced as uncaring and rejecting behavior, and that the therapy is better served by taking a more warm and active stance that allows a latitude of affective expression.* Most MPD patients come from backgrounds in which others who did not abuse them directly facilitated their abuse by their silence and passive complicity. In addition, many of the MPD patient's transferences are based on abusers and unconscious flashbacks (Blank 1985) of traumatic scenarios and may emerge abruptly. Therefore, the silent, passive, and neutral therapist is liable to be perceived in ways that lead the patient to misperceive the present as the past. This can be disruptive and dangerous. In my experience with all sorts of trauma victims, the cost-benefit ratio of such a stance is intolerable. It causes the patient tremendous distress and may jeopardize the safety of the treatment situation with MPD patients. I try to be warm and involved and to display a wide range of affect at a very low level of intensity.

There is another benefit to such a stance—it mutes many of a therapist's less egregious countertransference expressions. Work with MPD is exasperating (Coons 1986). Many therapists who attempt to be relatively neutral find themselves abruptly expressing their exasperation and anger at the patient. Conversely, therapists with a wider and more flexible range of affective expression within the treatment are more likely to have milder responses that they and the patient can manage with greater ease.

Case Study 1.   A patient came to me under the following circumstances. At 1:30 A.M., I received a call from a female colleague, who told me that a certain patient was intolerable, that she had been thrown out of therapy, and that she had instructed her to go to my office the following morning. She then hung up. The patient indeed arrived and was given an appointment for a few days later. I learned that the therapist was very neutral and spoke rarely. She and the patient had gotten into traumatic material, and the patient began to react to her as if she were an abuser. The patient vilified the therapist incessantly, and the therapist said very little.

One day the patient was showing the therapist her diary, full of negative reflections on the therapist, and asked to see some drawings done by child alters that the patient had left with the therapist. The therapist grabbed the paintings and tore them to shreds, and then she tore the diary apart. When the patient moved to intervene, the therapist raised her fist. The patient, who gave permission for my use of this vignette, admits to "being a royal bitch at times." However, the manner in which the therapy was conducted offered her little opportunity to mollify her projections. Without feedback or a sense of a reality anchor to which she could relate, she experienced the therapist as if the therapist had the quality of her abusers and was always ready to attack her. The transference assumed psychotic proportions. The therapist was growing more and more exasperated and containing this affect without processing it. Finally she exploded at the patient, with disastrous results. The patient was indeed demanding, but she has achieved integration and resumed a productive professional career.

12. Address and Correct Cognitive Errors

MPD is a condition in which the patient has developed many cognitive errors. *The therapy must address them and correct these cognitive errors on an ongoing basis.* The MPD patient lacks a unified and readily available observing ego, and many usually autonomous ego functions are compromised (Kluft 1984b). Furthermore, trauma disrupts the normal development of cognitive functions (Fine 1988, 1990). Because the MPD patient and the therapist may be processing their interactions and the material that emerges in the therapy in very different ways, there is ample opportunity for misunderstanding and mishap. This makes no small contribution to the difficulty of the treatment and to the likelihood of exasperation on the part of the therapist. It is not necessary to use the tools of formal cognitive therapy, but it is useful to have the patient share his or her thinking aloud and to model rational thought by sharing one's own reasoning process in judiciously chosen circumstances. Most MPD patients are sufficiently eager to please and so fearful of criticism that they will appear to agree with lines of thought that they cannot follow. If an appreciation of these problems escapes the therapist, the road may prove rocky.

Case Study 1.   An MPD patient appeared to agree with everything her therapist interpreted to her, yet therapy was stalemated. A consultant discovered that because the patient feared being disliked, she had endorsed everything the therapist had said. However, in the privacy of her own mind, she had developed a completely idiosyncratic understanding that was based on arbitrary inferences and the assumption of excessive responsibility.

Case Study 2. An MPD patient filled out an informational questionnaire in an extremely bizarre manner that suggested formal psychosis. Inquiry revealed that the patient, who had been told she was subhuman by her abusive parents, had answered the questions from the perspective of a lower animal.

It is difficult to overemphasize the problems that emerge when therapist and patient employ radically divergent cognitive strategies and schemata. I find it helpful to make what I call cognitive interpretations, in which I try to bring to the patient's awareness what I perceive to be the organizing logic of what I have been told. I find it impressive that patients who understand that I understand how their perceptions differ from my own often become much more active participants in therapy and are quite prepared to examine rather than act on their perceptions. One patient said recently, "Now that I can see how weird I think and that you understand what it is that I do, I have some hope of getting out of this maze."

Conclusions

This exploration of basic principles for the treatment of MPD discusses pragmatic rules of thumb that can be applied by most therapists in the context of most schools of therapy. They seem to address most of the problems discovered in consultations to therapists having difficulty in their work with MPD patients. A therapy that violates one of these rules is likely to be in difficulty; a therapy that violates more than one is likely to become stalemated or to fail completely. Although occasional successful therapies are encountered that defy these rules, the psychotherapist is well advised to avoid the assumption that he or she is the exceptional case, a stance fraught with innumerable countertransferential narcissistic traps and invitations to self-deception. Until controlled studies answer many of the unresolved questions in the field, these principles provide useful guidelines based on considerable clinical experience.

References

Allison RB: A new treatment approach for multiple personalities. Am J Clin Hypn 17:15–32, 1974

American Psychiatric Association: Diagnostic and Statistical Manual of Mental Disorders, 3rd Edition, Revised. Washington, DC, American Psychiatric Association, 1987

Beahrs JO: Unity and Multiplicity. New York, Brunner/Mazel, 1982

Bernstein E, Putnam FW: Development, reliability and validity of a dissociation scale. J Nerv Ment Dis 174:727–735, 1986

Blank AS: The unconscious flashback to the war in Viet Nam veterans: clinical mystery, legal defense, and community problem, in The Trauma of War: Stress and Recovery in Viet Nam Veterans. Edited by Sonneberg SM, Blank AS, Talbott JA. Washington, DC, American Psychiatric Press, 1985, pp 293–308

Bowers MK, Brecher-Marer S, Newton B, et al: Therapy of multiple personality. Int J Clin Exp Hypn 19:57–65, 1971

Braun BG (ed): Multiple Personality. Psychiatr Clin North Am 7, 1984

Braun BG: Issues in the psychotherapy of multiple personality, in Treatment of Multiple Personality Disorder. Edited by Braun BG. Washington, DC, American Psychiatric Press, 1986, pp 1–28

Coons PM: Multiple personality: diagnostic considerations. J Clin Psychiatry 41:330–337, 1980

Coons PM: The differential diagnosis of multiple personality. Psychiatr Clin North Am 12:51–67, 1984

Coons PM: Treatment progress in 20 patients with multiple personality disorder. J Nerv Ment Dis 174:715–721, 1986

Coons PM, Bowman ES, Milstein V: Multiple personality disorder: a clinical investigation of 50 cases. J Nerv Ment Dis 176:519–527, 1988

Fine CG: Thought on the cognitive perceptual substrates of multiple personality disorder. Dissociation 1(4):5–10, 1988

Fine CG: The cognitive sequelae of incest, in Incest-Related Syndromes of Adult Psychopathology. Edited by Kluft RP. Washington, DC, American Psychiatric Press, 1990, pp 161–182

Franklin J: Diagnosis of covert and subtle signs of multiple personality disorder through dissociative signs. Dissociation 1(2):27–33, 1988

Franklin J: The diagnosis of multiple personality disorder based on subtle dissociative signs. J Nerv Ment Dis 178:4–14, 1990

Greenson R: The Technique and Practice of Psychoanalysis—I. New York, International Universities Press, 1967

Janoff-Bulman R: The aftermath of victimization: rebuilding shattered assumptions, in Trauma and Its Wake: The Study and Treatment of Post-Traumatic Stress Disorder. Edited by Figley CR. New York, Brunner/Mazel, 1985

Kluft RP: Varieties of hypnotic intervention in the treatment of multiple personality. Am J Clin Hypn 24:230–240, 1982

Kluft RP: Treatment of multiple personality disorder: a study of 33 cases. Psychiatr Clin North Am 7:9–29, 1984a

Kluft RP: Aspects of the treatment of multiple personality disorder. Psychiatric Annals 14:51–55, 1984b

Kluft RP: On Making the Diagnosis of Multiple Personality Disorder (Directions in Psychiatry, Vol 5, Lesson 23). Edited by Flach FF. New York, Hatherleigh, 1985a, pp 1–11

Kluft RP: Treatment of Multiple Personality Disorder (Directions in Psychiatry, Vol 5, Lesson 24). Edited by Flach FF. New York, Hatherleigh, 1985b, pp 1–11

Kluft RP: The natural history of multiple personality disorder, in Childhood Antecedents of Multiple Personality. Edited by Kluft RP. Washington, DC, American Psychiatric Press, 1985c, pp 197–238

Kluft RP: Personality unification in multiple personality disorder: a follow-up study, in Treatment of Multiple Personality Disorder. Edited by Braun BG. Washington, DC, American Psychiatric Press, 1986, pp 29–60

Kluft RP: Making the diagnosis of multiple personality, in Diagnostics and Psychopathology. Edited by Flach FF. New York, WW Norton, 1987a, pp 207–225

Kluft RP: The simulation and dissimulation of multiple personality disorder. Am J Clin Hypn 30:104–118, 1987b

Kluft RP: An update on multiple personality disorder. Hosp Community Psychiatry 38:363–373, 1987c

Kluft RP: On giving consultations to therapists treating multiple personality disorder patients: fifteen years' experience, 1: diagnosis and treatment. Dissociation 1(3):23–29, 1988a

Kluft RP: On giving consultations to therapists treating multiple personality disorder patients: fifteen years' experience, II: the "surround" of treatment, forensics, hypnosis, patient-initiated requests. Dissociation 1(3):30–35, 1988b

Kluft RP: The phenomenology and treatment of extremely complex multiple personality disorder. Dissociation 1(4):47–58, 1988c

Kluft RP: What to bring to therapy. Many Voices, February 1989, pp 4–5, 1989

Kluft RP: Incest and subsequent revictimization: the case of therapist-patient sexual exploitation, with a description of the sitting duck syndrome, in Incest-Related Syndromes of Adult Psychopathology. Edited by Kluft RP. Washington, DC, American Psychiatric Press, 1990, pp 263–287

Kluft RP: Clinical presentations of multiple personality disorder. Psychiatr Clin North Am 14:605–630, 1991a

Kluft RP: Multiple personality disorder, in American Psychiatric Press Annual Review of Psychiatry, Vol 10. Edited by Tasman A, Goldfinger SM. Washington, DC, American Psychiatric Press, 1991b, pp 161–188

Kluft RP: The perspective of a specialist in the dissociative disorders. Psychoanalytic Inquiry 12:139–171, 1992

Kluft RP: The initial phases in the psychotherapy of multiple personality disorder. Dissociation (in press)

Langs R: The Bipersonal Field. New York, Jason Aronson, 1976

Langs R: The Therapeutic Environment. New York, Jason Aronson, 1979

Loewenstein RJ: An office mental status examination for complex chronic dissociative symptoms and multiple personality disorder. Psychiatr Clin North Am 14:567–604, 1991

Putnam FW: The treatment of multiple personality: the state of the art, in Treatment of Multiple Personality Disorder. Edited by Braun BG. Washington, DC, American Psychiatric Press, 1986

Putnam FW: The Diagnosis and Treatment of Multiple Personality Disorder. New York, Guilford, 1989

Putnam FW, Guroff JJ, Silberman EK, et al: The clinical phenomenology of multiple personality disorder: review of 100 recent cases. J Clin Psychiatry 47:285–293, 1986

Ross CA: Multiple Personality Disorder: Diagnosis, Clinical Features, and Treatment. New York, Wiley, 1989

Ross CA, Norton GR, Wozney K: Multiple personality disorder: an analysis of 236 cases. Can J Psychiatry 34:413–418, 1989

Schreiber FR: Sybil. Chicago, IL, Regnery, 1973

Schultz R, Braun BG, Kluft RP: Multiple personality disorder: phenomenology of selected variables in comparison to major depression. Dissociation 2:45–51, 1989

Solomon RS, Solomon V: Differential diagnosis of multiple personality. Psychol Rep 51:1187–1194, 1982

Steinberg M, Rounsaville B, Cicchetti DV: The structured clinical interview for DSM-III-R dissociative disorders: preliminary report on a new diagnostic instrument. Am J Psychiatry 147:76–82, 1990

Torem MS: Dissociative states presenting as an eating disorder. Am J Clin Hypn 29:137–142, 1986

Watkins H: Ego-state theory and therapy, in Encyclopedia of Psychology, Vol 1. Edited by Corsini RJ. New York, Wiley, 1984, pp 420–421

Watkins JG: The Therapeutic Self. New York, Human Sciences Press, 1978

Watkins JG, Watkins HH: Ego-state therapy, in Handbook of Innovative Therapies. Edited by Corsini RJ. New York, Wiley, 1981, pp 252–270

Chapter 4

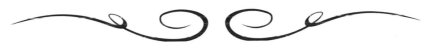

Posttraumatic and Dissociative Aspects of Transference and Countertransference in the Treatment of Multiple Personality Disorder

Richard J. Loewenstein, M.D.

Cornelia Wilbur is the originator of the modern conceptualization of multiple personality disorder (MPD; Schreiber 1973). All of us who work with MPD patients are her intellectual offspring. Connie Wilbur was the first to describe the complexity of the alter system in MPD patients. She also was the first to describe MPD as a developmental disorder related to childhood abuse and trauma. She was the first to formulate the modern view of dissociative defenses in MPD and the first to describe multiple transference reactions to the therapist

The author gratefully acknowledges the contributions to this work of his anonymous coauthors, his patients. Without their invaluable assistance, this chapter could never have been written.

51

among the alters in MPD patients (Wilbur 1984, 1988).

As I have described elsewhere (Loewenstein 1988), Connie Wilbur can be understood to have begun a "scientific revolution" in which a new "paradigm" for the dissociative disorders was formulated. According to Kuhn (1970),

> [A paradigm] define[s] the legitimate problems and methods and research in a field for succeeding generations. . . . The achievement [is] sufficiently unprecedented to attract an enduring group of adherents . . . [and] it [is] sufficiently open-ended to leave all sorts of problems for the redefined group of practitioners to solve. (p. 10)

A scientific revolution is defined by Kuhn as "a noncumulative developmental episode in which an older paradigm is replaced in whole or in part by an incompatible new one" (1970, p. 91).
Kuhn also states:

> During revolutions scientists see new and different things when looking with familiar instruments in places they have looked before. . . .
> In so far as their only recourse to that world is through what they see and do, we may want to say that *after a revolution scientists are responding to a different world.* (1970, p. 111; italics added)

Many of us believe that the apparent "explosion" in the diagnosis of MPD and dissociative disorders is really a result of the recognition of patients who have always been with us but simply were not "seen" before there was a paradigm to allow us to do so. This is the result of what might be called the "Wilburian Revolution" in the understanding of MPD. Although Kuhn (1970) does not focus extensively on the development of biological, medical, or social sciences in his discussion of the effects on perception of scientific revolutions, he notes that "skeptics" of his view "might remember that color blindness was nowhere noticed until John Dalton's description of it in 1794" (p. 192).

Kuhn's ideas also help us understand aspects of the battle between the "believers" and "skeptics" of the new paradigm in the study of MPD (see Dell 1988):

The proponents of competing paradigms practice their trades in different worlds. . . . Practicing in different worlds, the two groups . . . see different things when they look from the same point in the same direction. Both are looking at the world, and what they look at has not changed. But in some areas they see different things, and they see them in different relations one to the other. That is why a law that cannot even be demonstrated to one group of scientists may occasionally seem intuitively obvious to another. Equally, it is why, before they can hope to communicate fully, one group or the other must experience the conversion that we have been calling a paradigm shift. Just because it is a transition between incommensurables, the transition between the competing paradigms can not be made a step at a time, forced by logic and neutral experience. Like the gestalt switch, it must occur all at once (though not necessarily in an instant) or not at all. (1970, p. 150)

Transference, Countertransference, and MPD

In this chapter, I discuss aspects of transference, countertransference, limit setting, and boundary management in the treatment of MPD. To structure the subsequent discussion, I first briefly review basic concepts of transference and countertransference. I then review Connie Wilbur's contributions to this area. Next, I review some basic aspects of the post-Wilburian paradigm of MPD as a severe dissociative posttraumatic developmental disorder. Then, based on this review, I discuss aspects of transference and countertransference encountered in work with MPD patients.

Definitions of Transference and Countertransference

It would be impossible in this chapter for me to review completely the concepts of transference and countertransference in the psychoanalytic and psychotherapy literature (for such reviews, see Gill 1982; Greenson 1967; Laplanche and Pontalis 1973; Sandler et al. 1973).

Sandler and colleagues (1973) define transference thus:

a specific illusion which develops in regard to the other person, one which, unbeknown to the subject, represents in some of its features, a repetition of a relationship to an important figure in the person's past. It should be emphasized that this is felt by the subject not as a repetition of the past, but as strictly appropriate to the present and to the particular person involved. . . . [T]ransference need not be restricted to the illusory apperception of another person . . . but can be taken to include the unconscious (and often subtle) attempts to manipulate or to provoke situations with others which are a concealed repetition of earlier experiences and relationships. (pp. 49–50)

Classically, countertransference is defined as a homologue to transference (Greenson 1967; Laplanche and Pontalis 1973; Racker 1957; Sandler et al. 1973). That is, it represents unconscious activation in the therapist of blind spots, personality traits, and/or transference feelings toward the patient. These may be particularly aroused by certain patients or certain types of material or transference presented by patients (Sandler et al. 1973).

Currently, the view of countertransference has been expanded to define a variety of empathic phenomena that the therapist experiences about the patient's feelings, thoughts, reactions, and perceptions (Peebles-Kleiger 1989; Racker 1957). The therapist's empathic resonance with the patient is considered essential for understanding the patient (Kernberg 1984; Ogden 1979; Racker 1957; Searles 1979). Thus, the therapist must be sufficiently self-aware, and/or able to engage in sufficiently detached self-exploration, to be able to separate his or her own thoughts, reactions, conflicts, and feelings from those he or she empathically "takes in" from the patient (Racker 1957; Wilbur 1988).

A related notion is that the therapeutic situation is an interpersonal "field." In this view, manifestations of transference are generated from an interplay between the patient's reactions to the therapist and events in the actual therapeutic situation, in addition to the patient's unconscious reactions to important figures in his or her past and present life (Gill 1982; Langs 1977; Peebles-Kleiger 1989).

The therapist can not be uninvolved but rather influences the patient, who in turn influences the therapist; the drama that unfolds is always "created in the interaction." The therapist is no longer screen but instead is fellow-actor and codirector. The therapist learns the patient's past not as dispassionate audience, but as involved participant. (Peebles-Kleiger 1989, p. 520)

Countertransference can be "concordant," in which the therapist identifies with the patient and empathically internalizes the patient's feelings about him- or herself. Also, there is "complementary" countertransference, in which the therapist identifies with the patient's internalized version of significant others (Racker 1957). The process of projective identification may influence this process significantly. In projective identification:

A resonating field is set up with significant others in which the patient not only sees the other as having feelings not tolerable to the self, but also exerts an intense pull on the other to identify with and temporarily embrace those very feelings, however uncharacteristic they may be for that person. (Peebles-Kleiger 1989, p. 519)

Ogden (1979) points out that projective identification can represent

a pathway for psychological change by which feelings similar to those with which one is struggling are processed by another person, following which the projector may identify with the recipient's handling of the engendered feelings. (p. 371)

Peebles-Kleiger (1989) suggests that projective identification is common in those who have developed a dissociative response to childhood trauma. She argues that the psychological dividedness produced by the dissociative process readily facilitates this form of defense, especially when extreme forms of dissociative disavowal and denial are present. Thus, projective identification is common in MPD patients, especially very complex MPD patients with highly developed forms of layering and internal secrecy. Indeed, it may be that MPD patients demonstrate forms of "internal" projective identification from one dissociated part-self to another. As one MPD patient stated to her therapist: "You know, I'm finding out that the problems between you and me are really problems between me and me."

It may also be that an aspect of the abuse in MPD families involves a form of malignant projective identification from the abusive parent to the dissociation-prone child (Galdstone 1981). This may be an aspect of the process of formation of alters that appear as literal representations of abusive family members.

Cornelia Wilbur and Transference in MPD Patients

Connie Wilbur (1988) wrote the first systematic discussion of transference in the MPD literature. Here, she focuses on the various transferences manifested by the different MPD alters and the potential impact of these on the therapist:

> In [MPD] each individual alter within the complex develops its own transferential relationship with the therapist. Each transference relationship can become extremely complicated because it contains admixtures of many forms of transference. (Wilbur 1988, p. 73)

She discusses negative, dependent, and erotic transferences in MPD patients, as well as manifestations of transference as a resistance. She primarily relates these transference phenomena to the abuse experienced by the MPD patient and notes that therapists often fail to appreciate the subtlety and complexity of the transferences in MPD patients. She urges interpretation of the transference rather than either excessive gratification or retaliation against the patient for extreme positive and negative transferences, respectively.

Connie Wilbur describes frequent negative countertransference reactions to "very bright angry alters' persistent needlings and criticisms that provoke the therapist" (1988, p. 74). She also comments on actual erotic activity between therapist and patient as an unfortunately all-too-frequent transference/countertransference complication in the treatment of MPD.

Other Discussions of Transference/ Countertransference in the MPD Literature

Throughout his classic book, Putnam (1989) discusses transference/countertransference issues in work with MPD patients. He focuses on the multiple transferences of the MPD alters and the relationship of these patterns to childhood experiences with abusive and traumatizing figures. He points out the specific posttraumatic nature of transference phenomena in MPD. For example, apparently neutral aspects of the therapy situation, such as the configuration of chairs in the room, may trigger intense, often seemingly inexplicable emotional reactions related to dissociated traumatic experiences. Both Kluft (1984) and Spiegel (1986) have commented on the pervasive phenomenon of the "traumatic transference" in the treatment of MPD. Two related processes are subsumed under this concept. First, "the patient unconsciously expects that the therapist, despite overt helpfulness and concern, will exploit the patient for his or her own narcissistic gratification" (Spiegel 1986, p. 72). Because of this, virtually all aspects of therapy may be unconsciously understood by the patient to indicate abusive intent of some kind. Second, the term has been used to describe a perceptual illusion during therapy in which the therapist is literally experienced by the patient as a personification of a specific abuser (e.g., the father [Spiegel 1986]). I prefer to call this the "flashback transference." Briere (1989) makes a similar distinction.

Trauma-based transference issues also have been described in studies on the psychotherapy of combat veterans with severe forms of posttraumatic stress disorder (PTSD) and non-MPD survivors of incest and abuse (Briere 1989; Courtois 1988; Lindy 1988).

Putnam (1989) also discusses a variety of common countertransference issues in MPD treatment. These include basic problems in relating to the world of alters, such as reactions to the complexity and changeability of the MPD patient; difficulties in absorbing and working with traumatic memories; fantasies of reparenting the patient; omnipotent grandiosity in the therapist; problems handling erotic feelings toward the patient, as well as from the patient toward the therapist; and difficulties with reactions from colleagues.

Kluft (1984) also details the reactions of therapists working with MPD patients. These include "initial excitement, fascination, [and] overinvestment . . . yield[ing] to feelings of bewilderment, exasperation, and a sense of being drained by the patient" (p. 52). He describes the difficulties in working with MPD patients some of whose alters are abusive, demanding, intrusive, and controlling. He notes the empathic difficulties in working in the shifting landscape of the transference field of the MPD patient. He also comments on the problems therapists encounter working with the traumatic memories produced by MPD patients. He states that "empathizing with the MPD patient's experience of traumatization is grueling. One is tempted to withdraw, intellectualize, or defensively ruminate about whether or not the events are 'real'" (p. 53).

Lindy (1988), in a research study of intensive individual psychotherapy of Vietnam combat veterans with PTSD, described a number of countertransference reactions among the psychotherapists in the study. These included affects of rage, shame, fear, guilt, awe, horror, dread, voyeurism and excitement, disillusionment, and condemnation. Defensive avoidance, disavowal, "clinging to the professional role" (p. 255), isolation and intellectualization were common, especially in reaction to fear, anxiety, horror, and dread. Counterphobic overidentification and overprotection were also common. Therapists even noted PTSD symptoms such as nightmares, intrusive images, reenactments, amnesia, estrangement, alienation, irritability, excessive alcohol use, psychophysiological reactions, and survivor guilt. Briere (1989) describes similar countertransference phenomena in therapists of non-MPD incest survivors. "Secondary PTSD" has also been described in therapists and inpatient hospital staff working with MPD patients (Olson et al. 1987).

Overview of the Post-Wilburian View of
MPD and Its Relevance for Understanding
Transference and Countertransference

A review of some basic concepts in the modern study of MPD is helpful to focus the subsequent discussion of transference/countertransference in the treatment of MPD. The themes described here frequently occur in the transference of the MPD patient. Because of Connie Wilbur's pioneering observations, MPD is now understood as a complex form of posttraumatic dissociative disorder primarily related to severe, repetitive childhood abuse or trauma usually beginning before the age of 5 (Kluft 1988; Putnam 1989). Because most MPD patients have been traumatized in a family context, it is inevitable that a psychotherapeutic relationship will focus intense, overdetermined, trauma-related issues in the transference (Briere 1989).

In most cases, MPD patients report that the abuse has been perpetrated by family members. Less frequently, patients report that family members have been so neglectful, unnurturant, or emotionally unengaged with the patient that they ignored, minimized, and/or implicitly encouraged traumatization or abuse by those outside the immediate family or were unavailable to comfort the patient after nonabusive trauma such as repeated, painful medical procedures or near-death experiences (Kluft 1985; Wilbur 1988). In either case, MPD families provide little consistent nurturance or comforting, leaving the child to soothe and comfort him- or herself after being hurt (Kluft 1984; Marmer 1980).

Abuse in the histories of MPD patients is generally described as a mixture of recurrent sexual, physical, and emotional abuse usually of a highly sadistic, intrusive nature (Putnam 1989). MPD patients also frequently report histories of neglect, witnessing violence or murder in childhood, as well as other extreme forms of abuse such as confinement abuse; witnessing pets killed as punishment; denial of food as punishment; ritualistic abuse; recurrent bizarre "medical" procedures, such as frequent painful enemas; abuse as part of criminal activities of the perpetrators (e.g., child pornography or child prostitution); and being forced to perpetrate abuse on others (Putnam 1989).

Subtle or overt forms of psychological control and manipulation of the child's fears and emotional reactions to the abuse is also commonly reported. MPD patients often describe this as the most distressing aspect of the abuse. As one patient put it: "They could have my body if they wanted. It was when they went after my mind that things really got bad."

While growing up, the MPD child may also chronically experience bizarre, abusive double-binds and mixed messages; role reversal and "parentification"; secrets, denial, deceit, and "dual" realities (one inside the family and one outside); complete absence of interpersonal boundaries, often combined with rigid moralism; violence that may be planned and controlled or, alternatively, impulsive and wild; secret gratifications and power dynamics; attempts to invasively psychologically control or even "enslave" the child; family members who are so changeable, either due to their own dissociation or other factors, that they literally may appear to be "different people" at different times, especially to the child at the preoperational level of cognitive development; and family chaos with shifting partners, lovers, domiciles, and so on (Braun 1986; Briere 1989; Courtois 1988; Fine 1991; Fish-Murray et al. 1986; Kluft 1985, 1988; Putnam 1989; Spiegel 1986). In some MPD families, patients report that all adult family members, even multigenerationally, participate in and/or actively encourage and seek out abusive, exploitative, and perverse relationships with children. Children in these families may be actively encouraged to turn into perpetrators themselves at an early age, either with their siblings or other children.

In some ways, the MPD patient can be conceptualized as growing up in a different culture or a different "world" (R. P. Kluft, personal communication, February 1989), one in which abusive, exploitative relationships are the expected norm determining all basic aspects of the child's reality. In this world, the problem is not *whether* abuse will occur, but how to control, manage, and minimize its *inevitable* occurrence. As described by one highly complex MPD patient who reported an extensive history of physical, sexual, and psychological abuse by many family members and outsiders brought in by her parents:

> I never knew much about the outside world. I never went out except to school, and when I did well there, they tried to take that away from me too. I had to take care of the house and everything even when I was 4 or 5. I wasn't allowed to have friends or anything to do with anyone outside the family. They all lived together. That was all I ever knew. I was lucky to escape when I was 16. Otherwise I might never have gotten out of there.

Connie Wilbur was also the first to note that one function of the dissociation in MPD children is to preserve a relationship with the abusive parent (Putnam 1989; Schreiber 1973). Awareness of the abuse is dissociated into the "other" self that relates to the "other" parent. Thus, in many MPD patients, alters (or groups of alters) may be developed to contain, symbolize, and manage aspects of relationships to various family members, abusive or not. If an MPD patient's parent also had MPD, then some of his or her alters may specifically correlate with those of the MPD parent (Kluft 1985).

MPD Dissociativity and Transference

Recent studies suggest an important relationship between traumatization and dissociative and hypnotic capacities (Bliss 1986; Carlson and Putnam 1989). MPD patients frequently naturalistically display phenomena homologous to that seen in highly hypnotizable subjects without MPD studied in research hypnosis paradigms (Bliss 1986). These include intense absorption experiences, spontaneous trances, complex amnesias, hypermnesia, anesthesias, spontaneous negative hallucinations and age-regressions, dissociated motor actions, complex multimodal hallucinations and imagery, out-of-body experiences, hidden observer-like phenomena, and trance logic (Bliss 1986; Hilgard 1986; Kluft 1988; Loewenstein 1991; Loewenstein et al. 1988; Putnam 1989). A Spiegel eye-roll (Spiegel and Spiegel 1978) frequently accompanies switches in MPD patients, although this may be difficult to observe because of eyelid closure (Putnam 1988). Further, MPD patients usually manifest high scores on standard scales of hypnotizability (Bliss 1986).

Characteristics of the Dissociative/Posttraumatic Transference Field in Work With MPD Patients

The transference field in the treatment of MPD is fundamentally dissociative and posttraumatic. Abuse-related and trance-based phenomena are ubiquitous. In the following discussion, I will focus on transference "field effects," moving from the vantage point of the therapist to that of patient and back again. For simplicity, dissociative and posttraumatic aspects of the transference field will be discussed separately. In actuality, these processes are simultaneous and interactive in the treatment situation and are blended with more classical forms of transference.

Because of the nature of the dissociative defenses of the MPD patient, the therapist must be aware that core dynamic issues and critical historical information about the patient are usually shrouded in amnesia. Clarity about them may only emerge through problems, crises, and impasses, often primarily manifesting themselves in the transference.

For the most part, these transference/countertransference difficulties are unavoidable. It is the more-or-less successful *management* of them that leads to their eventual resolution over the long term. One very complex MPD patient summed up this process after years of recurrent problems and crises, each one eventually leading to increased understanding and mastery: "In the school of life, you get the test first and the lesson afterwards."

Properties of the Dissociative Transference Field

In this section, using a framework derived from the study of hypnosis, I outline the implications for the transference field of the high dissociativity of the MPD patient. I also discuss aspects of the therapist's experiences that may be clues to dissociation in the patient. Dissociative aspects of the transference field in MPD include absorption, focused attention, and amnesia; altered perceptions; and cognitive distortions such as literalness and tolerance and rationalization of illogic and contradiction (see Brown and Fromm 1986).

Absorption, Focused Attention, and Amnesia

Absorption, focused and/or selective attention, and amnesia are basic aspects of the hypnotic process (Brown and Fromm 1986). At least some degree of absorption in the imaginative creation of alter selves is characteristic of most MPD patients. Selective inattention to basic aspects of inner experience and major events in the life history also characterize the mental life of MPD patients. Clinically, this process ultimately results in gross amnesia experiences for many aspects of the life history and current interactions, including the therapeutic one.

MPD patients often describe intense discomfort in attempting to look at dissociated aspects of their experience or even to recognize their own propensity to dissociate. The selectively focused attention of the MPD patient often helps to maintain dissociation so intensely that any movement toward greater awareness may be experienced as dysphoric. The therapist may empathically experience the MPD patient's conflict about proceeding with therapy through concordant projective identifications. In this situation, the therapist may experience doubts about the correctness of the diagnosis of MPD (even though meeting alters on a regular basis), unnecessary concern about iatrogenic artifact, and excessive worries that the patient will be psychologically harmed by working directly with the multiplicity. This may also be seen in the psychiatric hospital milieu when patients with MPD are inpatients. Here, the common "belief-disbelief" split among staff often projectively mirrors a similar conflict about belief within the MPD patient.

It is useful for the therapist to bear in mind that the uncertainties he or she experiences about basic aspects of work with the MPD patient may at least partly reflect appropriate empathic attunement to the patient's conflicts about accepting the MPD diagnosis and opening up more fully in therapy. For example, if the therapist experiences preoccupation about the accuracy of the diagnosis or iatrogenesis, he or she may usefully inquire whether the patient has related concerns. Similarly, relating the hospital staff's struggles over belief in MPD to a similar process in the patient may be a helpful intervention in hospital treatment of MPD.

The most useful stance for the therapist is to help the patient begin to recognize and resolve such conflicts internally rather than by projection and externalization. The therapist may point out that it is up to the patient as a whole ultimately to resolve questions about the actual diagnosis, the utility of therapy, the meaning of the personal history, and so on. The therapist should be a facilitator and consultant to this process, not its final arbiter.

Similarly, therapists may become intensely absorbed, fascinated, and preoccupied with their MPD patients. In the countertransference, the therapist of the MPD patient may attend selectively to the dictates of basic clinical common sense, boundary issues, and realistic assessment of the MPD patient's pathology. This may lead to major distortions in the basic framework of treatment, such as length of sessions, fees, and the appropriate structure for therapist-patient interactions (Greaves 1988). The therapist's private life may become dominated by ruminations about the patient or intrusions by the patient into it via phone calls, emergencies, and the like. The therapist may become selectively inattentive to the personal and professional consequences of doing this and to the risk of his or her own enervation in this process. Some therapists even report developing a kind of dissociative split at such times. "Part" of them knows that there are countertransference problems but feels unable to stop another "part" that persists in conducting therapy in a maladaptive way. In extreme cases, the therapist's pathology is activated sufficiently that an extratherapy relationship develops between patient and therapist, invariably with disastrous consequences for the patient and often for the therapist as well.

In the transference field, the therapist and patient may unconsciously collude in not attending to a variety of important therapy issues and tasks. The therapist may not be able to "see" beyond the immediate clinical issues the patient presents in treatment. For example, a common therapeutic misalliance occurs in the treatment of MPD when the therapist and the patient focus only on gratifying certain alters, such as child alters, to the relative exclusion of all others. Similarly, therapists often conclude that the patient only has a few alters despite multitudes of unexplained symptoms and difficulties. The same therapist working with a non-MPD patient would hardly consider the limited mental contents of these few entities sufficient to account for the whole psychology of a person.

With respect to amnesia, the therapist of the MPD patient may frequently find difficulty in remembering what was said by the patient in previous sessions, even very important therapy material. Sudden amnesia during sessions may be also experienced by the MPD therapist. Similarly, Lindy (1988) has described amnesia and fragmentary recall for important clinical material in therapists working with traumatized Vietnam combat veterans.

It sometimes feels to the self-aware therapist in the MPD transference field that he or she has developed complete amnesia for the therapeutic skills that have worked effectively with patients with other diagnoses. Successful treatment of MPD seems partly to result from being able to remember and apply previously learned knowledge in the context of the dissociative transference field.

In this regard, it is helpful for the therapist to make conscious efforts to step back from the work with the MPD patient and take a broader perspective in order to try to overcome his or her selective attention and amnesia. Commonsensical, no-nonsense self-examination along the lines of "What would I do if this patient had bipolar disorder?" may be salubrious in this process.

Altered Perceptions and Trancelike Phenomena

Hallucinations in all sensory modalities, pseudo-hallucinations, illusions, anesthesias, negative hallucinations, and marked depersonalization experiences are all characteristic of deep trance. Clinically, most MPD patients display these phenomena on a routine basis. For example, in the flashback transference, some alters will continually "see" the therapist as someone else, usually an abusive figure from the past. Others will describe complex multimodal hallucinations in sessions or the ability to make the therapist "disappear."

On the other hand, some alters may report that they can provide misleading auditory and visual impressions about the therapist to other alters. Some alters may appear superficially to be relating adequately to contemporary reality in therapy. When questioned, however, they may admit that they do not know who the therapist really is and are unaware of basic orienting information about the contemporary situation such as the date or the purpose of the meeting.

It is useful for the therapist to have an index of suspicion that some or all of these phenomena are occurring continuously in the transference field. It is important to check and recheck with the patient about them, and it is helpful to convey to the patient the understanding that these phenomena are used at least in part as protective and restitutive measures.

For example, frequently these perceptual distortions have to do with (often covert) negative transference concerns about the therapist's trustworthiness, inherent dangerousness, and potential abusiveness. At one level, seeing an abuser instead of the therapist may be an attempt to warn vulnerable alters to "be careful." Also, the therapist may inadvertently trigger dissociated memories by words or gestures reminiscent of past traumatic situations. Thus, the therapy may stimulate flashback-based imagery on a continual basis in the patient.

It is most useful to identify these processes openly and to make them areas of focus for collaborative therapeutic work. Thus, the therapist might suggest that the patient's alter system as a whole might work more directly on the problem of pacing the therapy to avoid the untoward effects of too-rapid derepression. Negative transference feelings must be explored in detail within and among the different alters. Identification and detoxification of triggers for the purpose of their ultimate mastery is a vital therapeutic task for the MPD patient. This can be powerfully worked on directly in the transference situation, because so many basic triggers for the MPD patient are interpersonal.

Because of the intensity of the dissociative projective identifications, the therapist may also experience altered perceptions in work with MPD patients. These often-disconcerting phenomena include intense imagery, often with a sexual or aggressive content, negative hallucinations, depersonalization, trancelike experiences, countertransferential "spacing out" and sleepiness, and inability to think. Obviously, therapists must be extremely rigorous in accounting for their own idiosyncratic countertransference contributions to such phenomena. Also, it is critical for the therapist to inquire neutrally and tactfully when experiencing in the countertransference disquieting sexual or aggressive imagery that seems to be evoked projectively by the patient.

For example, I had the following experience in my early work with an MPD patient who had previously become overinvolved with several therapists. During a fairly routine session, I momentarily became flooded with an insistent visual image and tactile hallucination of touching the patient in an intimate manner. Although I felt intensely disquieted and disoriented by this experience, I managed to inquire neutrally if "something had shifted" within her at that moment. She replied: "Yes, the sexy one is here now. And do you know what? She's a child!" As this personality emerged and began to talk, my hallucinatory experiences ceased.

We were then able to discuss more openly various alters' fears that I would become involved with the sexual alter, who would be unable to refuse my advances. Also, we were able to discuss this alter's previous exploitation in several prior therapy and nontherapy relationships. The patient's more executive alters had been unaware that this alter was a child. Clarification of this led to better understanding of the particular sexual predicaments in which this patient frequently found herself. Ultimately, the patient was able to extricate herself from an abusive sadomasochistic sexual relationship that strongly evoked this alter.

With respect to negative hallucinations, a consultee of mine literally "forgot" to notice that in the middle of every therapy session for several months, an MPD patient's partner walked into the office to bring the patient a cup of tea. This was finally mentioned to me in passing during a consultation session. The consultee was amazed at having so successfully blocked from her own awareness the event and its meaning in terms of a variety of treatment issues.

Sudden countertransferential "spacing out," such as finding oneself thinking about something else and/or mild depersonalization, are often indicative of covert switching, passive influence, or dissociative processes "behind the scenes" in the MPD patient. At such times it is often useful to inquire whether something has just changed or shifted inside the patient or whether a covert switch or passive-influence experience has occurred.

One complex MPD patient began to describe intense dissociative spells in which she would "float away," both in sessions and at other times. She related these events to abuse involving deliberate induction of intense hypnotic states by those who had abused her. At other times, as she worked on abuse-related material, she would become uncontrollably sleepy. It eventually became a standing joke between us that episodes of my feeling sleepy, spacey, or preoccupied in her sessions (or even on the phone) almost invariably were empathically in tune with her own experiences. She said, "You didn't know that dissociation was contagious!"

At other times countertransferential sleepiness may be a response to covert conflict between alters over emergence and/or attempts by the patient to suppress painful material or unacceptable feelings in the transference. The therapist's sense that his or her thoughts are absent, blocked, or slowed may also be an empathic response to similar processes in the patient.

Occasionally, an alter describes direct control of such phenomena. For example, I began to feel very sleepy on a recurrent basis in work with another highly complex MPD patient. However, I did not feel sleepy in sessions scheduled right after hers. After several fruitless weeks of castigating myself and unsuccessfully attempting to analyze my countertransference responses, I asked her if *she* ever felt sleepy in sessions. She answered affirmatively. I asked if anyone "inside" caused this. The patient replied: "Oh, you mean Sandy? Does she do that to you too?"

"Sandy" was introduced and described her concern that too much was being revealed too quickly. She turned out to be very important in this patient's system, especially concerning titration of alters' tolerance for traumatic memories or full awareness of one another. My sudden sleepiness in sessions often signaled her arrival.

Cognitive Aspects of the Dissociative Transference Field in MPD
Trance logic—the tolerance and/or rationalization of logical inconsistency while in the hypnotic state—has been described as a core aspect of the cognition of MPD patients (Bliss 1986; Orne 1959). In addition, literal-mindedness and field-dependence characterize the cognition of the hypnotized person. The latter are also aspects of the unusual paralogical thinking of the MPD patient that may subtly infect the therapist.

Both patient and therapist may accept literally and uncritically the MPD patient's implicit or explicit premises about the nature of the patient's inner world. For example, therapists often readily believe that child or adolescent alters are *literally* the same in their needs and inner experiences as actual external children or adolescents. Cursory observation of real children is sufficient to demonstrate that the MPD child alter is an enacted representation of the childhood state, not its literal embodiment. Similarly, therapists may fail to examine critically the MPD patient's characterization of rageful alters, self-destructive alters, demonic alters, omniscient alters, robot alters, animal alters, and so on. The patient's view that some entities are part of "the system" and others alien to it is also often accepted by the therapist without question. Popular works such as *When Rabbit Howls* (Chase 1987) both illustrate and add to these difficulties by promulgating the unfortunate notion that the MPD alters are "separate people" rather than dissociated, concretely personified aspects of a single person.

Misguided ideas about this can lead to major therapeutic difficulties. For example, a worried therapist decided not to send the police to a suicidal patient's house because "the 16-year-old was out" and other alters refused to emerge to discuss hospitalization. The therapist had concluded that "an adolescent" would have been traumatized by the arrival of the police. Fortunately, the patient did not act on any suicidal urges. To be sure, the clinical naivete of the therapist is often important in such responses. However, I have seen mature clinicians make similar sorts of errors with MPD patients. Further, even naive or inexperienced clinicians usually do not make these types of errors with schizophrenic or bipolar patients.

These intensely projected dissociative distortions of logic may be part of the process that leads many therapists unquestioningly to attempt to provide external restorative experiences for the MPD patient rather than asking the patient to use his or her system's own resources to comfort and soothe those inside who are in difficulty. Patients are often partly gratified by this—partly relieved not to have to confront their own dissociativity, and partly resentful of the repetition inherent in having something "done" to them by a powerful external person who neglects the patient's inner experience and implicitly denies the patient's own resources. Thus, in the name of reparenting the patient, the therapist and patient reenact in a symbolic form a basic aspect of the abuse process that began the multiplicity!

The Posttraumatic Transference Field in Work With MPD

Introduction

Everything about the transference field in the treatment of MPD has a posttraumatic aspect. Indeed, much of what has been described in the previous section can be understood not only from the vantage point of dissociativity but from a posttraumatic one as well. The intensity of the traumatic transference in work with MPD patients is fueled by the shared trance experiences of both participants.

I will highlight a few major posttraumatic themes that commonly recur in work with MPD patients. They include management of boundaries and limit setting; the wish for a cure through love and nurturance; overt and covert flashbacks in the transference; lack of trust and the expectation of abusive intent; and action orientation.

Management of Boundaries, Limit Setting, and the Wish to Be Loved Into Health

Few topics command as much attention in consultation about the therapy of the MPD patient as those of boundaries and limit setting. Boundaries are particularly problematic in several ways in the treatment of patients with MPD.

First, the MPD patient has formed overabundant and overly rigid *internal* boundaries by using dissociative compartmentalization and creation of alter selves as a way of surviving childhood trauma (Fine 1989). Thus, much of the treatment is focused on altering the patient's internal boundaries by doing integrative therapy work (Kluft 1984). Overall, when treatment is successful, this process may be experienced very positively by the patient. However, many aspects of the work are experienced by the patient as excruciatingly painful, cruel, unfair, abusive, assaultive, and so on (Putnam 1989; Spiegel 1986).

Second, the patient's internal boundary problems have developed in response to family circumstances characterized by malignantly poor boundaries. In typical MPD families, parents could commit any known sexual perversion on their children with impunity, but the child was subjected to extreme punishment even for manifestations of normal development such as thumb-sucking or bed-wetting. The overt roles of the MPD patient's parents (and, later, other authority figures such as doctors, teachers, ministers, prior therapists, and others) did not predict their actual behavior. As Briere (1989) describes, the survivor of sexual abuse (and thus, most MPD patients) has been taught that relationship boundaries are "negotiable" and that the apparent role descriptions are relatively unimportant to what actually occurs in human interactions.

Also, children in MPD families may be press-ganged into age-inappropriate family roles. MPD patients report cooking, cleaning, doing laundry, and caring for other siblings even before the age of 5, with severe punishments frequently reported as a consequence of failing to follow parental demands. For example, one patient reported being physically disciplined at age 5 by her mother for phoning a neighbor when her slightly older brother (with whom she had been left home alone) developed a high fever. The mother was furious because she had returned home with her date after an evening out to find a male neighbor with whom she had also been involved tending to her sick child. She forbade the patient ever to call for help again in this manner.

Also, the MPD patient is often understandably desperate for love, nurturance, and comfort. This may manifest itself as a wish to be "loved into health" rather than do the painful therapy work of gaining self-understanding (R. P. Kluft, personal communication, October 1984). This wish is frequently unconscious to the whole MPD alter system and is often expressed indirectly through many alters. Thus it is often powerfully (and dissociatively) communicated to the therapist. The therapist who is unprepared to recognize this issue and deal with it by interpretation rather than action frequently reenacts the abuse relationship symbolically by breaking the therapy boundaries. It is almost inherent in the literal reparenting strategies for MPD patients that the childhood abuse-based themes of boundary transgression, inappropriate gratification, seduction, and abandonment are continuously replayed with the MPD patient.

The wish to be loved into health may have a number of determinants. First, it represents the patient's preservation of hope and the wish to get well despite the abusive past. Also, it is protective of the patient's current adaptation and positive feelings for his or her family. Thus it may represent a powerful resistance to forming a working alliance with the therapist in order to avoid the anguish that the patient senses will be a basic part of the therapy. The patient can therefore delay relinquishing dissociative dividedness and its protective numbing of pain, can keep at bay the shame and horror at the actual life history, can be spared the bitter task of giving up attachments to abusers and grieving the lost years and wasted time caused by the abuse and the multiplicity, and may suppress the intense feelings of rage at the unfairness of having to abandon numbing dissociative defenses despite having already endured years of difficulties because of abuse. All of these themes will be central to the work in the transference with most MPD patients.

At another level, the implicit (or explicit) requests for nurturance test the therapist. They test the therapist's standards and values and the therapist's willingness to go along with symbolic or actual violations of boundaries. They test the therapist's willingness to work with the angry, mistrustful, challenging alters who are usually concealed just behind the ones imploring for love. They test whether the therapist will risk disagreement with the patient on matters of principle and clinical judgment. They test whether the therapist will stand up for nonabusive values or will behave like a coabusive parent who coldly sanctions abuse while sanctimoniously claiming moral superiority.

Issues concerning boundaries will come up recurrently throughout the treatment of the MPD patient. They will be manifested continually and pleomorphically in the transference field. They will be linked intimately to the patterns of abusive relationships with past important figures.

It is likely that, at some point, even the most circumspect and experienced therapist will find him- or herself in some sort of boundary predicament in work with MPD patients. This is partly because of the inherent "pull" of the intense covert projective identifications in the dissociative field. Also, therapeutic work with MPD requires a mixture of well-defined boundaries and therapeutic creativity and flexibility. The tension between these may lead the therapist to allow the boundaries to become porous in some way.

If this occurs, it is useful for the therapist to openly address the difficulties that have arisen. He or she should then attempt to restore the appropriate boundaries without blaming the patient. It is useful to indicate that both parties have had a role in the creation of the current predicament, generally motivated to do something helpful or to resolve some problem. It may be fruitful to use the MPD metaphor in these discussions by suggesting that the issue has "come to ask for help" by manifesting itself in this way in the transference. Past errors cannot be changed; the issue becomes, how can we learn from them and go on from here?

In general, it is helpful early in treatment for the therapist of the MPD patient to discuss the importance of boundaries. All alters are asked to listen. The therapist can observe that the MPD patient's experiences historically with the boundaries of important people are likely to have been painfully confusing and traumatizing. Thus, in therapy, ongoing clarification and maintenance of boundaries will be a basic therapeutic task. It is also useful to introduce the notion that observation and reflection on the evocation in the transference field of past experiences, such as difficulties around boundaries, is the basic therapeutic approach. The purpose is to help the patient gain mastery through insight rather than stalemate or retraumatization through reenactment.

It is also useful to introduce the related notion that therapy involves developing improved internal strategies for coping, soothing, and internal growth, rather than relying on the therapist to provide this. Increased communication, coordination, and cooperation among alters is a central way that this internal boundary work is accomplished. Work to develop trance-based skills such as finding an internal "safe place" may also be introduced in this context (Kluft 1989).

I often point out that many alters are likely to mistrust my intent because, in the past, fine-sounding phrases have often been tricks that have preceded abuse. I urge that protective alters be present as much as possible in treatment to monitor whether my behavior is consistent with my words. I urge them to question me if they feel I am not practicing what I preach. I state clearly that I believe that trust is earned over time and should not be awarded without good reason.

Conflicts over dependency among the MPD alters frequently may be embedded in problems around boundaries. For example, some alters may quickly develop a dependent attachment to the therapist. Protective alters may experience this as a dangerous situation, because the pain of abuse is even worse if it is accompanied by a betrayal by someone to whom the MPD patient is attached. The protectors may not be able to manifest themselves in a way that has prevented such hurts in the past.

In my experience, many situations of apparently intractable self-destructive behavior or battles with the therapist in treatment relate to attempts on the part of protectors to stop the easily attached alters from becoming too dependent. Therapists who merely attempt to nurture or gratify the latter alters without gaining a clear understanding of the whole transference field unwittingly amplify these internal battles and the resultant self-destructiveness. Generally it is best for the therapist to indicate quickly his or her understanding that there are vigilant alters who are panicked at the attachment they see developing. In many cases, this is one covert motivation of alters who manifest themselves as malign, persecutory, provocative, angry, self-punishing, and so on. These alters are frequently quite surprised that the therapist recognizes their basic protectiveness and that he or she wishes to recognize and support their efforts.

A related problem occurs when, despite the patient's desperate need for nonabusive, comforting relationships, the therapist's positive qualities have a paradoxical posttraumatic meaning. Thus, one patient routinely provoked me into angry battles with hostile, derisive alters who continually distorted my communications, especially after sessions in which therapeutic movement was made. Ultimately, she understood that she was experiencing me as her father in the transference. When things with her father had been "nice," he was more likely to molest her. If she provoked him, she was punished and hit, but at least she was less likely to be sexually abused.

Similarly, a number of patients experience the positive qualities of the therapist as indicating only a more clever concealment of abusive intent than the patient has encountered previously. In this situation, the patient expects that the therapist is sadistically manipulating the patient's attachment to enjoy his or her pain at betrayal when the abuse finally occurs. Provocations of the therapist by unreasonable, disagreeable, or exasperating alters may be an unconscious attempt to take control of this anticipated abusive process and at least "get it over with." These patients often describe that the moment of actual physical or sexual abuse in childhood was "not that bad" compared to the uncertain agony of waiting for its inevitable occurrence.

Issues around control of abuse often account in part for the development of active sexual alters who sought out or initiated sexual experiences with abusers in childhood. The appearance of these entities in treatment often relates to the patient's fears of abuse or abandonment by the therapist and attempts to handle these feelings by familiar methods of controlling the situation. It is vital to understand the nonsexual purposes of these alters (see also Briere 1989 for additional discussion of related issues).

Overt and Covert Flashbacks in the Transference

Most MPD patients meet criteria for PTSD and experience frequent flashback experiences (Armstrong and Loewenstein 1990; Kluft 1988; Putnam 1989). Putnam (1989) following the typology of Blank (1985) enumerates four types of flashbacks in MPD patients:

> 1) vivid dreams and nightmares of the traumatic events; 2) vivid dreams from which the dreamer awakens still under the influence of the dream content and has difficulty making contact with reality; 3) conscious flashbacks in which the subject experiences intrusive recall of traumatic events, accompanied by vivid multimodal hallucinations, and may or may not lose contact with reality; and 4) unconscious flashbacks, in which the individual has a sudden, discrete experience that leads to an action that recreates or repeats a traumatic event, but the subject does not have any awareness at the time or later of the connection between this action and the past trauma. (p. 237)

In the unconscious flashback, Blank (1985) states:

Manifest psychic content is only indirectly related to [traumatic experiences]. The individual's state of consciousness, outwardly observed, may or may not be altered. Memories, affects and impulses come . . . without conscious visual or other registration. The subject . . . [carries] out complex integrated actions based on past experiences that are not consciously remembered, with no awareness that he [or she] is repeating anything. . . . As in post-hypnotic suggestion, the subject invents rationalizations for his or her behavior. (pp. 297–298)

Conscious flashbacks are commonly recognized in MPD patients and frequently manifest themselves in therapy, often in response to triggers or cues in the therapy session or setting (Putnam 1989; Spiegel 1986). Frequently the behavior of the MPD patient in therapy is related to attempts to suppress or control these experiences and the alters who bear them. At other times, appearance of flashbacks may be related to many issues, including attempts by alters to punish or suppress one another, to resist attempts at working together, to warn others about the therapist, and as an attempt to unload rapidly all painful material at the therapist's office in the hope that it will remain there permanently.

It is less commonly realized, however, that unconscious flashback experiences permeate the life of the MPD patient and are frequently omnipresent in the therapy. In addition, projective identifications in the dissociative transference field may give rise to an uncanny phenomenon in which the patient and therapist appear to have "walked into the flashback together," as one of my patients described it. Although this can be a very awkward and uncomfortable situation, some MPD patients bring important material into therapy in just this way.

Putnam (1989) describes more extreme forms of the same phenomenon in which "abuse equivalents" (p. 178) occur in the treatment of MPD, often as an attempt by the therapist to handle dangerousness to self or others by the patient. Putnam cites the case of an MPD patient who in childhood had been tied down and forced to fellate her father. In hospital, she was eventually placed in four-point restraints and force-fed for long periods of time because of intractable self-destructive and anorexic symptoms. In my experience, this extreme concretized recreation of abusive experiences occurs frequently in the inpatient management of more disturbed MPD patients with significant issues around dangerousness to self and/or others. In the hospital context, this can be a complex issue to resolve.

Case Study 1. My earliest experience with recognizing a shared unconscious flashback occurred with one of my first MPD patients. In my beginning work with MPD, I was much less aware of the critical importance of boundary issues. This patient had a happy-go-lucky alter who had asked me to go for a walk with her "sometime" when she came out. I had frequently done such peripatetic therapy when I had worked with schizophrenic patients, so I assented readily. At that time, I assumed that the "primitive character structure" of MPD patients required such concrete responses. I thought that this intervention would be helpful in managing the patient's anxiety in therapy and in providing a tangible restorative experience to overcome the patient's early deprivations.

Thus, when this alter emerged one day, I felt little compunction in suddenly suggesting that we go for a walk. This process was repeated several times, with our always taking the same walk through town. However, while walking one day, several additional alters emerged who described that a walk through precisely the same area, at precisely the same time of year, during treatment with a previous long-term therapist had ended with her going home to bed with him. This was a major hidden trauma that had affected this patient profoundly.

As therapy progressed, the patient reported having had sexual relationships with many previous "helpers" throughout her life, including teachers, ministers, guidance counselors, therapists, and others. This was a major issue in establishing a workable therapeutic alliance.

Subsequently, I became far more circumspect in altering the usual boundaries of MPD patients' treatment, insisting instead that, in general, work on issues be confined to talking in the office and that urges to do otherwise (in either patient or therapist) needed exploration, not gratification.

Case Study 2.   Another patient switched to alters who were intensely rageful, accusatory, and regressed in therapy whenever seemingly neutral and nondirective remarks (e.g., "Tell me about that") were uttered. Therapy sessions came to a standstill as this process unfolded. The patient then redoubled her accusations that everything I said made her "worse" and that I was preventing therapy from going forward because of the way I talked. Attempts at interpretation failed utterly to change this process. In fact, doing so only seemed to make things worse. In many other respects, the patient worked extremely hard in treatment. Thus, the whole situation was painfully bizarre. Eventually, I was provoked to fury. This frightened me and the patient as well. Consultation with several MPD experts did little to increase my understanding of this process. These puzzling, excruciating interactions gradually became less frequent, although they recurred periodically.

After much additional work, in a very powerful abreaction, the patient finally described that as part of her abuse, she was made to explore with her abusers her "thoughts and feelings" about looking at photos of the abuse. She quoted them as saying: "Tell me about all your thoughts and feelings about these photos. Are you sure you've told me all your thoughts and feelings about the pictures?" Later still, several alters stated that when I had been furious it was a relief to them, because the abusers had spoken in soft voices. It was easier to tell that I was not one of them when I raised my voice in exasperation!

Case Study 3.   A complex MPD patient and her therapist consulted me because of an impasse in therapy in which the patient had become upset over a somewhat sexualized remark the therapist had made in talking with one of her alters. Attempts at resolution were unsuccessful over several sessions. Eventually, the therapist told the patient, "I'm not going to walk on eggshells with you" in reference to this problem. The patient was intensely triggered by this, because these were the exact words family members had used with her when she was exhausted and ill after being abused.

The patient and the therapist both found it helpful to use the construct of "walking into the flashback together" to break the impasse in treatment. They were now freer to do additional work on the patient's abusive childhood. In addition, it was suggested that the uncharacteristic gaffe made by this otherwise circumspect therapist might also partly reflect the covert appearance of previously unknown material about the abuse. Further exploration suggested that this was also likely.

In conceptualizing the shared unconscious flashback, the therapist must become aware of the kind of projective identifications that can manifest themselves in this way. Frequently, the therapist will reenact the role of the abuser or coabuser in this process. However, simultaneously, the therapist may have experiences concordant with those of the patient. In Case Study 2, I partly represented the helpless patient who, in childhood, could do nothing right, whose words and thoughts were controlled, and whose most innocent behavior was a cause for punishment and abuse. In addition, I was provoked into behavior that was like one of the patient's most important alters who was explosively rageful in response to abuse. Finally, I represented a hope for something different in that, despite everything, some alters perceived me as someone other than the abusers in the transference.

However, before introducing the concept of the shared flashback into the treatment, the therapist must rigorously explore the extent of his or her own personal, "classical" countertransference contribution to the situation. I do intensive self-exploration to identify ways in which my own conflicts or blind spots may be provoking or perpetuating these transference field phenomena. I will not discuss these in detail with patients. I will, however, acknowledge to patients in a general way when I feel that my own difficulties have contributed to problems in the therapy.

In bringing up the issue of the shared unconscious flashback, I point out our *mutual* contribution to the process, especially when I feel I could clearly have handled things better. In discussing the shared unconscious flashback experience, I will often say that, like a new alter, the flashback is "coming for help," asking for resolution and mastery, knowing no other way to come forward. Like an alter, the flashback can be understood as trying to help the whole system master the abusive past and to struggle for healing. Indeed, once the flashback is overtly abreacted, additional alters who hold the relevant memories are frequently revealed.

Early on in the therapy of an MPD patient I find it helpful to introduce the concept of "living in the flashback world" and the importance for the patient of gaining freedom from a life determined by flashbacks. I emphasize that the patient who is continually reliving flashbacks, consciously and unconsciously, has little freedom to choose reactions to current situations. I may or may not be an abusive therapist, but in the dissociative posttraumatic transference world of the MPD patient, he or she is not able to freely choose whether I am or not.

Through ideomotor signals, internal vocalization, "talking over," or direct contact, I am usually quite active in attempting to reach alters who perceive the therapy from flashback perspectives. I regard this work in the transference as crucial in helping the patient gain mastery intrapsychically and interpersonally. In particular, I work actively to acknowledge, account for, understand, and communicate with the most angry, suspicious, mistrustful, and apparently negative alters, as well as those who are literally experiencing the flashback transference.

The "Holding Environment" for the MPD Patient: Limits, Boundaries, and the Treatment Frame

D. W. Winnicott (1965) defined the concept of "the holding environment" in the treatment of very disturbed patients in intensive psychotherapy. This concept is related to hypothesized early physical and psychological "holding" functions provided for the infant by the mother. Winnicott hypothesized that holding processes are crucial in the infant's development of differentiation of self and other, symbolizing capacity and secondary process thought. Psychotherapists often characterize the holding environment for the disturbed patient as a similar kind of receptive, supportive stance in which an intense regressed dependency in the patient is tolerated in the hope of overcoming deficits in the patient's psychological development (Winnicott 1965).

In MPD it is more useful to conceptualize the supportive, containing, holding functions of the therapist in terms of the traumatic transference. Here, the MPD therapist is very active in anticipating abuse-related transference themes. These include the patient's expectation that all relationships will be abusive, including the one with the therapist. The therapist should anticipate the concerns about his or her potential abusiveness and be active in discussing them with the alters.

In addition, however, the therapist needs to be active in addressing the patient's abusiveness to self and others, including overt and covert aggression against the therapist. Most experienced MPD therapists begin treatment with a very clear articulation of expectations, boundaries, and limits about dangerousness to self and others, internal punitiveness among alters, abusiveness toward the therapist, and clarity about the structure of treatment. MPD patients frequently test these structures very creatively, particularly in the early phases of treatment. The therapist should be prepared to defend the concept of nonabusiveness vigorously. Getting "safe" from self- or other-destructive behaviors and abusive relationships is the cornerstone of treatment of MPD patients. The therapist needs to be a clear, articulate spokesperson for nonabusive values.

In general, it is helpful to frame discussion of these issues in transference terms. The patient has had little in the way of nonabusive formative relationships, so it is hardly surprising that the alter system has created an adaptation based on the anticipation of abusive situations. Alters' behaviors invariably constitute responses to and efforts to overcome the impact of past abuses. Some of their efforts are misguided. Methods such as self-mutilation, eating disorders, and suicide attempts must be differentiated from the goals that they are trying to achieve. Thus a patient who has alters with bulimia related to oral sexual abuse will be congratulated on their refusal to "swallow" the abuse. On the other hand, the therapist should take a firm stand about the need to find alternative methods to solve these problems.

It is common in the early phase of MPD treatment for intense crises around self-destructiveness or abusiveness to arise, with one or more alters refusing to relinquish some form of unsafe behavior. Almost invariably, the situation is ameliorated with firm limits by the therapist who insists on nonabusive values, even to the point of threatening to discontinue treatment unless the behavior is stopped. The MPD patient will experience more passive approaches by the therapist either in terms of past coabusers who were permissive about abuse or in terms of his or her own inability to effectively combat abuse and aggression. Unfortunately, many MPD patients feel the need to push these limits as far as possible to test that the therapist will not act as an abuser or facilitator of abuse. Ultimately, full explication of the dynamics of these issues are only understood through analysis of the traumatic and flashback transferences once a safe container has been created in the therapy.

Conclusions

In this chapter, I have discussed a few basic aspects of the dissociative, posttraumatic transference field in work with MPD patients. It is the combination of these two elements that contributes to the full intensity of transference/countertransference processes in work with these patients. The combination of the abuse-based dynamics propelled by the intense hypnotic energy of the MPD patient may be overwhelming, particularly for the therapist just beginning to work with such a patient. Obviously, volumes could be written explicating all aspects of these issues, because they are so basic to understanding the psychodynamics of MPD.

Connie Wilbur began a revolution that has given us a powerful paradigm to frame our study of MPD and the dissociative response to trauma. The breadth of the Wilburian revolution in the study of the dissociative disorders is exemplified by the issues of transference and countertransference. Here, the basic human processes at work in MPD are most clearly illustrated in the complex relationships that develop in the therapy of the MPD patient. Connie Wilbur showed us that these relationships contain the extremes of human pain as well as the capacity for healing and redemption in the face of suffering.

References

Armstrong JG, Loewenstein RJ: Characteristics of patients with multiple personality and dissociative disorders on psychological testing. J Nerv Ment Dis 178:448–454, 1990

Blank AS: The unconscious flashback to the war in Viet Nam veterans: clinical mystery, legal defense, and community problem, in The Trauma of War: Stress and Recovery in Vietnam Veterans. Edited by Sonnenberg SM, Blank AS, Talbott JA. Washington, DC, American Psychiatric Press, 1985, pp 293–308

Bliss EL: Multiple Personality, Allied Disorders and Hypnosis. New York, Oxford University Press, 1986

Braun BG (ed): The Treatment of Multiple Personality Disorder. Washington, DC, American Psychiatric Press, 1986

Briere J: Therapy for Adults Molested as Children: Beyond Survival. New York, Springer, 1989

Brown DP, Fromm E: Hypnotherapy and Hypnoanalysis. Hillsdale, NJ, Lawrence Erlbaum, 1986

Carlson EB, Putnam FW: Integrating research on dissociation and hypnotizability: are there two pathways to hypnotizability? Dissociation 2(1):32–38, 1989

Chase T: When Rabbit Howls. New York, Dutton, 1987

Courtois CA: Healing the Incest Wound: Adult Survivors in Therapy. New York, WW Norton, 1988

Dell P: Professional skepticism about multiple personality disorder. J Nerv Ment Dis 176:131–137, 1988

Fine CG: Thoughts on the cognitive-perceptual substrates of multiple personality disorder. Dissociation 1:5–10, 1988

Fine CG: Treatment errors and iatrogenesis across therapeutic modalities in MPD and allied dissociative disorders. Dissociation 2(2):77–82, 1989

Fine CG: Treatment stabilization and crisis prevention: pacing the therapy of the MPD patient. Psychiatr Clin North Am 14:661–675, 1991

Fish-Murray CC, Koby EV, van der Kolk B: Evolving ideas: the effect of abuse on children's thought, in Psychological Trauma. Edited by van der Kolk B. Washington, DC, American Psychiatric Press, 1986, pp 89–110

Galdstone R: The domestic dimensions of violence. Psychoanal Study Child 36:391–414, 1981

Gill MM: Analysis of Transference, Vol 1: Theory and Technique. New York, International Universities Press, 1982

Greaves GB: Common errors in the treatment of multiple personality disorder. Dissociation 1(1):61–66, 1988

Greenson RR: The Technique and Practice of Psychoanalysis, Vol 1. New York, International Universities Press, 1967

Hilgard ER: Divided Consciousness: Multiple Controls in Human Thought and Action, Expanded Edition. New York, Wiley, 1986

Kernberg O: Severe Personality Disorders. New York, Jason Aronson, 1984

Kluft RP: Aspects of the treatment of multiple personality disorder. Psychiatric Annals 14:51–55, 1984

Kluft RP: Childhood multiple personality disorder: predictors, clinical findings, and treatment results, in Childhood Antecedents of Multiple Personality. Edited by Kluft RP. Washington, DC, American Psychiatric Press, 1985, pp 167–196

Kluft RP: The dissociative disorders, in The American Psychiatric Press Textbook of Psychiatry. Edited by Talbott JA, Hales RE, Yudofsky SC. Washington, DC, American Psychiatric Press, 1988, pp 557–584

Kluft RP: Playing for time: temporizing techniques in the treatment of multiple personality disorder. Am J Clin Hypnosis 32:90–97, 1989

Kuhn TS: The Structure of Scientific Revolutions, 2nd Edition, Enlarged. Chicago, IL, University of Chicago Press, 1970

Langs R: The Therapeutic Interaction: A Synthesis. New York, Jason Aronson, 1977

Laplanche J, Pontalis JB: The Language of Psychoanalysis. New York, WW Norton, 1973

Lindy JD: Vietnam: A Casebook. New York, Brunner/Mazel, 1988

Loewenstein RJ: The spectrum of phenomenology in multiple personality disorder: implications for diagnosis and treatment. Proceedings of the Fifth International Conference on Multiple Personality Disorder/Dissociative States. Edited by Braun BG. Chicago, IL, Rush University Department of Psychiatry, 1988, p 7

Loewenstein RJ: An office mental status examination for chronic complex dissociative symptoms and multiple personality disorder. Psychiatr Clin North Am 14:567–604, 1991

Loewenstein RJ, Hornstein N, Farber B: Open trial of clonazepam in the treatment of posttraumatic stress symptoms in MPD. Dissociation 1(3):3–12, 1988

Marmer S: Psychoanalysis of multiple personality disorder. Int J Psychoanal 61:439–451, 1980

Ogden TH: On projective identification. Int J Psychoanal 60:357–373, 1979

Olson J, Mayton K, Kowal-Ellis N: Secondary posttraumatic stress disorder: therapist response to the horror. Proceedings of the Fourth International Conference on Multiple Personality Disorder/Dissociative States. Edited by Braun BG. Chicago, IL, Rush University Department of Psychiatry, 1987, p 29

Orne MT: The nature of hypnosis: artifact and essence. J Abnorm Soc Psychol 58:277–299, 1959

Peebles-Kleiger MJ: Using countertransference in the hypnosis of trauma victims: a model for turning hazard into healing. Am J Psychother 48:518–530, 1989

Putnam FW: The switch process in multiple personality disorder and other state-change disorders. Dissociation 1(1):24–32, 1988

Putnam FW: Diagnosis and Treatment of Multiple Personality Disorder. New York, Guilford, 1989

Racker H: The meanings and uses of countertransference. Psychoanal Q 26:303–357, 1957

Sandler J, Dare C, Holder A: The Patient and the Analyst: The Basis of the Psychoanalytic Process. New York, International Universities Press, 1973

Schreiber FR: Sybil. Chicago, IL, Regnery, 1973

Searles HF: Countertransference and Related Subjects. New York, International Universities Press, 1979

Spiegel H: Dissociation, double binds, and posttraumatic stress in multiple personality disorder, in The Treatment of Multiple Personality Disorder. Edited by Braun BG. Washington, DC, American Psychiatric Press, 1986, pp 61–78

Spiegel H, Spiegel D: Trance and Treatment. New York, Basic Books, 1978

Wilbur C: Treatment of multiple personality disorder. Psychiatric Annals 14:27–31, 1984

Wilbur C: Multiple personality disorder and transference. Dissociation 1(1):73–76, 1988

Winnicott DW: The Maturational Processes and the Facilitating Environment. New York, International Universities Press, 1965

Chapter 5

Multiple Posttraumatic Personality Disorder

David Spiegel, M.D.

Multiple personality disorder (MPD) is a mental disorder that by its very nature seems to mock reality and common sense. Patients claim to be inhabited by a series of personalities, each of which occupies the center of consciousness for varying periods of time and has a complex set of relationships (some supportive, some hostile) with the other personality states. In a formal sense, many of these patients could be said to meet DSM-III-R (American Psychiatric Association 1987) criteria for schizophrenia (Kluft 1987). They have the bizarre delusion that their body is inhabited by more than one independent personality. In addition, they often have auditory hallucinations (e.g., the perception of the voices of other personalities speaking to the overt one personality that is apparently in executive control).

Why pay attention to such symptoms? Is the syndrome itself unreal? Or is it in fact a response to trauma that is so overwhelming that such patients doubt the veracity of their own perceptions? Is the fact that many therapists, psychiatrists, and psychologists doubt the existence of MPD a reflection of the fact that these patients often doubt themselves, are unsure that their own perceptions of physical and sexual abuse by trusted people could possibly be real, and are troubled that the terrifying incidents of torture that flash through their minds could possibly have occurred? What would it take to cause such extreme fragmentation of a personality, to call into question the Cartesian proof of existence and transform it from "I think, therefore I am" to "We think, therefore we must be"?

Pioneers in this field, beginning with Morton Prince (1905), William James (1890), Pierre Janet (1920), and more recently with Cornelia Wilbur (1984, 1985), have been keen observers of the unusual. They have been willing, first of all, to stand against the denial that surrounds victims of trauma. They have brought to our attention a discrete syndrome that is often misdiagnosed as schizophrenia or some form of personality disorder. They have encouraged the development of the dissociative disorders field and provided information and support to therapists who undertake the difficult task of treating MPD.

But what is MPD? And why take it seriously? What happens if we fail to recognize this entity? Clearly, there are dangers associated with labeling any patient with any psychiatric diagnosis. However, the fact is that most MPD patients earnestly seem to seek the correct diagnosis and are misdiagnosed, on average, for more than 6 years before their condition is recognized (Putnam 1985; Putnam et al. 1986). Interestingly, they do not respond to the negative suggestions that they do not have the disorder or believe that they have another illness. They tend to be misdiagnosed as schizophrenic or borderline patients or as patients with bipolar disorder, and each of those diagnoses carries with it its own set of adverse consequences. Rather than accept misdiagnosis and mistreatment, many patients with dissociative disorders persist in seeking additional evaluations. Furthermore, MPD is one of the few serious psychiatric illnesses for which a record of success with appropriate psychotherapy is developing (Kluft 1986). At a time when most psychiatric problems are either being dismissed as problems of living or treated solely as biological disorders to be dealt with pharmacologically, it is important to recognize that MPD is an anomaly—a serious psychiatric disturbance that responds to psychotherapy.

Dissociation as a Defense Against Trauma

MPD is a failure of self-integration in which individuals isolate or separate one component of memory from another, usually for defensive purposes. As an example, one MPD patient who was raped as a teenager dissociated to a new personality during the rape whom she called "No One." This enabled her to experience the rape as having happened to "no one." Most such imaginative defenses are complex. Her defensive response also conveyed another meaning: that she had been made to feel like a "nobody" during the rape.

Another MPD patient reported that the first time she dissociated was the first time her father took off his necktie, tied her to the bed, and raped her. The alter said to her, "You don't want to be with that bastard. You come and be with me." Thus, the dissociation serves to make victimization less than complete, allowing the victim of assault to say, in essence, "He may be raping part of me but he is not getting all of me." This defense allows the victim to state in the strongest psychological terms her fervent wish to distance herself from what was happening. Very often, such victims experience themselves as floating above their bodies or as going to a peaceful mountain meadow during assaults. These extreme acute dissociative symptoms may actually help patients to maintain their sanity during their exposure to a reality that is intolerable and incomprehensible.

But how is one to maintain one's sense of self worth while at the same time being aware of intense memories of a loved one, especially a trusted parent, having tortured one physically? The pictures of such events, self-contained in these two diverse percepts—normal parental support and physical abuse—seem incompatible to the patient, who must then make them become compatible with one or the other. In this sense, the MPD patient "becomes" the double-bind imprint placed on him or her by sadistic parents or others: the "good" child who is forced to often care for parents and must do everything right, and the "evil" child who in his or her mind deserves the victimization imposed on him or her. Consistent with double-bind theory, such children are forbidden ever to comment on the paradox (Bateson et al. 1956; Spiegel 1986b).

Are these reports true? Herman and Schatzow (1987) found that of 53 women alleging incestuous abuse, 74% were able to obtain corroborative evidence such as a direct confession, and another 9% of accusations were supported by highly suggestive ancillary data. In a later study, Herman and colleagues (1989) found that a history of abuse in childhood was strongly associated with higher scores on the Dissociative Experiences Scale (Bernstein and Putnam 1986). Bliss (1984) investigated 14 MPD patients who reported abuse, and with only 1 of the 14 did collateral evidence not confirm the patient's assertion of abuse.

Although their intense ability to fantasize and their willingness to pursue a thought single-mindedly without judging it makes reports made by hypnotizable individuals open to question (especially when they are hypnotized), there do seem to be convergent lines of evidence of an association between high hypnotizability and traumatic experiences. Josephine Hilgard (1970) originally observed that one of the factors in childhood associated with later high hypnotizability in college students was a history of punishment in childhood that was uncorrelated with parental warmth. She noted that hypnosis may have been mobilized spontaneously as an escape from unpleasant reality, although it must be borne in mind that this was the third variable in her regression equation. The first two (and more powerful) variables were histories of imaginative involvements and identification with the opposite-sex parents, both positive developmental variables. Nash and Lynn (1986; Nash et al. 1984) found that a majority of students with a history of abuse were more highly hypnotizable than control subjects, and Rhue and Lynn (1987) found that students with a history of abuse were not more hypnotizable than nonabused students but were better fantasizers. Wilson and Barber (1983) found that those who were lonely and isolated as children used fantasy to help them cope with the loneliness, and that physical abuse was not uncommon in their histories.

The link between hypnotizability and trauma in adults has been confirmed in two separate studies of Vietnam veterans with posttraumatic stress disorder (PTSD). Stutman and Bliss (1985) tested veteran respondents to a newspaper advertisement for hypnotizability with the Stanford Hypnotic Susceptibility Scale, Form C (Weitzenhoffer and Hilgard 1962) and classified them in terms of high or low symptomatology of PTSD. The veterans higher in PTSD symptomatology were significantly more hypnotizable. Spiegel and colleagues (1988) found that the hypnotizability of 65 Vietnam veterans hospitalized for PTSD was significantly higher on the Hypnotic Induction Profile (Spiegel and Spiegel 1978) than comparison populations of patients with schizophrenia, generalized anxiety disorder, or affective disorders, and even a sample of control subjects.

Dissociation: A Computational Model

In the ensuing discussion, I use the metaphor of the computer to describe and discuss several aspects of the phenomena and function of MPD. Computational models of consciousness, while necessarily simplistic, are providing intriguing insights into the organization of mental function.

The dissociation of memories may be understood as being analogous to the structure of various directories in a DOS-type computer system. One can be working away happily in a word processing directory when the need for a command safely stored in another directory arises. One tries to execute a program and it fails, the more intelligent computers complaining that a required program is unavailable. The user knows the file is there; he or she *put* it there. But the computer has a dissociative disorder. It acts as though it (the file) were not there. To allow things to proceed, one must go back to the main directory, enter the other directory, and retrieve the needed information. Thus, the computer acts as though the directory the user is in were its entire store of memory, when in fact it has other memories as well. Only in the main directory does the computer lack this dissociative disorder. Similarly, when the patient with a dissociative reaction to trauma remembers it, he or she relives it with such intensity that it is as though all other information about the individual and how he or she has been loved, valued, and respected did not exist. Further, knowledge that the patient did indeed survive life-threatening trauma is unavailable. Once again, in reliving the assault, the possibility of proximate death becomes subjectively real.

To pursue this computing analogy further, one can draw on the exciting theoretical work of McClelland and Rumelhart (1985), McClelland and colleagues (1986a, 1986b), and Rumelhart and McClelland (1986). They hypothesize the processing of perception in memory to involve a series of nets, defined by relationships among components of the net that may be expressed as "weightings," or shared patterns of activation. That is, when one unit is on, what is the probability that another unit is on? These relationships may be expressed as a kind of correlation matrix that in essence constitutes a memory. New information, which involves a new pattern of relationships among these units, can be processed in the net, changing the overall pattern of relationships—and thus the net "learns."

Among the interesting properties of this parallel distributed processing model is the fact that it can accommodate pattern recognition and partial information better than a digital system. Most simple computers are so obtuse and frustrating because a single error in a long string of commands renders the entire string useless, whereas in a parallel distributed processing system a near-miss does not frustrate the entire endeavor. A net can recognize input patterns that are close to but not identical to previously learned patterns. McClelland and Rumelhart (1985; McClelland et al. 1986a, 1986b) note that such nets can approximate aspects of functional amnesia for two reasons. First, they can act as though they have learned something without having a given instance of exposure to the information because of the weightings in the net; and second, a single strong aberrant input does not impede the net's ability to learn to any great degree. In other words, the fact that individuals with traumatic amnesia may consciously forget the traumatic experience but act as though they remembered it all too well is quite consistent with the behavior of this neural net model (Li and Spiegel 1991). This model also has a kind of bottom-up contentiousness, in which overreaching or complex and integrated knowledge is composed of a series of lower-level interactions, the outputs of which make up larger nets. Patterns are constructed bottom-up, rather than in a top-down system in which a given, highly integrated center is activated and places in context or provides meaning for inputs from lower down. That means that the problem for consciousness in the system is integration. How does one extract a coherent overall pattern of reaction from a series of contentiously interacting subunits?

Self-Integration Disorder

As Sir Charles Sherrington (1950) elegantly said, "That our being should consist of two fundamental elements offers, I suppose, no greater inherent improbability than that it should rest on one only."

This perspective may be useful because it makes MPD seem less strange. The issue is not how can it be that certain individuals have MPD; rather, it is why more people do not have it, since the experience of personal unity is seen as an achievement rather than a given. Other writers have raised this fascinating issue, ranging from Jaynes' (1976) conception that consciousness arose out of the developmental need to reconcile the often conflicting functions of the left and right hemispheres, to Galin's (1974) observation that the relationship between the hemispheres may constitute the workings of repression, to the studies of split-brain researchers who can document comparatively independent functioning of left and right cerebral hemispheres in commissurotomy patients (Gazzaniga et al. 1965). All of this suggests that the brain is not only capable of but also prone to doing numerous things at once. It suggests that the development of an overreaching sense of personal identity is an achievement made possible in part by the fact that these different subunits are able to communicate with one another and that the contents of one are not inimical to the contents of another.

Dissociation and PTSD

From this point of view, an analogy can be drawn between the symptoms of PTSD and the primary phenomena associated with hypnosis: absorption, dissociation, and suggestibility. Absorption, a crucial aspect of hypnosis, is very much analogous to the phenomena described in Section B of the DSM-III-R description of PTSD—the persistent reexperiencing of the traumatic event—including "sudden acting or feeling as if the traumatic event were recurring (includes a sense of reliving the experience, illusions, hallucinations, and dissociative [flashback] episodes . . .)."

These are not simple memories of the trauma but intense experiences analogous to hypnotic age-regression, in which a previous event is not merely remembered but relived. Furthermore, the event is so intensely experienced that awareness that it is now over and that the patient is currently safe is suspended.

The second major component of hypnosis, dissociation (Hilgard 1977), is analogous to the phenomena described under Section C of the description in DSM-III-R:

> Persistent avoidance of stimuli associated with the trauma or numbing of general responsiveness. Examples include avoidance of thoughts or feelings associated with the trauma or situations that arouse recollection of it; psychogenic amnesia, the inability to recall an important aspect of the trauma; feeling detached or estranged from others; and feeling a restricted range of affect.

In other words, a gap in the traumatic memories is accomplished at the expense of (or perhaps for the purpose of) warding off feelings or memories associated with the trauma at other times. Indeed, many PTSD patients may alternate between intense and painful absorption in the memory and a kind of numbing or withdrawal more typical of the dissociative component of hypnosis. Material that should be conscious is no longer conscious, and an amnesic barrier is constructed, interfering with the normal continuity between memory and present experience.

Section D of the DSM-III-R description describes persistence of increased arousal or stimulus sensitivity, including hypervigilance and physiologic reactivity on exposure to events reminiscent of the trauma. This is a kind of heightened responsiveness to environmental cues that is similar to the suggestibility of hypnotized individuals. They respond as if the mere similarity to the trauma means that the trauma is recurring. Thus, many of the symptoms of PTSD are quite analogous to the phenomena associated with hypnosis. Indeed, it is of great interest that historically there have been resurgences of interest in hypnosis during wars, when the prevalence of PTSD symptoms suddenly increases (Kardiner and Spiegel 1947).

Hypnosis in Treatment

The psychotherapy of posttraumatic dissociative disorders involves establishing access to and eventually control over these dissociated states, often facilitated with the formal use of hypnosis (Kluft 1985). MPD can be understood as an uncontrolled hypnotic state in which patients have trouble staying out of rather than getting into hypnotic states.

As I noted previously, hypnosis has three main components: absorption, or intense focus of concentration with a relative suspension of peripheral awareness, something like looking through a telephoto lens; dissociation, or the compartmentalization of experience; and suggestibility, an enhanced responsiveness to external cues (Spiegel 1988; Spiegel and Spiegel 1978). When MPD is understood as a chronic PTSD (Spiegel 1984, 1986a), it may seem that these patients replace the physical helplessness they experience during repeated episodes of trauma with a sense of psychological helplessness and inability to control their own state of mind. They thus maintain the fantasy that somehow they could have controlled their physical state (e.g., by being an even better child, or by avoiding provoking a sadistic parent) while acting out the sense of helplessness in being victimized now through the experience of their own personalities. They thus act out psychologically what they once experienced physically. The therapy requires helping them psychologically face, acknowledge and put in perspective, or grieve for their physical helplessness during episodes of victimization, while enhancing their here-and-now sense of psychological control. Thus, the psychotherapy involves recognition of the dissociative disorder, gaining increasingly controlled access to these dissociated states, working through their traumatic origins, and negotiating and altering the complex relationships among the dissociated states.

In this sense, the psychotherapy of MPD can be seen as analogous to writing path commands in a DOS-type computer system. A path command is another way to help the computer with its dissociative disorder, rather than going back to the main directory and finding what is inaccessible. Writing a path command tells the computer that it may find the necessary information even if it is in a different directory. In this sense, the computer is allowed to become aware of a broader body of information even though it is working actively in one directory. In the same way, trauma victims reexperiencing sexual or physical assault may also access memories of their own courage in resisting the assault or in enduring it in order to protect younger siblings. They thus emerge from the memory with a more complex and integrated view of what has occurred, which helps them work through their memories rather than simply be retraumatized by them. It is in this sense—conceptualizing the illness as a multiple posttraumatic personality disorder—that the origins of this fragmentation of personality can be faced and worked through, enabling patients to bear, master, and integrate the traumatic memories.

The treatment of this disorder therefore involves a confrontation with its traumatic origins. The effort, in essence, is to help patients work through the traumatic experiences and to restructure their memories. They are essentially helped to write path commands, linking the isolated and terrifying experiences of relived trauma with a wider variety of life experiences and self-perceptions. A patient reliving an episode at age 5, when she was strangled by her mother in a jealous rage over the daughter's close relationship with her estranged husband, smiled when her therapist said, "You are a brave little girl." She said, "I never thought of myself as brave. I am bad!" Patients who blame themselves for "provoking" attacks of abuse can learn to face the events as an effort to protect younger siblings from abuse; that is, they emerge, on the one hand, facing and bearing their helplessness at the hands of an abusive parent or stranger, and at the same time see themselves as attempting to transcend the situation to salvage their safety or to afford some protection for someone else.

This involves complex and intense transference and countertransference issues as well. Patients often identify the therapist as an assailant during regressions, particularly regressions to a personality state of a younger age. This traumatic transference happens in more subtle forms in all of the psychotherapy of trauma victims. The therapist comes to be identified with the assailant, especially if the assailant is a parent. This must be recognized and its effects minimized by emphasizing the patient's sense of control over access to and use of the traumatic memories. Furthermore, consolation for a patient's suffering with intense emotional experiences should be offered in professionally appropriate ways, so that the patient's sense of being unacceptable and ruined by the traumatic experience is not reinforced by his or her perception of the therapist's avoidance or withdrawal. Furthermore, the therapist must be cautious not to tend to favor the subset of personality types that tend to be passive and somewhat masochistic at the expense of the more assertive and sometimes frankly aggressive ones. Clearly, limit setting is important in terms of violent actions or acting out; yet the assertiveness of these personalities and their propensity to be rather protective at times must be reinforced.

In this sense, the neutral system orientation of the couples therapist or family therapist may be helpful. These therapists consider themselves a therapist to the family system rather than to any one member. In a sense this analogy holds well for the therapist of the MPD patient who really wants to improve communication among the elements of the system rather than reinforce any one component of it. The ultimate goal of such interventions is congruence—helping these patients to integrate and bear the shared experience of the disparate personality states, to transcend the discontinuities in their history by mastering their ability to integrate memories, and to tolerate their view of themselves, even while their traumatic memories are present in their consciousness.

References

American Psychiatric Association: Diagnostic and Statistical Manual of Mental Disorders, 3rd Edition, Revised. Washington, DC, American Psychiatric Association, 1987

Bateson G, Jackson D, Haley J, et al: Toward a theory of schizophrenia. Behav Sci 1:251–264, 1956

Bernstein E, Putnam FW: Development, reliability and validity of a dissociation scale. J Nerv Ment Dis 174:727–735, 1986

Bliss EL: A symptom profile of patients with multiple personalities including MMPI results. J Nerv Ment Dis 172:197–202, 1984

Galin D: Implications for psychiatry of left and right cerebral specialization: a neurophysiological context for unconscious processes. Arch Gen Psychiatry 31:572–583, 1974

Gazzaniga MS, Bogen JE, Sperry RW: Observations on visual perception after disconnection of the cerebral hemispheres in man. Brain 8:221–236, 1965

Herman JL, Schatzow EJ: Recovery and verification of memories of childhood sexual trauma. J Psychoanal Psychol 4:1–14, 1987

Herman JL, Perry JC, van der Kolk BA: Childhood trauma in borderline personality disorder. Am J Psychiatry 146:490–495, 1989

Hilgard ER: Divided Consciousness: Multiple Controls in Human Thought and Action. New York, Wiley, 1977

Hilgard JR: Personality and Hypnosis: A Study of Imaginative Involvement. Chicago, IL, University of Chicago Press, 1970

James W: The consciousness of self, in Principles of Psychology, Vol 1. New York, Holt, 1890, pp 387–388

Janet P: The Major Symptoms of Hysteria. New York, Macmillan, 1920

Jaynes J: The Origin of Consciousness in the Breakdown of the Bicameral Mind. Boston, MA, Houghton Mifflin, 1976

Kardiner A, Spiegel H: War Stress and Neurotic Illness. New York, Paul Hoeber, Inc, 1947

Kluft RP: Aspects of the treatment of multiple personality disorder. Psychiatric Annals 14:51–55, 1985

Kluft RP: Personality unification in multiple personality disorder: a follow-up study, in Treatment of Multiple Personality Disorder. Edited by Braun BG. Washington, DC, American Psychiatric Press, 1986, pp 29–60

Kluft RP: First-rank symptoms as a diagnostic clue to multiple personality. Am J Psychiatry 144:293–298, 1987

Li D, Spiegel D: A neural network model of dissociative disorders. Psychiatric Annals 22:144–147, 1992

McClelland JL, Rumelhart DE: Distributed memory and the representation of general and specific information. J Exp Psychol 114:159–188, 1985

McClelland JL, Rumelhart DE, Hinton GE: The appeal of parallel distributed processing, in Parallel Distributed Processing: Explorations in the Microstructure of Cognition, Vol 1: Foundations. Edited by Rumelhart DE, McClelland JL. Cambridge, MA, MIT Press, 1986a

McClelland JL, Rumelhart DE, Hinton GE: A distributed model of human learning and memory, in Parallel Distributed Processing: Explorations in the Microstructure of Cognition, Vol 2: Psychological and Biological Models. Edited by Rumelhart DE, McClelland JL. Cambridge, MA, MIT Press, 1986b

Nash MR, Lynn SJ: Child abuse and hypnotic ability. Imagination, Cognition and Personality 5:211–218, 1986

Nash MR, Lynn SJ, Givens DL: Adult hypnotic susceptibility, childhood punishment, and child abuse: a brief communication. Int J Clin Exp Hypn 32:6–11, 1984

Prince M: The Dissociation of a Personality. London, Longmans, Green and Company, 1905

Putnam FW: Dissociation as a response to extreme trauma, in Childhood Antecedents of Multiple Personality Disorder. Edited by Kluft RP. Washington, DC, American Psychiatric Press, 1985, pp 65–97

Putnam FW, Post RM, Guroff JJ, et al: The clinical phenomenology of multiple personality disorder: review of 100 recent cases. J Clin Psychiatry 47:286–293, 1986

Rhue JW, Lynn SJ: Fantasy proneness: developmental antecedents. J Pers 55:121–137, 1987

Rumelhart F, McClelland JL (eds): Parallel Distributed Processing: Explorations in the Microstructure of Cognition, Vol 1: Foundations. Cambridge, MA, MIT Press, 1986

Sherrington C: Introductory, in The Physical Basis of Mind: A Symposium. Edited by Laslett P. New York, Macmillian, 1950

Spiegel D: Multiple personality as a post-traumatic stress disorder. Psychiatr Clin North Am 7:101–110, 1984

Spiegel D: Dissociating damage. Am J Clin Hypn 29:123–131, 1986a

Spiegel D: Dissociation, double binds, and post-traumatic stress in multiple personality disorder, in Treatment of Multiple Personality Disorder. Edited by BG Braun. Washington, DC, American Psychiatric Press, 1986b, pp 61–78

Spiegel D: Hypnosis, in American Psychiatric Press Textbook of Psychiatry. Edited by RE Hales, SC Yudofsky, JA Talbott. Washington DC, American Psychiatric Press, 1988, pp 907–928

Spiegel D, Hunt T, Dondershine HE: Dissociation and hypnotizability in post-traumatic stress disorder. Am J Psychiatry 145:301–305, 1988

Spiegel H, Spiegel D: Trance and Treatment: Clinical Uses of Hypnosis. New York, Basic Books, 1978

Stutman RK, Bliss EL: Posttraumatic stress disorder, hypnotizability and imagery. Am J Psychiatry 142:741–743, 1985

Weitzenhoffer AM, Hilgard ER: Stanford Hypnotic Susceptibility Scale, Form C. Palo Alto, CA, Consulting Psychologists Press, 1962

Wilbur CB: Multiple personality and child abuse. Psychiatr Clin North Am 7:3–7, 1984

Wilbur CB: The effect of child abuse on the psyche, in Childhood Antecedents of Multiple Personality Disorder. Edited by Kluft RP. Washington, DC, American Psychiatric Press, 1985, pp 21–35

Wilson SC, Barber TX: The fantasy-prone personality: implications for understanding imagery, hypnosis, and parapsychological phenomena, in Imagery: Current Theory, Research, and Applications. Edited by Sheikh AA. New York, Wiley, 1983, pp 430–390

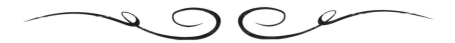

Chapter 6

Clinical Approaches to the Integration of Personalities

Richard P. Kluft, M.D.

The most distinguishing characteristic of multiple personality disor-
der (MPD) is the presence of alters that recurrently influence
behavior and assume executive control of the body. The first personalities develop in the course of an overwhelmed child's efforts to
contend and to cope with overwhelming circumstances. They enact
alternative strategies and approaches to the handling of difficult
events, serve protective and self-soothing functions, and internalize
the constellation of events and relationships in which they are involved (Kluft et al. 1984). In many patients, both the alters and the
process by which they are formed rapidly attain secondary autonomy, and what had proved adaptive under duress may become an
ongoing and increasingly elaborated way of responding to life's
events and challenges.

Although this method of responding to difficulties begins as an
heroic effort that may well be necessary to preserve the life and/or
sanity of a beleaguered child, its persistence beyond the actual period of duress may prove more a liability than an asset. Removed
from the circumstances under which such an adaptation was func-

tional, the individual with MPD is condemned to reiterate the circumstances of his or her childhood misfortunes within the world of the alters and mirror them in the alters' interactions. All too often this proves dysfunctional and subjects the MPD patient to a kaleidoscopic array of symptoms, difficulties in relationships, and considerable personal anguish. Most of those who have MPD initially seek treatment for symptoms and circumstances that are epiphenomena of their MPD, which may remain unnoticed despite years of treatment within the mental health care delivery system (Putnam et al. 1986).

When MPD was regarded as a possession state of supernatural origin, and the personalities understood as intrusive entities, the exorcism of those entities was considered a proper therapeutic goal (Ellenberger 1970; Kluft 1991). The first secular psychotherapy in which the entities were brought into accord and then unified reached its successful conclusion in June 1835, when Despine facilitated the blending of the normal and "magnetic" alters of 11-year-old Estelle (Ellenberger 1970; Fine 1988; Kluft 1984a). Although many unique and curious approaches to the treatment of MPD have been advocated between then and the present, the vast majority have recommended bringing the alters to a state of unification.

> The unification of the MPD patient is only one aspect of the treatment of [the individual] and may be only an incidental consideration in some cases. . . . The tasks of the therapy are the same as those of any reasonably intense change-oriented approach. However, these tasks are pursued in an individual who lacks a unified personality (and hence observing ego). The several personalities may have different perceptions, memories, problems, priorities, goals, and different degrees of involvement with and commitment to the treatment and one another. It usually becomes essential to replace dividedness with unity, at least of purpose and motivation, for any treatment to succeed. Work toward this goal and the possible integration of the personalities distinguishes the treatment of MPD. (Kluft 1984b, p. 11)

My studies have demonstrated that integration is a reasonable goal for the majority of MPD patients, and that stable retention of integration is feasible for this patient group (Kluft 1984b, 1986a).

Although the majority of therapists who treat MPD patients attempt to help their patients attain unification, there is general agreement that this goal may not be achieved (or in fact achievable) by some patients (e.g., Putnam 1989). In certain circumstances, treatment of sufficient expertise, intensity, and duration may not be available. In others, patients decline to work toward this objective for a variety of motives, or they seem unable to attain it because of the severity of their dissociative and concomitant psychopathology.

Thoughts on Controversies Surrounding Integration

As MPD is diagnosed and studied with increasing frequency, voices have been raised the question the wisdom of attempting to bring about integration. Three types of arguments have been put forward. They may be understood respectively as arguments based on advocacy and apology, theoretical considerations, and concerns about available resources.

Advocacy and apology.   A small but vocal minority of MPD patients are vehemently opposed to any change in their system of alters. Some perceive the alters as real people, and they are appalled at any attempt to reason to the contrary and "do away" with members of their inner families (see Chase 1987). Others appreciate that work with the alters involves dealing with the painful materials that they sequester or block, and they refuse (and/or perceive themselves as unable) to face the discomfort attendant on such efforts. Many patients admit that they find the world so threatening that the idea of dealing with it directly on an ongoing basis is terrifying and oppose integration on these grounds. In some areas an unofficial "MPD community" has developed—a community whose members perceive themselves as a mistreated minority that should be respected and accepted rather than asked to change.

Theoretical considerations.   Hilgard (1977) offers impressive testimony to the presence of ongoing separate cognitive systems in the mind. He concludes that the unity of the mind is an illusion. Beahrs (1982) and Watkins and Watkins (1979; see also Chapter 14) argue eloquently that the mind is a family of selves and that its harmonious orchestration rather than its unification should constitute mental health. From this perspective, the attempt to bring about unification is paradoxical and counterproductive.

Adaptationalism.   Many therapists prioritize function rather than integration. They point to the scant therapeutic resources available to treat MPD patients; some doubt the average therapist's ability to help a patient toward integration. They thus see integration as an ideal but unlikely outcome, the pursuit of which is overly consuming of available therapeutic assets, and elect to focus their efforts elsewhere.

It is difficult to address the arguments based on advocacy and apology in an objective manner. Many of those who oppose integration on these grounds are quite vehement in their beliefs, and they are unwilling to consider that their stance may be one of resistance and based on apprehension (of dealing with life directly and of facing the traumata that led to the MPD). Although no controlled studies demonstrate the clear superiority of one approach over another, sufficient information is available to allow the tentative statement that integration is a sufficiently desirable goal to be pursued whenever possible. In my study of 210 MPD patients (Kluft 1985a) and my follow-up of 52 patients successfully treated to integration (Kluft 1984b, 1986a), I found that 94% of the 52 patients ($n = 49$) who were treated to integration reported enhanced quality of life and continuing gains. Only two of the integrated patients took efforts to reinstitute their MPD. Conversely, most patients I have assessed who achieved a resolution that left them still with MPD found that they often relapsed into dysfunctional dividedness under stress or as painful material that they had not yet addressed entered their awareness. More than 70% of this group (unpublished data) returned to work for integration, and all of this group achieved and sustained integration.

Therefore, although any study based on the experience of one practitioner and without controls and external validation must be regarded with caution, on the basis of the track records of these two groups, the data available (however tentative) suggest that integrated patients did far better and were more content with their lot. That more than 70% of the unintegrated group returned for integration, but only 4% of the integrated group elected to restore their dividedness, offers poignant testimony to this perspective.

Furthermore, the use of dissociative defenses renders those who use them vulnerable (Kluft 1990a, 1990b). Because dissociation involves the segregation of sets of information from one another in a relatively rule-bound manner (Spiegel 1986), those who dissociate may not have access to data that would facilitate their decision making and commit egregious errors of judgment that lead to undesirable consequences (Kluft 1990a, 1990b). This causes many MPD patients to manifest what has been called the "sitting duck syndrome" (Kluft 1989, 1990a). Despite the benefits of integration, it must be acknowledged that patients can rarely be treated toward a goal that they do not accept, because no true therapeutic alliance exists toward that end.

The theoretical arguments against integration are fascinating but appear overstated. Hilgard himself, whose work (1977) is often used to justify such stances, cautioned against such extensions of his research (Hilgard 1984). However, he inadvertently encouraged them by presenting data that transcended the cognitive aspects of his research (on which he focused) and by neglecting to address the implications of these data. It seems undeniable that aspects of multiplicity are encountered in nondissociating as well as dissociating individuals (Beahrs 1982; Hilgard 1977; see also Chapter 14). However, the normal spectrum of such phenomena does not lead to differences in the dimensions that distinguish true MPD from them. In normal shifts, other aspects of the mind do not assume executive control, although they may influence behavior. In normal shifts and complexities of human experience, there is no change of identity— there is a sense of continuity as to who and what one is. Second, there is no change in self-representation. One may feel very different without perceiving oneself as a different entity with a different appearance. Third, there are no major barriers (such as amnesia) for important aspects of self-referential memory. Fourth, there is no loss of the sense of ownership for what one has done (Kluft 1991). A close inspection reveals that, although many multiplicity-spectrum phenomena are normative and will not be eliminated by the integration of alters, the phenomena of true MPD are beyond the pale of what is normative and can be resolved without an implicit violation or nonrecognition of the normal spectrum of human multiplicity. Although true MPD phenomena are part of the same spectrum of phenomena as normative multiplicity, their characteristics are inconsistent with normal unimpeded mental function.

With regard to the adaptationalist argument, although it is true that limited resources may dictate the provision of suboptimal treatment, it is crucial to avoid self-deception and convince oneself that the constricted treatment that is provided is what should be understood as desirable. The preservation of function and work toward integration need not be seen as incompatible, although they may in fact be irreconcilable at certain times in the treatment of particular patients. What is needed is increased sophistication with regard to the pacing of therapy (see Chapter 7), therapeutic tact, patience, skill in ego-building and supportive measures, and a keen appreciation of the toleration of each individual patient for anxiety-laden materials. Elsewhere I have outlined certain considerations in the preservation of function in the course of therapy (Kluft 1986b, 1991). The success of increasing numbers of therapists in their work with MPD patients indicates that integration-oriented treatment is not the province of a few exceptional individuals.

On the basis of the information available at this time, it appears that integration is a goal worthy of pursuit and is attainable in whole or in part by most motivated MPD patients. Although there are egregious exceptions, integrated patients are, on the whole, more likely to be stable, make further gains, and be less vulnerable than patients who pursue alternative objectives.

When Should the Therapist Advocate for Integration?

Putnam (1989) has observed that it is the patient's right to remain an individual with MPD. The late David Caul wisely observed: "It seems to me that after treatment you want to end up with a functional unit, be it a corporation, a partnership, or a one-owner business" (quoted in Kluft 1984b, p. 11). It is indeed possible for *some* MPD individuals to cope well while divided, and many patients are sure or want to believe that they are members of this group. When confronted with an MPD patient, especially one who expresses misgivings about integration, the therapist may have serious questions as to whether to advocate such a goal. What follows are empirical guidelines based on more than 20 years' work with MPD patients.

The therapist confronted with a patient who raises issues regarding integration early in therapy often does best if he or she is told that it seems to be desirable for most patients, but that decisions about what will occur at a later stage of his or her treatment are premature—what is best will emerge as treatment progresses. Early arguments about and pressures toward integration stiffen resistances at a stage when the patient may still hold relatively naive and reified notions about the personalities as "real people" with different ages, genders, orientations, and values. Under such circumstances, the patient's alters almost invariably conceptualize integration as their death or elimination. The same discussion at a more advanced stage of treatment often will be much less troubling, because the alters will be more aware of what they share in common and less narcissistically invested in separateness. One patient observed:

> When I came to treatment I was sure I would never integrate. As work got under way, I came to see integration is nothing to fear, no more than being there all of the time. Now that I have been integrated for a year, I think of being multiple as something that is archaic for me.

Less frequently, resistance toughens as treatment goes on. In my experience, age and life circumstances play a major role in determining whether one should press for integration (Kluft 1991). The integration of children with MPD is universally desirable, because it protects the child from the adverse consequences of a life with MPD. Several children in my series have maintained their integration for more than a decade and done well. However, the treatment of children with MPD should remain supportive until their protection against further abuse is assured. The MPD offers some protection against adversity until external stressors can be controlled. Premature efforts to work toward integration may lead the overwhelmed child to become more rather than less complex. Many adolescents with MPD provide a unique challenge, because many of their normative developmental tasks and thrusts are at odds with treatment toward integration. Many of them combat or decline therapy. Often it is more critical to address pressing age-appropriate issues and attempt to protect the potential trajectory of their lives against deterioration. Building the foundation for a more definitive future therapy may be all that is possible.

Some adults' life circumstances preclude definitive therapy for MPD. Their energy and attention may be so consumed by here-and-now concerns that it is pointless and unrealistic to impose the additional burden of an arduous type of treatment. That qualification aside, for the patient who is or who may become a parent, integration is highly desirable. I studied 75 mothers with MPD (Kluft 1987a). Although 38.7% ($n = 29$) were good or exceptional parents, the remainder, who universally described themselves as good mothers, gave self-reports divergent with reality. A minority, 16% ($n = 12$), were frankly abusive. Alters exploited the children or injured them. Sometimes they were deliberately hurtful to the children, but at times they hurt their children while misperceiving them for others. However, the remainder—nearly half ($n = 34$)—were sufficiently impaired by their amnesias and inconsistencies across alters to be quite compromised as parents, despite their conviction this was not the case. They absented themselves, failed to protect the children, and often injured them by their inconsistency and MPD-oriented behaviors. Furthermore, for a child to build his or her psychic structure via identification with an MPD parent is suboptimal.

For the MPD patient without parenting responsibility or ambitions, there are less compelling grounds to press for integration, even if it is objectively more desirable. For the older or medically infirm MPD patient, the type of treatment necessary to bring about integration may be too demanding and unsettling to be endured. A focus on quality of life may be more appropriate.

It is helpful to bear in mind that the decision as to whether to move toward integration is one that is not made once and for all at the start of therapy. Many patients' vehement objections are mollified in the course of treatment; still others grudgingly accept its inevitability. It is most important to decline to engage in arguments over integration with the patient, because this course of action almost inevitably heightens narcissistic investment in the wish to avoid integration and introduces an adversarial tension into an already difficult treatment. My personal style is to encourage a wait-and-see attitude. Usually by the time integration becomes an issue, it is in the process of occurring and perceived as inevitable. The argument is then irrelevant.

Integration, Fusion, Unification, and Resolution

In general, alters either cease to be separate or can be brought together when their unique reasons for being cease to be relevant. However, with a substantial minority of entities, their narcissistic investment in separateness or the patient's fear of ceding multiplicity outlives the alters' functions. Within the field, the terms unification, fusion, and integration are often used as synonyms and are contrasted with resolution, which refers to any improved, stable outcome that enhances the patient's comfort and function, whether or not the alters come together. However, each of these terms (which are used both as synonyms and in their special senses in different contexts in this communication) has a more specialized meaning as well.

Unification is an overall, general term and encompasses both fusion and integration. Integration refers to an ongoing process of undoing all aspects of dissociative dividedness that begins long before there is any reduction in the number or distinctness of the personalities, persists through their fusion, and continues at a deeper level even after the personalities have blended into one. It denotes an ongoing process in the tradition of psychoanalytic perspectives on structural change. In contrast, fusion refers to the moment in time at which the alters can be considered to have ceded their separateness

(Kluft 1986b; Wilbur and Kluft 1988). The definitions herein stem from research findings on the stability of what appears to be the ending of separateness (Kluft 1982, 1984b, 1986a). An alter that is believed to have ceased being separate is considered "apparently fused." However, many apparent fusions do not hold; rapid relapses are common. Any alter, or the patient as a whole, actually should not be considered to have fused until there have been 3 stable months of the following:

1. Continuity of contemporary memory;
2. Absence of overt behavioral signs of MPD;
3. Subjective sense of unity;
4. An absence of alters (or the particular alter) on reexploration (preferably involving hypnotic inquiry);
5. Modification of the transference phenomena consistent with the bringing together of the personalities; and
6. Clinical evidence that the unified patient's self-representation includes acknowledgment of attitudes and awarenesses that previously were segregated in separate personalities.

When these criteria have been fulfilled for 2 years after the 3 months, one can use the term "stable fusion." My unpublished data on patients followed from 5 to 12 years after fusion indicate that less than 1% of alters that have been absent for 27 months will make a reappearance.

Many clinicians question the virtue of such stringent criteria. The rationale for such a "high threshold" is based on both research findings and clinical pragmatics. Patients (and unfortunately many therapists) are prone to overdramatize fusion. It is not uncommon for celebrations to be made and profuse congratulations to be offered. Profound pressures to sustain apparent fusion are imposed on a patient who has received special praise for having achieved his or her unification. To lose the fusion may be perceived as a sign of failure or weakness, of having taken back a gift to the therapist, of being a bad patient, and so on. The patient may be plunged into despair, feel pressures toward self-harm, and anticipate the therapist's anger, disappointment, and withdrawal of caring. Under such circumstances many patients deny or dissociate emerging evidence that all is not well, placing themselves and the therapy in jeopardy (Kluft 1984b).

However, my research (1984b, 1986a) is consistent with Bennett G. Braun's terse clinical dictum: "The first final integration usually isn't" (personal communication, May 1981). Alters may reappear for a variety of reasons (reviewed in Kluft 1986a). More than 90% of relapses occur in the first 3 months after apparent integration. With that knowledge, using the criteria enumerated previously and dedramatizing fusion is protective of the patient. He or she is socialized to understand signs of relapse as no more than an indication that there is additional work to be done before a stable situation is reached and is encouraged to be alert for any signs that the fusion is in trouble. The 3-month waiting period throws cold water on undue fusion ardor in therapist and patient alike. It builds in a delay that confounds the thrust toward drama, and it encourages the patient to think about therapy in a longitudinal, problem-solving perspective rather than an instant and magical frame of reference.

An additional benefit of such terms is to discourage the patient's premature flight from therapy. Relatively few MPD patients are ready to discontinue treatment upon apparent fusion. In bringing more than 140 adult MPD patients to integration, I have seen this occur only 4 times, each in a very strong patient with a small number of alters. In contrast, in following up 20 patients who left treatment against my advice immediately or within a month after apparent fusion, I found that 19 had relapsed into MPD and that their leaving therapy was a flight into health, defending against dealing with further material. The last patient was lost to follow-up. A significant minority of MPD patients feel pressures to leave treatment upon apparent integration; any factors that discourage this will be in their best interests (Kluft 1984b).

Moving Toward Unification

Every aspect of the therapy contributes toward unification; several efforts to define the stages of treatment have been offered (Braun

1986; Kluft 1991; Putnam 1989; Ross 1989). The consensus is that explicit and overt efforts to move toward integration follow upon rather than precede the formation of a solid therapeutic alliance, attention to the issues of the individual personalities, reconciliation of many of the conflicts among the alters, and metabolism of the traumatic antecedents of the personalities' reasons for being and their subsequent experiences.

Greaves (1989) and I (1991) have emphasized the importance of the therapist's consistency across alters as a major contribution toward integration. If the therapist is relatively the same to all the alters, the patient's switching does not alter the patient's experience of the therapist overly much—a continuity of experience and a similarity of perception across the alters begins to erode the dissociative barriers (see Chapter 3). Greaves observes: "Integration begins at the moment when variously cathected parts of the patient's fragmented personality begin to cathect to the therapist as a commonly recognized external object" (1989, p. 225).

Many techniques are specifically designed to pave the way toward integration. Efforts to have alters listen in on one another in sessions; to comment upon and react to one another's experiences; to move toward mutual collaboration, communication, empathy, and identification—these and other interventions bring the alters to appreciate rather than avoid, combat, or disparage one another. In addition, the therapist may bring about copresence to allow alters to be "out together;" facilitate arrangements for inner communication and the respecting of one another's priorities; suggest a common diary, journal, or bulletin board; and intercede in any number of ways limited only by the ingenuity and determination of the therapist-patient dyad.

If the therapist succeeds in treating all alters with respect and consistency and insists that the alters maintain a "golden rule mentality" of not doing unto others as they would not be done to by others, the alters come to see that there is little secondary gain within the treatment for their continued separateness. As the work of therapy proceeds, boundaries begin to blur and become porous where they once had been relatively rigid and impermeable. The alters begin to change and to become more alike. The profound and previously "impossible" differences among the alters involving age, gender, race, religion, sexual orientation, and so on prove accessible, subside spontaneously, or are amenable to alteration.

The neophyte therapist is often discouraged by what appears to be the passage of time without any superficial sign that integration is occurring in the sense of the alters joining. It is not uncommon for impatience to dictate premature efforts to "do something." Sensitive to this clinical dilemma, Greaves (1989) contributed an extremely valuable article, "Precursors of Integration in the Treatment of Multiple Personality Disorder."

Greaves listed 13 markers of integration as well as 3 ambiguous markers that at times indicate progress but are not unequivocal. I have revised some of his wording to be consistent with the vocabulary of this chapter.

1. *Convergence phenomena* are those that require a focusing of attention and effort that implicitly require the cooperation of several alters, such as keeping appointments regularly and promptly, working well in therapy, and completing assigned projects.
2. The *spontaneous appearance of alters* in the course of sessions indicates sufficient trust to abandon dissimulation and to talk in session.
3. The *presentation of vague physical symptoms without a clear medical origin* may indicate the early loosening of repressions and the emergence of "body" or "somatic memories," which often are precursors of the recovery of traumatic events in a fuller form. This should not be read to understand that the MPD patient's physical complaints should not receive a conscientious medical evaluation!
4. The *spontaneous appearance of a hostile alter* is a major landmark, because usually these alters exert their impact within the world of the alters and are loath to acknowledge or to commit themselves to the therapy process. Closely related is
5. *Signs of cooperation by a formerly hostile alter.* This indicates an enhancement of the therapeutic alliance, a growing tendency to value the therapist and is an implicit statement that some hope for and anticipation of integration is at work. When, in a patient who never before has heard the alters' voices,

6. *The presenting or host personality begins to hear voices for the first time,* this indicates that previously dense amnestic barriers are eroding, and that communication among the alters is being prioritized over the maintenance of the previously isolating patterns of interaction.
7. *Increased internal communication,*
8. *Increased coconsciousness,* and
9. *Copresence* are clear signs that the initial relative isolation of the alters is changing. These are often followed by situations in which
10. *Major alters cannot be distinguished by the therapist,* and
11. *Personalities cannot distinguish themselves from one another.* At this point, integration of some sort is near, and
12. *The patient may request integration of two or more of his or her parts,* and/or may manifest
13. *Spontaneous unification.*

Less reliable indicators, the meaning of which must be determined by the clinical context in which they occur, are 1) *flooding of memories,* 2) *redissociation,* and 3) *prolific reports of previously unknown personalities.* Any of these may occur in either a patient whose dissociative barriers are crumbling (and being temporarily overwhelmed) in the course of a constructive therapeutic process, or in one who is simply overwhelmed and regressing because of too rapid a pace of treatment or a failure of the patient's ego strength to effect necessary restabilizations.

When Should a Unification Occur?

Therapists must be empathically attuned to the purposes served by alters, and they should not anticipate that an alter will integrate or can be integrated until it is willing to do so and its function has ceased to be of use or is assumed by another alter. When a particular separateness no longer serves a meaningful function in the patient's ability to adapt to environmental and intrapsychic pressures, and its separateness is no longer the focus of narcissistic investment, it may be ceded without adverse consequences. This is usually the case when the alters in question identify and empathize with one another, are willing to cooperate, and accept not only one another but also one another's memories and feelings.

[A fusion, whether spontaneous or facilitated,] will not substitute for the hard work of other aspects of the therapy, and is not a potent technique in and of itself. It is no more than an agreed-upon formalization of work already accomplished. . . . The timing of a fusion should emerge from the intrinsic process and momentum of the therapeutic endeavor. It should never be undertaken because the therapist or patient is eager to see fusion achieved, or hopes to find some sort of short cut. In essence, it is a permissive and positive intervention that is understood as tentative, and framed in a manner that clearly states that if the fusion does not hold it is not a failure, but more an indication that there is more work to be done before a fusion would be appropriate. For this reason, it is not helpful to bypass resistances to fusion. They should be dealt with straightforwardly. A bypassed resistance or a procedure perceived as coercive virtually guarantees a rapid relapse into dividedness. In the long run, going slower and more gently speeds therapy and reduces both crises and failure experiences for both clinician and patient. (Kluft 1986c, pp. 4–5)

Often the apparent failure of a fusion is due to the intervention of an alter that is not a party to the proposed fusion but that feels strongly that it should not occur. Other common causes are an alter's wish to fuse before facing some painful material it contains (so that the fusion is actually a flight into health rather than the mark of the conclusion of a piece of work) or an alter's having repressed within itself material that has not yet been the focus of the therapy.

It is not common for fusions to occur rapidly in the course of treatment, although this may occur in simple and highly cooperative cases and in patients who are beginning with a new therapist after having done good preliminary work with another treating professional. In 1977, I saw a motivated dual-personality patient fuse in her first session and remain integrated on 10-year follow-up, but I have not seen a similar case since. I have reported many cases with six or fewer alters that reached integration in a few months (Kluft 1984b,

1986a). It is not uncommon for a patient who has received good prior outpatient treatment and is hospitalized at a specialized unit to work on material that could not be managed on an outpatient basis to arrive "ready to burst" and abreact material very rapidly with the prompt integration of the alters involved in what has been abreacted.

There are two procedures that are used infrequently, and only by a small number of experts, that may be confused with the types of unification being described here. For several years, Bennett G. Braun, M.D., has described in workshop settings, but not in the literature, the technique of forced fusion. In certain crises or therapeutic impasses, during which all conventional interventions are unavailing, Braun may attempt to force a fusion to destabilize the pathological configuration that prevails and appears impervious to routine measures. The goal is not to achieve a fusion—any results will be transient. Instead, it changes the characteristics of the alter system for a brief period of time, during which the patient may become more accessible to other interventions. For example, when confronted with an absolutely intransigent situation with a chronically suicidal inpatient in whom one alter was unmanageable, I attempted such a procedure. It suppressed the alter for 5 minutes but upset it so much that it entered into the therapeutic dialogue.

A second specialized procedure is temporary blending, described by Fine and Comstock (1989). Alters are brought together for a time-limited period in the hope that their individual cognitive schemes, disrupted by trauma (Fine 1990), can be enriched by the experience of one another's perspectives. This may be more similar to the hypnotic technique of having alters copresent to enhance their mutual acceptance and empathy (Kluft 1982) than it is to actual fusion or integration.

The Patient's Beliefs and the Therapist's Maps: The Influence of Myths on Unification

Before discussing the pathways and patterns by which MPD patients unify, it is useful to digress briefly to consider the impact of subjective beliefs upon this process. Many MPD patients have no particular feelings about the way integration proceeds. Their general stance is a reluctant and begrudging acknowledgment (after considerable initial resistance) that the painful past must be dealt with in a tactful manner and at a tolerable pace. The alters that become accessible for work and integration do so in a manner unique to each patient. But often the first are some alters containing relatively minor burdens of memory and affects, and some alters involved in traumata that do not cast aspersions upon those traumatizers who are also being defensively idealized.

However, many MPD patients (and/or their alters) have very distinct ideas as to how the process should occur. These protocols vary from the fantastic to the astute, from the vague to the obsessively meticulous. Although many are useful in combination with the therapist's observations, many contain within their structure the wish to postpone indefinitely the encounter of certain alters with pain. The MPD patient as his or her own therapist is not immune to countertransference! Because so many MPD patients have covert agendas and unstated objectives that they manage to convince themselves that they are entitled to withhold from the therapist, it is essential that the therapist not become infatuated with the proposals of helper personalities to the detriment or abdication of his or her clinical judgment. In the last few months before this book went to press, four MPD patients in the final stages of integration acknowledged that their inner-self helper alters' plans included suicide if the pain of the last material was perceived as intolerable to the alters they most wanted to defend. Two others, after failed integrations, confessed that they had withheld information about the abuses done by family members that the host had defensively idealized and wished to continue to visit.

Therapists, too, develop ideas of how integrations should proceed. It is not uncommon for even experienced therapists to mistake the maps they have made of the patient's system of personalities for the clinical realities of those systems. Therapists far too sophisticated to reify alters may unwittingly impute undue significance to the schemes they and their patients have derived. They attempt to work within the structures of the schemes to the neglect of the dynamic and/or thematic connectedness of alters from different groups and systems. They thereby treat an abstraction rather than the human being before them. Those who use maps best are those most sensitive to their limitations and most prepared to either revise or abandon them in the face of emerging clinical realities.

In sum, clinical experience cautions us that the structured protocols for integration that both we and our patients are inclined to evolve for our own guidance and (perhaps more realistically) our own security may prove more myth than mentor in the crucible of therapy. Although they often prove useful guides, it is essential to avoid overestimating their importance and reliability.

Pathways to Unification

Alters cease to be separate in a number of ways. No data are available to help us define either what actually occurs at such times or whether alters who apparently have come together in different ways have undergone similar or separate types of processes. With each alter, as for the MPD patient as a whole, the process begins before the moment of apparent fusion and continues thereafter. Here I will attempt a crude classification of pathways to unification. I appreciate that they are no more than metaphoric approximations based on my patients' and my own subjective experiences, and I hope that in the future they will be superseded by more substantial explanations.

The most commonly reported pathways to unification involve descriptions of alters gradually merging in the course of therapy and alters joining in the course of therapeutic rituals involving imagery, the latter often facilitated by hypnosis. In the first, gradual merging, the involved alter reports and is reported by other alters to be gradually fading and becoming less distinct, or as slowly blending or joining into another alter or alters. This is the most common pathway in therapies that involve little formal hypnosis. The apparent fusion may be with the whole or with particular alters. As psychotherapy erodes the dissociative boundaries across and between alters, they become more aware of one another, feel along with one another, share more and more, and sense their strength, distinctness, and individuality becoming muted. They may begin to experience identity diffusion and confusion, or they may retain their identity as they fade. At times it is quite difficult to ascertain when they have fused (usually when the alter is represented as integrating with the whole or all alters); in other instances, the other alters suddenly become aware that such an event has occurred (usually when the merger has been completed with a specific alter or alters). In my experience as a consultant, I have become aware of many instances in which, though an alter is believed to have integrated in this manner, the alter in question remains separate and accessible to hypnosis, although it experiences itself as a mere shadow of what it had been. The patients in whom I found this phenomenon were referred because they were believed to be integrated, but they were still uncomfortable and had a vague sense that there was more to be done. The implicit lessons of these observations are that the patient treated without hypnosis may merit hypnotic exploration to ascertain whether all is as it seems to be, and that some MPD patients may require hypnotic interventions to bring about the complete resolution of their multiplicity.

A second pathway is the most common in those patients whose treatment has been facilitated with hypnotic interventions. Imagery and suggestion is used, usually in conjunction with formal hypnosis, but often deliberately or unwittingly relying on the patient's autohypnotic capacities to bring about the joining of alters. As Braun (1983) has demonstrated, this process may have psychophysiological correlates. Many patients become fascinated with the apparent drama of such experiences. They may become subjectively convinced that such procedures are essential for them and will hear of nothing else, hamstringing the best efforts of therapists who do not use such interventions routinely. However, as noted previously, there is anecdotal experience to indicate that such ceremonies may be necessary in work with some patients.

Fusion rituals are ceremonies at a discrete point in time which are perceived by some MPD patients as crucial rites of passage from the subjective sense of dividedness to the subjective sense of unity. . . .

Because such ceremonies are obvious and memorable landmarks in the treatment, they are often accorded an unfortunate overemphasis and unnecessarily invested in drama by both patient and clinician alike. (Kluft 1986c, p. 4)

As noted previously, these rituals merely formalize the subjective experience of the work that therapy has already accomplished, have more inherent drama than intrinsic potency, and are unlikely to have a salubrious impact if done out of context or if poorly timed.

Clinical experience demonstrates that individualized images rather than cookbook repetitions of those demonstrated by well-known therapists are most helpful. In addition, images that suggest merger, union, and rebirth, in which it is suggested that all aspects of all alters are preserved, are much more likely to be accepted than those that suggest elimination, subtraction, death, or going away. I have recently seen in consultation a series of MPD patients allegedly treated with amazing rapidity by practitioners of Neurolinguistic Programming (NLP) who used such "extrusive" or "riddance" images. In all cases, all of the original alters remained separate but had remained unavailable and apparently "gone" in sessions with the NLP therapists. (At the end of this section, a verbalization illustrating an integration ceremony has been appended.)

Much as those who omit the formal use of hypnosis may miss subtle residual dividedness, those who use hypnosis may inadvertently create demand characteristics within their therapies that encourage the patient to represent him- or herself as ready for such a procedure before this is in fact the case. Most relapses after such interventions are the result of insufficient working-through, and, in retrospect, are appreciated to have been undertaken prematurely (Kluft 1986a).

Third, many alters spontaneously cease to be separate after they have shared the materials that they encapsulate with another alter(s). In a typical scenario, an alter that holds the memory of a particular trauma may, after the abreaction of that trauma, be inaccessible to the therapist's efforts to reach it once again and may be reported by other alters to have ceased to be separate in the course of or at the finale of the abreactive episode. This is most common in rather complex MPD cases in which certain alters are specialized to hold specific painful material, entities that Braun (1986) has called "memory trace fragments." It is quite uncommon in major alters with wide ranges of functions.

A fourth pathway is demonstrated when alters who represent themselves as having reached a decision that it is time for them to cease being separate. Sometimes these alters experience themselves as integrating, but they may feel they are dying or going away. However, it is not uncommon for alters to try to avoid treatment by telling other alters that they are going: the therapist is told the alter is gone. Hence, such reports should be studied carefully. If all of the psychological work that the therapist thought that the alter in question had to accomplish has not been completed, it is most likely that the report is inaccurate, if not deliberately evasive. Nonetheless, this is not an uncommon way for alters to depart. Usually they will tell the therapist and other alters that they feel it is time to go, that they have done what they had to do, and that their functions are now being carried out to their satisfaction by others or have become unnecessary. It is almost universal in patients who cannot be convinced that integration is a coming together rather than a death; in such cases, the alters may insist on elaborate rituals of farewell.

A fifth pathway might be termed a "brokered departure." In such cases, an alter's ceasing to be separate is virtually negotiated within the alter system. Such alters may report or be reported to have joined with one or several alters in a planful way. For example, one patient decided among her alters that Joe, a strong protector alter, would integrate with Felicia, a traumatized child, so that she would not be as hurt when she dealt with the traumata that had befallen her. In another patient, a strong young male alter with specific skills was reported to have given those skills to a young female alter, his strength to another protector, and his specific male attributes to another male alter, because none of the female alters felt prepared to accept these aspects of him. It is difficult to know what to make of such reified internal myths; but it is a clinical fact that many MPD patients report such inner experiences, and the alters involved in the arrangement thereafter comport themselves as if these events in fact have come to pass.

A sixth pathway has recently been described to me by C. G. Fine (personal communication, October 1992). In this pathway, once a series of temporary blendings of personalities (Fine 1991; Fine and Comstock 1989) has been undertaken in order to attain a series of therapeutic objectives, the personalities involved may indicate that they have become so much alike in the course of the temporary blendings that they elect to become and remain one. This appears to be a gentle approach to integration that is worthy of further study.

Illustrative Hypnotically-Facilitated Fusion Ritual

The following verbalizations were used with a female MPD patient, Claire (a pseudonym), who had already integrated many alters. The imagery had been developed with the patient across her system of alters in a series of discussions more than a year previously, and all alters had found it congenial. On this day, alters Joan and Anne had already been elicited. Both had affirmed that they had no more work to do and were ready to join. The patient had been asked if any other alters believed that Joan and Anne had more left to do than they realized and if any alters objected. No alter thought that necessary work had been avoided, but one objected to these integrations. This alter agreed not to interfere when it was reminded that its freedom of decision was being respected and that Joan and Anne deserved similar consideration. This established, I said:

> Please allow your eyes to role up and your eyelids to flutter down and close. [The student of hypnosis will recognize the eye role induction attributed to Herbert Spiegel, M.D. (Spiegel and Spiegel 1987)]. Let yourself go deep at the count of three—one, two, three. If at any time you want to stop or tell me about something, raise your right index finger. And now, deeper at the count of four . . . [deepening by count until eight, and then] . . . as deep as you've ever been at the count of nine, and now deeper still at 10. That's right. Nod if you're ready. [Patient nods.]
>
> O.K. You are all in a beautiful clearing in the woods, a place of complete privacy and safety. All stand in a circle, take one another's

hands, and now move toward the center of the circle. You'll find you have to let your arms slide gently around one another as the circle grows smaller. And as you get closer, already you can feel a pleasant sense of warmth from the closeness, a sense of warmth and closeness that feels good to you all, even those who have no plans to join with one another today. Above the center of the circle, a point of light is seen, which rapidly becomes brighter and more radiant—a warming, comforting, and healing form of light that rapidly becomes so beautiful, bright, and radiant, that although it does not hurt your eyes at all, is so luminous that each of you, no matter where you look, all you see is a beautiful field of light that engulfs you all. No matter where you look, there is no evidence of detail or separateness, only beautiful healing light. And now the light seems to enter you as a warming current and flows throughout the circle, back and forth, forth and back, sharing with you all the experience of peace and well-being. And now the current flows to Joan and Anne alone, back and forth between you. Back and forth, forth and back, and soon it takes with it all the memories, feelings, and qualities of Joan into Anne, and of Anne into Joan [this is elaborated]. Nothing is withheld, nothing is omitted [elaborate on back-and-forth motif].

And now that all from each has flowed into the other, and all from the other has flowed into each, it seems so pointless to be separate. At three, the barriers between Joan and Anne gently crumble, and peacefully are washed away. All that was Anne flows into Joan, and all that was Joan into Anne. .. . And that's so easy and gentle because you already have become the same. Everything blending, joining, and mixing [elaborate]. And now everything settles gently and peacefully, joined now and forever at the count of two. . . . That feels so natural, so right. . . .

And now the light recedes. All of you look around. Everyone feeling better, stronger, safer. Where there were Joan and Anne, there is a single individual, stronger, more peaceful, more resilient, and unified now and forever at the count of one. How do you feel? [The patient opens her eyes and says it went well.] O.K. Close your eyes and rapidly go as deep as you were. You had said that the unified person would be called Joan. Joan, nod if you are there and O.K. [Nods.] Anne, nod if you remain separate. [No nod.] Everyone else, raise the right index finger if anyone senses or knows Anne remains separate or notices anything amiss. [No signal.] O.K., let this fusion be sealed and solid, now and forever, at the count of three. . . . One, two, three. [The patient opened her eyes, and volunteered that she felt good.] (Kluft 1986c, p. 5)

In the final few integrations with this patient, as she approached total unity, the imagery at the end of the ceremony was modified so that the light, instead of receding toward the point, completely entered the patient and remained within her as a source of ongoing healing and renewal.

Patterns of Integration

Most alters' integration processes are ongoing simultaneously at some level, but most alters' moments of apparent fusion appear to occur one at a time or in small clusters. The fusion events are the most dramatic evidences of the overall integration process. If the therapy is more process-oriented and less structured, it is not uncommon for many alters to be undergoing rather gradual parallel routes toward fusion. Conversely, if the therapy is more structured, with more discrete and controlled interventions, while the former process goes along (usually at a slower pace because of the thrust of the therapy), specific alters or constellations of alters are frequently the subject of more focused efforts to bring about the completion of their work and to facilitate their fusions. Elsewhere I have discussed the differences between these approaches, which I have called strategic and tactical integrationalism, respectively (Kluft 1988a; see also Chapters 3 and 7). The remarks that follow describe phenomena that are more clearly evident in more structured therapies but occur in more process-oriented ones as well.

Personality-by-personality patterns may proceed along any of the pathways described in a previous section. In general, the alters that are most alike are those that are likely to come together first in this manner. Single personality fusions may dominate the treatment of simple cases and instances in which each alter's investment in separateness is intense. They also are characteristic of the earliest integrations in any treatments, before one sees clusters of alters joining simultaneously. The patient's first steps toward facing painful affect and materials and moving toward integration are tentative, and the fate of the first alter to work toward fusion and the nature of the therapist's dealings with that alter are scrutinized with care. After it has become clear to the patient that the therapy and the therapist can be trusted, and the evidence of change in the alters into whom others have fused makes it apparent that those who have fused were not eliminated, but remain present although in a changed form, momentum may accelerate and groups of alters coalesce at once in more complex cases.

It is almost always a major error to urge the patient to condense experiences across alters from the first, although this may be possible for the bulk of the therapy. This is because if the therapist does so, he or she may be experienced as trivializing the pain of the individual alters, and this may intensify resistances and be perceived as a reenactment of the indifference of significant others to the patient's pain. On the other hand, after the patient has seen that the issues of each alter are treated with consummate respect, the alters often "hitch a ride" on the therapist's work with alters that are facing analogous issues. When this happens, the impact of the therapy may widen and become more generalized, and either more than one will fuse at a time, even if not requested to, or subsequent alters with analogous issues may require far less time in treatment. This is another illustration of the observation that the alters that are most alike often are those who are most readily integrated with one another.

Patterns of fusion often are perforce dependent on both likeness, as indicated previously, and upon the patterns by which alters were formed. For example, if a patient reacted to severe trauma by the formation of a cascade of alters, each of which is related to a temporal period of the trauma, it is conceivable that after work with the first, it might join the second, and so on, or remain separate until the event was processed completely, after which all might be ready to join at once. If a patient adapted to a traumatic situation by dividing the perceptions of the various sensory modalities into different alters, or by segregating in different alters each aspect of their complex reactions toward those involved in hurting them, in some instances all alters may appear to "need" to remain separate for the overall event to be reconstructed and worked through, after which all might be able to join.

At times alters cannot join until other alters, who contain aspects of the experiences with which they are connected, are worked with. For example, the alters associated with the death of a sibling could not integrate until the patient was able to tolerate depression and grief, which were encapsulated in alters that had sequestered these feeling states from the others' awarenesses. Sometimes the patient may come to the realization that a defensive pattern is no longer needed and make rapid internal changes in short order. In an extreme case, one patient who had been severely hurt over a good many years had developed approximately 300 entities that held the memory and pain of these events, and a protector alter for each. All of the protectors were very similar, and none held information not present in other alters. When the patient became secure in the therapy, the protector alters declared that they were redundant and asked to be condensed into a single entity. This was rapidly accomplished with hypnosis. After a few of the alters that held the pain and memory were addressed individually, the remainder "hitched rides" and fused in clusters of from 2 to more than 10 entities. The 600 entities (300 protectors and 300 with fragments of memory) were fused within a few months. In another case, the male personalities concluded that the patient had become strong enough to do without their being males and blended with strong female counterparts in short order.

In some patients, alters work toward fusion in the order in which they became separate, or in the reverse order. In others, alters are clustered according to the period of time in which they were created or most active, and they may fuse as the issues of that time are addressed. Eras of life, events, affects, functions, and relationships within the world of the alters may be powerful determinants of how a pattern of fusion takes shape. Some complex MPD patients have elaborate inner worlds and become so concrete about their sense of reality that their inner myth dictates the course of the therapeutic process. For example, in one patient, several alters believed themselves to be sisters, and none would integrate and "abandon" the others. Although as each dealt with its issues it served no ongoing function, the strength of the patient's belief was such that the alters' fusion was deferred until all were ready to integrate at once.

In my experience, integrations of many alters are no less likely to succeed than integrations of single alters if the preparatory work has been adequate. It is interesting to observe that in mass integrations, the failure of one or more alters to integrate may indicate either that the issues of that alter are unresolved, that the remainder is emblematic of the need for more general and thorough working-through of the issues that the group had shared in common, or that the recalcitrant alter is the door to work with another alter or system of alters to which the integrating group had some relationship.

The Patient's Reaction to the Experience of Unification

Patients' degrees of concern with fusions and the integration process are often more an intermittent interest than an ongoing preoccupation. Their attention instead is usually directed to their symptoms, the painful nature of the material that they confront, and the state of their relationships. Although there are some who are so fervid in pursuit of integration or sufficiently fanatic in resisting it that these concerns dominate the treatment, in most cases patients are more concerned with unification at particularly poignant moments (i.e., the time the first apparent fusion occurs, when particularly major alters yield their separateness, at apparent total fusion, at times of relapse, and as they come to grips with the vicissitudes of living with single personality disorder and are tempted to regress). In many cases, a time in which many fusions occur may be noteworthy for the patient's relative disinterest in the overall process in which he or she is engaged.

The blending of single personalities that do not play major roles in day-to-day life often is attended with minimal disruptive consequences, especially if the blending has been with another alter that does not have a great impact on current functioning. The alter that emerges from the blending may be transiently overwhelmed by the impact of the material of the alter that has just ceded separateness and may undergo a period of adjustment if the alter with which it has blended is significantly different from it in a major characteristic, such as attitude, gender, or age. Alters in executive control may be affected by the feeling states of the newly fused entity, which they may experience as a made feeling "from behind the scenes" (Kluft 1987b).

When major personalities that play substantial roles in the world of the personalities fuse and when total fusions occur, the impact on the patient may be quite marked. Braun (1983) has described some typical responses. It is not uncommon for patients to go through a period of time in which their senses and perceptions are particularly vivid and "new." A certain number of MPD patients are joyous and find a deep spiritual relevance in the fusion experience. In some cases, major symptoms change or disappear, and medication need and tolerance must be monitored carefully, because they may be modified. I am impressed by the frequency with which my patients become acutely hypersomnolent after a major or final integration, especially if it follows close on intense psychotherapeutic work with painful material. On the other hand, I have observed that when such integrations occur some time after the affective component has been addressed and worked through, the patient's perception of the fusion experience and its aftermath may be mundane, undramatic, and anticlimactic. The patient's conviction that major change has occurred may be related to having had a striking subjective experience.

It can be quite impressive to observe and interview MPD patients as they reconfigure subsequent to fusions. It is not uncommon to find one is contending with a veritable blend of the alters that integrated, although often the contribution of one member of the pair or cluster that fused clearly dominates the new appearance. It often takes several days or longer for the completely integrated patient (or the fusion product of two or more major alters) to come to a new equilibrium and make a consistent and stable presentation.

Although most well-planned and well-timed fusions hold, it is rare for all the fusions that lead to a first apparent final fusion to have fulfilled these criteria. A host of factors combine to make MPD patients vulnerable to destabilization and inclined to withhold crucial materials as long as possible. Therefore, it is commonplace for the emergence of additional information and/or layers of alters to lead to relapses, a subject discussed in detail elsewhere (Kluft 1986a). The clinician should expect to encounter such phenomena and should be prepared to deal with them without becoming angered and exasperated with the patient. One of the best safeguards against countertransference excesses is the systematic effort to recheck the state of a patient's integration on a periodic basis. A protocol for such efforts has been published (Kluft 1985b). Most relapses are readily addressed and achieve a stable resolution.

In my experience with more than 140 integrated MPD patients, the majority simply go on working with their issues and make further gains. In one paper (Kluft 1988b), I reported on the issues encountered in the treatment of 91 of these integrated patients:

1. Coping with the physiologic changes associated with integration;
2. Coping with the psychological changes associated with integration;
3. Working-through;
4. Abandoning autohypnotic evasions;
5. Modifying adaptive and coping mechanisms;
6. Making interpersonal adjustments; and
7. Making major life changes.

Some unusual phenomena are infrequently encountered in integrated MPD patients but are sufficiently disconcerting as to require special attention. I cannot offer precise statistics, because some patients left therapy immediately after integration. Even though I have follow-up on all but one of these, I could not observe them over the period in which these phenomena were seen in the patients who remained under continuous observations. Approximately 1 patient in 20 will attempt to rerepress all of the traumatic material that has been unearthed, as an attempt (in effect) to be "born anew." These patients try to convince themselves that they have put their past behind them. This group consists of two types of patients, in approximately equal proportions. The first group behave like patients with repression hysteria—they do not reestablish their MPD (but they might have were they not under observation and able to receive very prompt intervention), the repression is readily undone, and the material then must be worked through anew. I have only seen one repeated major rerepression, and this collapsed within 2 weeks. The second group of patients reconstitute MPD after a period of rerepression. They may reactivate one or more prior alters or form one or more new ones. One type of new alter is isomorphic with the apparently fused personality but contains all of the suppressed memory and affect.

Another type of reaction was seen in approximately 1 out of 50 patients, a prolonged period (days to weeks) of confusion in which the unified individual is overwhelmed by what has been integrated and regresses into altered states, may regress to and relive past events, and may have periods of disorientation. The few patients who showed such reactions were found to have held back from complete working-through of their traumata. Despite having done arduous work, at some point each had decided in one or several alters "That's enough!" and had withheld this determination from the therapist, who continued to believe that all necessary work had been completed. Interestingly, on follow-up, some of the patients who did this repeated the process in further therapy and went through decompensation after apparent stabilization once again. Furthermore, after some of their decompensations, two such patients also formed additional alters, apparently isomorphic with the integrated personality, to handle overflows of affect.

A profound dyssynchrony between unification and true integration was noted in one patient, who was unified for more than a year before the memories, assets, knowledge, and talents that had previously been sequestered in her separate alters became accessible once again to the unified individual. This woman had had several alters with professional levels of musical talent both in singing and in playing instruments, but she had had no access to these abilities for years after the integration of the alters that had these talents, despite deliberate and sustained therapeutic efforts to help her do so. One and a half years after the final unification of the alters, her musical and other skills gradually made their reappearance. The recurrent themes in her therapy during the period the talents remained inaccessible suggested that conflictual issues in her family and church (the main locus of her musical activities) were major determinants in her difficulties, which may have been conversion phenomena only tangentially related to her MPD. With the restabilization of her family and her changing her affiliation to a less stress-ridden congregation, her talents gradually returned to a level equal to or surpassing those she had treasured.

A final complication is one that I have seen once in another therapist's patient but that I am told was seen more than infrequently by some of the older pioneers in the field. It occurs when the alters integrate into an entity believed to represent the original personality, and the integrated entity represents itself as young (perhaps even a baby or child) or as having forgotten or never known important personal and procedural knowledge, and as needing to be taught things all over again. The patient gradually reacquires the lost knowledge and skills. This type of outcome appears to emerge from either unique demand characteristics in the treatment, idiosyncratic and strongly held beliefs in the patient, and/or the wish to convince oneself that one can make up for or replace a difficult childhood (in effect, a rebirth fantasy). In the case that I observed and intervened with, age-progression suggestions administered under hypnosis over a brief series of session were quite successful, and hypnoanalytic explorations suggested that the behavior reflected a wish to be born again in a literal sense, much as the patient firmly believed she had been born again in a religious sense.

Conclusions

Our understanding of what occurs when alters yield dividedness is incomplete; our best theories and descriptions are painfully rudimentary. We can hope that the next decade will witness both research and clinical efforts to better understand these phenomena and processes and to render the contents of this discussion dated, or even obsolete. Although we cannot yet grasp what we witness and behold, we can be confident that the process of unification can provide a valuable window into both the study of structural change in psychotherapy and the interface of brain and mind, of psyche and soma. The implications of this study will far transcend the field of MPD and the dissociative disorders.

References

Beahrs JO: Unity and Multiplicity. New York, Brunner/Mazel, 1982

Braun BG: Neuropsychological changes in multiple personality due to integration: a preliminary report. Am J Clin Hypn 26:84–92, 1983

Braun BG: Issues in the psychotherapy of multiple personality disorder, in Treatment of Multiple Personality Disorder. Washington, DC, American Psychiatric Press, 1986, pp 1–28

Chase T: When Rabbit Howls. New York, EP Dutton, 1987

Ellenberger HF: The Discovery of the Unconscious. New York, Basic Books, 1970

Fine CG: The work of Antoine Despine: the first scientific report on the diagnosis of a child with multiple personality disorder. Am J Clin Hypn 31:33–39, 1988

Fine CG: The cognitive sequelae of incest, in Incest-Related Syndromes of Adult Psychopathology. Edited by Kluft RP. Washington, DC, American Psychiatric Press, 1990, pp 161–182

Fine CG: Treatment stabilization and crisis prevention: pacing the therapy of the multiple personality disorder patient. Psychiatr Clin North Am 14:661–675, 1991

Fine CG, Comstock C: Completion of cognitive schemata and affective realms through temporary blending of personalities, in Dissociative Disorders 1989—Proceedings of the Sixth International Conference on Multiple Personality/Dissociative States. Edited by Braun BG. Chicago, IL, Rush University, 1989, p 17

Greaves GB: Precursors of integration in multiple personality disorder. Dissociation 2:225–231, 1989

Hilgard ER: Divided Consciousness: Multiple Controls in Human Thought and Action. New York, Wiley, 1977 (expanded edition 1986)

Hilgard ER: The hidden observer and multiple personality. Int J Clin Exp Hypn 32:248–253, 1984

Kluft RP: Varieties of hypnotic intervention in the treatment of multiple personality. Am J Clin Hypn 24:230–240, 1982

Kluft RP: Multiple personality in childhood. Psychiatr Clin North Am 7:121–134, 1984a

Kluft RP: Treatment of multiple personality disorder: a study of 33 cases. Psychiatr Clin North Am 7:9–29, 1984b

Kluft RP: The natural history of multiple personality disorder, in Childhood Antecedents of Multiple Personality Disorder. Edited by Kluft RP. Washington, DC, American Psychiatric Press, 1985a, pp 197–238

Kluft RP: Using hypnotic inquiry protocols to monitor treatment progress and stability in multiple personality disorder. Am J Clin Hypn 28:63–75, 1985b

Kluft RP: Personality unification in multiple personality disorder: a follow-up study, in Treatment of Multiple Personality Disorder. Edited by Braun BG. Washington, DC, American Psychiatric Press, 1986a, pp 29–60

Kluft RP: High-functioning multiple personality patients: three cases. J Nerv Ment Dis 174:722–726, 1986b

Kluft RP: The place and role of fusion rituals in treating multiple personality. Newsletter of The American Society of Clinical Hypnosis 26:4–5, 1986c

Kluft RP: The parental fitness of mothers with multiple personality disorder: a preliminary study. Child Abuse Negl 11:272–280, 1987a

Kluft RP: First rank symptoms as diagnostic indicators of multiple personality disorder. Am J Psychiatry 144:293–298, 1987b

Kluft RP: Today's therapeutic pluralism. Dissociation 1(4):1–2, 1988a

Kluft RP: The postunification treatment of multiple personality disorder: first findings. Am J Psychother 42:212–228, 1988b

Kluft RP: Treating the patient who has been sexually exploited by a previous therapist. Psychiatr Clin North Am 12:483–500, 1989

Kluft RP: Incest and subsequent revictimization: the case of therapist-patient sexual exploitation, with a description of the sitting duck syndrome, in Incest-Related Syndromes of Adult Psychopathology. Edited by Kluft RP. Washington, DC, American Psychiatric Press, 1990a, pp 263–287

Kluft RP: Dissociation and subsequent vulnerability: a preliminary study. Dissociation 3:167–173, 1990b

Kluft RP: Multiple personality disorder, in American Psychiatric Press Review of Psychiatry, Vol 10. Edited by Tasman A, Goldfinger SM. Washington, DC, American Psychiatric Press, 1991, pp 161–188

Kluft RP, Braun BG, Sachs RG: Multiple personality, intrafamilial abuse, and family psychiatry. International Journal of Family Psychiatry 5:283–301, 1984

Putnam FW: The Diagnosis and Treatment of Multiple Personality Disorder. New York, Guilford, 1989

Putnam FW, Guroff JJ, Silberman EK, et al: The clinical phenomenology of multiple personality disorder: review of 100 recent cases. J Clin Psychiatry 47:285–293, 1986

Ross CA: Multiple Personality Disorder: Diagnosis, Clinical Features, and Treatment. New York, Wiley, 1989

Spiegel D: Dissociating damage. Am J Clin Hypn 29:123–131, 1986

Spiegel H, Spiegel D: Trance and Treatment (1978). Washington, DC, American Psychiatric Press, 1987

Watkins JG, Watkins HH: The theory and practice of ego-state therapy, in Short Term Approaches to Psychotherapy. Edited by Grayson H. New York, National Institute for the Psychotherapies and Human Sciences Press, 1979

Wilbur CB, Kluft RP: Multiple personality disorder, in Treatments of Mental Disorders: A Task Force Report of the American Psychiatric Association, Vol 3. Washington, DC, American Psychiatric Press, 1988

Chapter 7

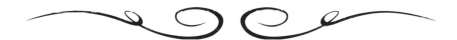

A Tactical Integrationalist Perspective on the Treatment of Multiple Personality Disorder

Catherine G. Fine, Ph.D.

In this chapter, I review diverse treatment philosophies that have been considered in the treatment of multiple personality disorder (MPD) since Cornelia Wilbur was instrumental in reviving interest in its diagnosis and treatment. I introduce and develop the tactical integration perspective in the treatment of MPD and explore the cognitive foundation of this model. I then present the conceptual foundation of the tactical integration model and the intervention modules that have evolved to dilute the affect and facilitate abreactions. In the last section, I present a composite case study to illustrate a few representative interventions.

The rising index of suspicion among therapists with respect to the diagnosis of dissociative disorders in general and of MPD in particular, combined with more specific and readily accessible diagnostic criteria (DSM-III-R; American Psychiatric Association 1987) and newly developed clinical interview schedules and specialized mental status examinations (Bernstein and Putnam 1986; Loewenstein 1991; Ross et al. 1989; Steinberg et al. 1990), have jointly contributed to its "derarification." As these conditions were recognized with increased frequency, a number of treatment strategies evolved to aid the recovery of patients with dissociative disorders. Philosophies espoused by therapists treating these patients have ranged from theory-based perspectives to novel, even opportunistic, atheoretical views created on the spur of the moment or amidst a crisis.

Overview of Treatment Philosophies in Work With MPD Patients

In his editorial "Therapeutic Pluralism," Kluft (1989b) categorized approaches to treatment in seven major groups. These ranged from the confused and desperate attempts of overwhelmed therapists to thoughtful protocols for well-planned interventions.

The first (whimsically named) approach to treatment is the "Nantucket Sleigh Ride" therapy. It encompasses efforts to ride out a chaotic situation and apply any technique or approach that the therapist may feel inspired to use at the moment. Another approach is "Modality Maven" therapy, in which what occurs between the patient and the therapist is limited to and by the therapist's modality of choice. A third therapy approach focuses on the use and contribution to the therapeutic process of specific personalities or personality types. Therapists who subscribe to this approach often preferentially empower certain personalities in their patients whom they perceive or construe to be insightful guides and more knowledgeable than other personalities in some special way. The risk for the therapist-patient dyad in preferring this approach is the potential of the relinquishing by the therapist of the responsibility of the treatment process to a personality who by its very nature is decontextualized and incapable of carrying out the responsibilities it may have sought.

A fourth approach to the treatment of MPD is the adaptationalist stance. Working from this perspective, the therapists support the patients' attempts to be more functional within a societal context;

they help the patient survive in the here and now and may collude with the patient's wish to ignore major dissociative pathology so as to avoid painful and/or overwhelming affect. A fifth treatment philosophy is often espoused by the therapist who is ambivalent or skeptical about the diagnosis of MPD; it is the "leave it alone and it will go away" stance. However, Kluft (1985) reports that without treatment addressing the dissociative defenses, MPD patients will still have MPD on follow-up. The aftermath of this stance of benign neglect has a negative impact on the MPD patient, who is typically pessimistic about the future, and who may come to believe that therapy is not to be counted on to acknowledge and address his or her difficulties.

A controversial therapy modality not amply reported on by Kluft (1989b) is the reparenting model. Supporters of this model rely on the belief that a patient can be loved into health. Though not an atheoretical perspective, it nonetheless leads the MPD patient down a very tenuous path. The reparenting model presupposes that giving an MPD patient a real and/or fictional and/or metaphorical breast/baby bottle will help the patient enjoy a corrective emotional experience; this experience is intended to "undo" or decrease dissociation. In reality, the reparenting model falls more within the realm of misguided efforts to gratify the patient's wishes to avoid negative affects and to take flights into tenuous approximations of health rather than actual recovery.

A few therapeutic modalities seem, nonetheless, to have survived the test of time and have allowed a substantial number of MPD patients to achieve successful and robust integrations. These are the strategic and the tactical integration models. The strategic integration therapist focuses more specifically on undermining the dissociative defenses that support the multiplicity; this erosion is ongoing and relentless so that the dissociative structure collapses from within. The strategic integration model has been widely described (Kluft 1984; Wilbur 1984) and has been the most acceptable and respected treatment modality to date. It is implicit in the treatment conducted by Cornelia Wilbur herself (Schreiber 1973). A more recently developed therapeutic stance for the treatment of MPD has been called tactical integration (Fine 1991, 1992; Kluft 1989b). The treatment premises for the tactical integration therapist are similar to beliefs held by the strategic integrationalist; but they carry with them a technical preference for mounting many specific planned avenues of intervention addressing a number of deliberately chosen short- and long-term goals at the onset of treatment, rather than initiating a more broadly based attack on the dissociative defenses in general.

Throughout the remainder of this chapter, I will consider issues of interest for those therapists who work within the tactical integration perspective. Initially, the cognitive foundation of the tactical integration model is reviewed, followed by a description of how the therapy itself would be structured. Various aspects of the therapy are discussed in detail in the final section of the chapter, along with a more particularized illustration of some tactical integration techniques.

Cognitive Foundation of the Tactical Integration Model

The tactical integration model subscribes to the view that the therapy for MPD involves a collaboration between a consistent, predictable, and empathic therapist and an affectively overwhelmed patient who struggles with issues of trust, shame, and responsibility. The tactical integration model fosters the development of an evolving yet sturdy cognitive foundation that can serve as an anchor for the patient and the patient's personalities during the processing of powerful affect-laden material. Planned and openly anticipated rather than serendipitous or opportunistic cognitive interventions help establish an atmosphere of safety and predictability in the treatment as MPD patients learn to use an experimental model to hypothesis-test the validity of their established beliefs (Fine 1988).

Once explored, patients' beliefs will either remain unchanged or be modified to conform to a newer and/or better assessment of present reality. It has been established elsewhere that MPD patients are noteworthy for the delusional quality of some of their beliefs as well as for the number and rigidity of their cognitive distortions (Fine 1988; see also Chapter 19). Therefore, the verification of cognitions should be understood not only as essential, but also as a difficult and often confusing aspect of the therapy for MPD patients. These cognitive distortions serve as defenses to maintain dissociation and to continue the warding off of unbearable affect. Because of their configuration, these distortions not only reflect difficulties in the patients' perceptual experiences, but also interfere repeatedly with the patients' capacity to derive appropriate learning from abreactions. For the tactical integrationalist, the extent and elaborateness of the cognitive groundwork is primarily in preparation for abreactive work. Abreactions are considered necessary and painful treatment components; they involve the reconnecting affect to cognition, but they are helpful only if they reconnect affect to a corrected, nondistorted (or less distorted) cognitive foundation. This means that patients' distorted thinking must be modified through cognitive restructuring as a prerequisite to their being able to engage in effective abreactive work. Only with the achievement of the capacity to "think straight" can MPD patients finally begin to learn to reality-test.

Therefore, in the course of therapy, the tactical integration therapist can anticipate needing to challenge cognitions in an ongoing manner and to modify, slowly but effectively, the posttraumatic/abuse schemata that are at the origin of the patient's distorted globalized cognitions (Spiegel 1986). Appropriate changes in the cognitions, and eventually in the personality's/patient's beliefs, will effectively redress inexact self-attributions and begin, in combination with the therapeutic abreactions, to reequilibrate the personality's/patient's worldview. The tactical integrationalist will alternate the cognitive-affective interventions to create gentle dissonances within each personality that will, taken as a whole, lead to the MPD patient's eventual correct recontextualization of his or her experiences and perceptions.

Indeed, it is important to remember that most personalities within an MPD patient exist within a contextual void (Fine 1988, 1990; Kluft 1990). They do not have and often never have had access to all the cognitive and/or affective information necessary to make sense of their present circumstances. If their dissociative barriers remain unchallenged, MPD patients become increasingly unable to formulate helpful decisions for the future, because decisions based on "war zone" beliefs (i.e., traumatic anticipations) are likely to maintain a warlike atmosphere. A systematic consideration of MPD patients' and their personalities' cognitive realities requires careful planning and preparation; it also calls for caution and respect in making efforts to jar their false (but often ego-syntonic) assumptions. Therefore, it becomes important for the therapist to be clear on how and when to establish cognitive dissonance in MPD patients so that treatment can proceed successfully and with minimal disruptions (Fine 1991). This treatment flow will only proceed as smoothly as the therapeutic alliance is strong and the structure of the tactical integration work is clearly delineated.

Structuring for Tactical Integration

The tactical integrationalist approach to the therapy of MPD can be divided into two general phases: the preunification phase of treatment and the postunification phase of treatment. The goals of the preunification phase of the treatment for MPD is the returning of all the different personalities and their unique contents to the mainstream of consciousness. This implies that all pathologically dissociated aspects of knowledge, affect, sensation, and behavior must come together and unify (Braun 1988; Fine 1991). The postunification phase of treatment (which will not be the focus of this chapter) begins after the last final integration of the last personality (Kluft 1984).

The preunification phase of treatment for the tactical integrationalist consists of two contiguous and overlapping stages. These stages are 1) a suppression of affect stage, followed by 2) a dilution of affect stage. This two-stage model is based on the premise that the different personalities are differentially ready and differentially able to engage in the therapy process. Therefore, at a particular moment in treatment, it is possible to be working with personalities who cannot easily contain strong affect and must remain in a suppression of affect mode for long periods of time, whereas other personalities may be involved in the therapy who have mastered overwhelming affect more rapidly. The latter group can begin the more advanced process of diluting the affect. In my experience, personalities who can navigate more easily through affective storms can also more readily work through the traumatic experiences that must be faced and processed.

The Suppression of Affect Phase

The initial aspect of treatment involves getting to know the MPD patient through his or her defensive vehicle of choice: the personalities. As in any other therapy, the patient and the therapist cooperate on establishing a working relationship. With MPD patients, the therapeutic alliance must be grounded not only in the relationship with the patient as a whole but also must be extended to encompass all personalities of that patient (Kluft 1984). Patient and therapist alike need to build a strong therapeutic foundation with clearly delineated roles (Fine 1989a). This foundation is a necessary but insufficient condition to foster safety in the midst of arduous processing and powerful abreactive events. An atmosphere of safety is additionally rooted in the therapist's willingness to get to know each of the personalities individually and to take an interest in their personal histories and their perspectives, as well as to inquire about their understandings of the therapeutic process. The therapist must be prepared to take a psychoeducational stance as well as to pursue the completion of the extensive cognitive groundwork. If this preparatory stage is ignored by either the therapist, the patient, or both, the patient is likely not to be helped. Instead, he or she is likely to be thrown prematurely into remembering the early and/or more recent traumas of his or her life at a time when he or she would have to face affect that is difficult to manage.

Getting to Know the MPD Patient: Mapping of the Personalities

In one of the initial sessions, the MPD patient is often asked to take a large sheet of paper and to place the name of the host personality in the center. The patient is then invited to have the respective personalities place their names on the paper "in a meaningful way." The therapist may clarify further by specifying that the names be placed in a way that would describe "how similar or dissimilar the personalities feel toward or about one another." Depending on 1) the total number of personalities, 2) the number of personalities in conscious awareness, or 3) the patient's overall investment in the psychotherapy, the page may remain virtually blank or resemble a scattergram. This initial mapping represents a baseline against which all subsequent mappings can be compared; it can also be understood as an introduction to the personalities on the patient's own terms. Therefore, from the beginning of treatment, the therapist is empowering the patient and respectfully supporting the patient's involvement in the therapy process. Through their mapping of their system of personalities, MPD patients invite their therapists to join them in the cautious explorations of their dissociated inner realities.

These mappings commonly reveal groups of personalities clustered together for reasons foreign to them. Continued probing often unveils common core conflictual relationship themes (CCRT [Luborsky 1984]) among the members of each cluster. The mapping of personalities in combination with the therapist's clinical interview constitutes a first unifying step in the MPD patient's treatment. It is also an invitation to all who are part of the patient's mind to join in the therapy.

Discovering the Cognitive World of the MPD Patient

The personalities who are originally delineated in the mapping become a point of entry (a psychological wedge) into the system of personalities and an opportunity to better understand the patient. As "all parts of the mind" are invited to listen, the personalities are asked to tell their stories, to talk about themselves, and to describe what they know and remember without going into the details at this point. The MPD patients' autohypnotic abilities (which may be at the basis for the formation of personalities [Bliss 1984]) make them nicely responsive to "distancing" suggestions such as "All that you need to do at this time is talk about what happened as if you were watching from a distance—way far away from you." Using the patients' dissociative abilities to their benefit rather than to their detriment will facilitate mutual acknowledgment between the different parts of the mind and foster recognition of their respective needs. It will cultivate an atmosphere where they can compare histories respectfully and learn to agree to disagree. By patiently asking questions about the personalities, by keeping an open mind, and by not having preconceived expectations, the therapist models for the patient (and for the various personalities) what is expected in treatment.

Therefore, uncovering the "story lines" with the various personalities has a twofold benefit for the therapy. It establishes a treatment philosophy for the patient as a whole and serves as a distraction from the affect at a time at which the intensity of the affect would feel unmanageable. "Mapping the system of the personalities" encourages the development of a road map for the exploration of the life events that need to be faced by all personalities. This map makes available to the therapist both additional time and opportunities to challenge the cognitive distortions present in all personalities. The requisite correction of these distortions will facilitate thorough abreactive work and will favor a corrective emotional experience rather than a retraumatization. This contrasts with following the red thread of the person's affective reality that is tied to victimization in childhood and very much linked to childlike thinking and perceiving.

The Dilution of Affect Phase

The dilution of affect phase of treatment overlaps with the suppression of affect phase when the therapist asks the various personalities to describe their lives "from a distance." As stated previously, this strategy takes advantage of the MPD patient's ability to dissociate and uses this well-rehearsed skill to the patient's present advantage. Each personality needs to adjust to the sheer horror of its individual story line before it can possibly face the knowledge that other personalities' story lines are also part of its life experience.

Work Within Like-Clusters of Personalities
A review of the mapping of the personalities may be helpful at this time, because the preferred aggregation of the groups/clusters of personalities may currently be more conceptually meaningful. Each personality cluster may connect in the knowledge about particular events, or else the link among the personalities in the cluster may be an affective one. Thus, clusters may group according to cognitive or

affective themes. Some groupings of personalities may be the concomitant accumulation of both cognitive and affective experiences.

The tactical integrationalist will initially prefer to work with the affect shared within the same cluster of personalities, rather than across clusters or between a cluster and the host. Structuring the therapy work in this fashion is designed to make abreactive work less traumatizing to all personalities. It will also reduce patients' feelings that they are being revictimized by their therapist. Therefore, the affect initially is contained, retained, and processed within clusters and among similar personalities. As a consequence, by the time the affect seeps to other personalities outside the original cluster or to the host, it will be more diluted and less "raw."

Use of Fractionated Abreactions

A second precaution to dilute affect and decrease the patient's fear of doing abreactive work is to do fractionated abreactions rather than full abreactions. This approach was developed by Kluft (1989c) to avoid overwhelming medically compromised and vulnerable MPD patients.

Abreactions are necessary in the treatment of the MPD patient. An abreaction helps personalities reconnect their perceptions of reality formed in the past to the present reality. The purpose of the abreaction is therefore to inform, educate, or reeducate, to release the repressed affect, and to complete content and reformulate cognitive schemata and beliefs as well as to release somatically encapsulated traumata (Comstock 1986). Abreactions are necessary to reconnect the behavioral, affective, sensory, and cognitive dimensions of events (Braun 1988; Fine 1989b), to ward off further amnesia, and to achieve continuity of life experiences (Fine 1989b, 1992). The detailed course of abreactions in the treatment of MPD is best described elsewhere (Comstock 1986), but what is essential is that these abreactions be done systematically and completely.

The fractionated abreaction involves achieving this goal in small increments (Kluft 1989c). Rather than doing a complete abreaction in one (extended) session, the feelings are slowly reconnected to discrete aspects of the history. Each partial abreaction precedes and follows cognitive restructuring as more knowledge and affect become reconnected. This process parallels the use of systematic desensitization to achieve gradual mastery over a phobic stimulus, rather than presenting a powerful stimulus, as is done in flooding procedures.

The fractionated abreaction enhances MPD patients' feelings of control and self-efficacy as they become increasingly able to pace the necessary therapeutic work by diluting the affect rather than becoming entangled in and chronically overwhelmed and depleted in powerful affective storms.

Collaborative Abreactions Through Blending of Personalities

An additional method to dilute affect is through "blending of personalities" (Fine and Comstock 1989). Blending involves the temporary integration and sharing, in part or in whole, of cognitions, affects, sensations, and/or behaviors among personalities. A time-limited blending between two or more personalities can be helpful to facilitate abreactions by decreasing anxiety, fear, and terror associated with some of the memories. Personalities who have achieved a certain degree of affective or cognitive mastery over an event may blend with a personality or personalities that are new to the experience, to help the novice personality or personalities better navigate their ways through these feelings. By means of blending, personalities learn to slowly absorb, contain, and retain powerful and/or painful feelings. They learn that they need not feel all the affect in one moment; but more importantly, they come to understand the importance of cooperation and mutual support in the face of adverse circumstances.

In addition, blending of personalities can help different personalities experience an alternative to their often all-or-none perspectives and points of view. Blending of personalities may help mollify rigidly encapsulated beliefs and powerfully upheld feelings by letting personalities test them for themselves in the context of an alternative experience. Blending teaches the personalities that they can "think and feel" differently. It demonstrates to them the worth of hypothesis testing. They learn that they need not respond in a purely reflexive way.

Blending of personalities is a safe intervention when used judiciously and with various personalities' permission. However, there are a few caveats. Blendings should never be forced. Indeed, an imposed blending may leave an alter more fearful, devastated, and decided in attempts to avoid or reduce communication with other personalities. In addition, certain personalities would do better *not* to merge, because the intensity of the potentially destructive emotion might culminate in inappropriate actions, such as in the case of abusive and suicidal alters.

In summary, the three tactics to dilute affect (working within similar clusters of personalities, doing fractionated abreactions, and blending personalities) can be used concurrently within the MPD patient as the therapist works with an increasing number of personalities and their respective conflicts.

Neither the tactical integration therapist nor the MPD patient will know the complete hierarchy of cognitive-affective building blocks until the end of therapy. However, a slow, cooperative, and studied approach to the personality system, combined with a systematic elicitation of all cognitions and affects contained within all personalities, will allow the MPD patient to approach therapy (and ultimately life) with an increasing sense of control and self-efficacy, as well as with steadfast purpose. The tactical integration approach will help the MPD patient recontextualize his or her life experiences and live in one rather than in multiple realities.

Case Study

History

Carmen (a pseudonym) is a 30-year-old woman, divorced and childless, who presented for treatment with symptoms of anxiety, only partially relieved by anxiolytic medication. She stated, "Something is not right—I don't know what's wrong; I'm just unhappy. . . . At times everything just goes wrong . . . like my relationships." Further questioning revealed that Carmen was involved in a number of concurrent sexual relationships from which she derived little satisfaction; this had been her pattern for the last 10 years. Carmen had terminated five pregnancies; her reactions had been a combination of regret and relief. Her former husband had been no more important to her than the other men in her life ("except for all the legal complications!"). Despite a rather chaotic personal life, she was able to maintain a growing career with some degree of success.

Carmen was the eldest of three children and the first girl, born to an upwardly mobile middle-class family with established religious principles. The parents have been described in a confusing manner, but Carmen's nonverbal behaviors (facial and postural) suggest a wish for distance from them. Both parents were reported to be perfectionists; demanding, exacting, unreliable, and critical. Carmen said they are intrusive, yet unavailable. Carmen's mother was described as "flaky" and "out to lunch." Her father has a long history of alcohol abuse that (according to the patient) has not affected his professional life; he is also prone to fits of anger. Carmen struggles with understanding her shifting alliances with her parents and is perplexed about their alliances with one another against her.

Her relationships with her siblings have been tenuous. Carmen felt responsible for them when they were young, and she was angry at them because she had to maintain a parental role toward them. Yet she experienced them as competitors for what scant parental attention and recognition was available. Currently, she has little to do with them; but her unresolved sibling rivalry is repeatedly reenacted in her professional life with her co-workers.

Carmen initially presented as a neurotic patient with few signs of dissociative disorder. However, her vagueness about her childhood, the presence of many somatic problems of unexplained origin, and recurrent contradictions in her perceptions of her parents led me to pursue a more detailed and thorough childhood history than would ordinarily be indicated. This revealed large gaps in her memory beyond the normative childhood amnesias. A review of some journals she had kept during childhood and adolescence suggested incest with her father, starting in early childhood. Through those journals, she described her mother as unavailable, or at least inaccessible to her.

Course of Treatment

As Carmen and I gently explored her history, Carmen became more symptomatic. She changed in her behavior, her dress, her words, and her ability to remain grounded as an adult. She identified parts of the mind ("aspects of myself") that "are still living in the past" and "don't feel grown up at all." She reported, "I still feel as if I am looking for a daddy—a real daddy."

The spontaneous emergence of a child personality in the course of a session convinced me to shift Carmen's diagnosis from anxiety disorder with dissociative features to MPD. Once welcomed into treatment, many child personalities wanted to "speak up." I witnessed many incidents of rapid switching that were later to be understood as reflecting a conflict among the personalities over revealing "the secret."

Carmen became increasingly distressed and dysfunctional. It was agreed that, for the moment, the personalities would be welcomed to "come out" completely during the therapy sessions in my office but that they would talk with one another inside Carmen's head outside of the therapy sessions. This was a compromise that we were temporarily willing to strike.

The alters were invited to put their names on a sheet of paper; many eagerly identified themselves as wanting more and more attention as the sessions progressed. Some were lonely and had a strong desire to know other parts of the mind; others were tired and hurting and were hopeful for some relief; others still remained cautious and quiet, simultaneously wishing and fearing that I would go away. A relatively complete mapping of the personalities was possible early in treatment. I became acquainted with many of the personalities and their stated problems. No formal abreactive work was initiated by either the patient or me at this point.

One particular session proved to be a landmark in the therapy. An "older," more stable personality within the personality system whose name had always intrigued me felt that "it was time" to meet her. Her name was Pandora; she said she had been helping all along and would continue to do so.

I asked Pandora to explain the inner world of the personalities through their mapping. She acknowledged having helped regroup the child personalities according to those who remembered similar events; the adolescent and adult personalities had followed her lead and also clustered according to cognitive dimensions. By this time, many of the different personalities knew (or at least, knew of) one another. It was time to prepare more thoroughly for doing abreactive work. The remainder of this case study will follow one of the clusters of personalities in Carmen through interventions that illustrate the aforementioned three methods to dilute affect.

Working Within Like-Clusters

I encouraged some of the older child personalities (8-year-old to 9-year-old group) to begin the abreactive work and be role models. This particular group seemed both motivated and cognitively able to engage in the necessary work. They were the ones who knew about the abuse by Carmen's father during the elementary school years. Initially, they knew who Carmen's father was, but they did not fully understand that this man was their father, too. Their motivation was based on the wish to be a "big girl," to be a "good girl," and also to no longer have to be scared all the time. They knew that Carmen's father had touched their "private parts" and that when they remembered him, they hurt "down there" and had trouble breathing; they also as a group remembered shaking and feeling "real, real cold." They wanted to spend more time playing and reading and going out with Carmen, instead of hurting.

The Fractionated Abreactions

Pandora volunteered to help oversee the sharing of the feelings among these child personalities. The alters and I agreed that the imagery that would be used to do the fractionated abreactions should be meaningful to all the child alters in that cluster. I remembered the alters speaking of "shaking and being real cold"; I also recalled how the personalities described being thrown into a cold lake by one of Carmen's boyfriends. It was decided that these particular abreactions would be like slowly stepping into the cold water of the lake and adjusting to the temperature. The personalities kept open the option of running out of the water if it were unbearably cold, but they promised to return to it eventually. This implied that the child alters would try to feel the feelings associated with the abreactions for as long as they could, but could stop when necessary, as long as they would go back to the feelings when the time was right.

This cluster of personalities went to the lake together. They sat on the shore and talked about their life; they then joined hands as they stood in a row and slowly dipped their toes in the water. By analogy, this is how they began to feel one another's feelings. They discovered going into the water as a group, all together at once, seemed less frightening to them than each one going into the lake individually. Thus, feeling the feelings about Carmen's father together as a group seemed less terrifying to the alters than the prospect of each facing the feelings individually. This group of child alters and I made many trips to that (hypnotic) lake until the alters could tolerate the temperature of the water and swim with confidence within it, knowing that they would not drown. The alters became increasingly able to tolerate the affect associated with the memories of Carmen's father. Eventually, swimming at the lake allowed the children to "play mermaid" and "be magical" and for them to fuse with one another as they matched their breathing with their swimming strokes. This occurred for all but two of the child personalities in this cluster.

Blending of Personalities

Upon inquiry, I discovered that the two unintegrated children from this cluster differed in the following way: one of them knew that Carmen's father was also her father, the other one remained ignorant of this. The first one knew that he wasn't just a "mean man"; she knew that "this mean man was suppose to love [her] and take care of [her] and protect [her]," and she was terrified. Pandora, these two child alters, and I decided to have the child alters blend during the therapy sessions only while the alters remained in my office. Being aware of their surrounds allowed them to learn from one another as they remained oriented to place, person, and time. Using a more formal hypnotic induction, I had both child personalities step front and center as all other parts of the mind stepped back. I paced and timed for the children their stepping together (blending), which they could initially tolerate only for seconds. Repeated blendings led to the children's mutual acceptance and mutual identification. Eventually, they felt that the blending could become a fusion, and they refused to step apart because "together we feel stronger."

The previous section described the work with one of the many clusters of personalities within Carmen. It should be noted that I had to divide her time among all the clusters, though few of the others would consider abreactive work until they were assured that the 8-year-old to 9-year-old cluster had safely negotiated their task. I consistently proposed dilution of affect techniques to the various personalities, utilizing the patient's own imagery. The retrieval of memories of abuse were paced to be tolerated by the alters and by Carmen, who needed to function as a professional. The course of Carmen's therapy has been punctuated by many stumbling blocks; these often involved some personality's unwillingness to "get [his or her] feet wet" and the subsequent rise in suicidal ideation and suicidal impulses.

Two years into treatment, Carmen reported struggling with having to face feelings and having difficulty dissociating them away. She became flustered that her sexual life was so calm, and she put complete responsibility for this "mishap" on me. However, she does acknowledge that she is more demanding in her selection of sexual partners: "Now, I sound so conservative!" Carmen is not yet integrated, but her observing ego is more developed and healthier. She is making plans for the future and feels confident about her ability to complete therapy successfully.

This brief case study reveals a careful pacing of the therapy work and a collaboration between patient and therapist to avoid unnecessary crises. The cognitive strategies within the tactical integration model allow for the exploration of conflicts, detailing of the affect associated with the conflicts, and their eventual integration into the mainstream of consciousness. In this model, the patient assumes an increasing responsibility for treatment and is clearly expected to monitor and interpret the progress in the therapy work. This example also clarifies how important cognitive reframing is for the host personality, as is the restructuring of cognitions for the personality clusters. Indeed, Carmen, to appreciate her therapy accomplishments, had to struggle with the concept that having fewer sexual partners meant that she was getting better, not worse. The slowness (thoroughness) of the reintegration of the feelings allowed Carmen to better understand some of the driving influences in her life and to make choices about future paths. Carmen had also learned about the importance of trial and error and that, unlike in her family of origin, things did not have to work out perfectly on the first try to achieve ultimate success.

What Carmen has learned in her self-explorations is not unlike what therapists working with MPD patients have learned in the last 20 years. They have learned that a concerted attention and respect for the ground rules of therapy, an awareness of symptoms without an overreaction to them, and a steadfast undermining of the dissociative barriers will let the MPD patient develop continuity of past and present memory and will foster an ongoing sense of self. The tactical integration model follows these principles. It is one of the effective treatment possibilities for the MPD patient who is willing to take control of his or her life in a planful way.

References

American Psychiatric Association: Diagnostic and Statistical Manual of Mental Disorders, 3rd Edition, Revised. Washington, DC, American Psychiatric Association, 1987

Bernstein MA, Putnam FW: Development, reliability and validity of a dissociation scale. J Nerv Ment Dis 174:727–735, 1986

Bliss EL: Spontaneous self hypnosis in multiple personality disorder. Psychiatr Clin North Am 7:135–148, 1984

Braun BG: The BASK model of dissociation. Dissociation 1(1):4–24, 1988

Comstock CM: The therapeutic utilization of abreactive experiences in the treatment of multiple personality disorder, in Dissociative Disorders 1986. Edited by Braun BG. Chicago, IL, Rush University, 1986, p 105

Fine CG: Thoughts on the cognitive-perceptual substrates of multiple personality disorder. Dissociation 1(4):5–10, 1988a

Fine CG: Treatment errors and iatrogenesis across therapeutic modalities in MPD and allied dissociative disorders. Dissociation 2:77–82, 1989a

Fine CG: Cognitive aspects of hypnotherapeutic interventions with dissociative disorders patients. Paper presented at the 32nd annual meeting of the American Society of Clinical Hypnosis, Orlando, FL, March 1989b

Fine CG: The cognitive sequelae of incest, in Incest-Related Syndromes of Adult Psychopathology. Edited by Kluft RP. Washington, DC, American Psychiatric Press, 1990, pp 161–182

Fine CG: Treatment stabilization and crisis prevention: pacing the therapy of the MPD patient. Psychiatr Clin North Am 14:661–675, 1991

Fine CG: The cognitive therapy of multiple personality disorder, in Comprehensive Casebook of Cognitive-Behavior Therapy. Edited by Freeman A, D'attilio FM. New York, Plenum, 1992, pp 347–360

Fine CG, Comstock CM: Completion of cognitive schemata and affective realms through the temporary blending of personalities in the treatment of multiple personality disorder, in Dissociative Disorders 1989. Edited by Braun BG. Chicago, IL, Rush University, 1989, p 17

Kluft RP: Treatment of multiple personality disorder: a study of 33 cases. Psychiatr Clin North Am 7:9–29, 1984

Kluft RP: The natural history of multiple personality disorder, in Childhood Antecedents of Multiple Personality Disorder. Edited by Kluft RP. Washington, DC, American Psychiatric Press, 1985, pp 197–238

Kluft RP: Making the diagnosis of multiple personality disorder, in Diagnostics and Psychopathology. Edited by Flach FF. New York, WW Norton, 1987, pp 207–225

Kluft RP: Playing for time: temporizing techniques in the treatment of multiple personality disorder. Am J Clin Hypn 32:90–98, 1989a

Kluft RP: Today's therapeutic pluralism. Dissociation 1(4):1–2, 1989b

Kluft RP: Playing for time: temporizing techniques in the treatment of multiple personality disorder. Am J Clin Hypn 32:90–98, 1989c

Kluft RP: Incest and subsequent revictimization: the case of therapist-patient sexual exploitation, with a description of the sitting duck syndrome, in Incest-Related Syndromes of Adult Psychopathology. Edited by Kluft RP. Washington, DC, American Psychiatric Press, 1990, pp 263–286

Loewenstein RJ: An office mental status examination for chronic complex dissociative symptoms and multiple personality disorder. Psychiatr Clin North Am 14:567–604, 1991

Luborsky L: Principles of Psychoanalytic Psychotherapy: A Manual for Supportive-Expressive Treatment. New York, Basic Books, 1984

Ross CA, Heber S, Norton GR, et al: The dissociative disorders interview schedule: a structured interview. Dissociation 2:169–189, 1989

Schreiber FR: Sybil. Chicago, IL, Regnery, 1973

Spiegel D: Dissociation, double binds and post-traumatic stress in multiple personality disorder, in Treatment of Multiple Personality Disorder. Edited by Braun BG. Washington, DC, American Psychiatric Press, 1986, pp 61–77

Steinberg M, Rousainville B, Cicchetti D: The structured clinical interview for DSM-III-R dissociative disorders: preliminary report on a new diagnostic instrument. Am J Psychiatry 147:76–82, 1990

Wilbur CB: Treatment of multiple personality. Psychiatric Annals 14:27–31, 1984

Chapter 8

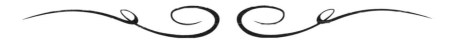

Aids to the Treatment of Multiple Personality Disorder on a General Psychiatric Inpatient Unit

Bennett G. Braun, M.D.

The therapist who treats patients with multiple personality disorder (MPD) may have to arrange for their hospital treatment under certain circumstances (Braun 1986; Kluft 1984, 1985, 1991). Unless the therapist has admitting privileges to a specialty unit for patients with MPD or dissociative disorders, the admission is most likely to be to the general psychiatric unit of a local hospital or to a freestanding psychiatric hospital.

Such hospital stays may be relatively smooth if the staff of the unit to which the patient is admitted have experience with MPD patients or have been trained to work with MPD patients. Otherwise, these admissions may result in problems that can be perceived as retraumatizing by the patient and split the unit's staff into opposing factions.

Kluft (1984, 1991) has observed that it is not necessarily the patient that splits a staff. Rather, the staff splits itself when differing views about this controversial condition are allowed to influence professional behavior. In addition, staff members come to feel incompetent and helpless, and resentment begins to build against both the patient and the psychiatrist or other mental health professional who brought the patient into the hospital. Other patients may respond to staff splitting by playing into it and by turning against the patient. The end result can be disastrous for all concerned—the MPD patient, the therapist(s), the other patients, the hospital staff, and the hospital administration.

Therapists who work regularly with MPD patients are familiar with the difficulty of obtaining good inpatient care for this group of patients. Despite the growing number of hospitals with special MPD/dissociative disorder units, space on these units continues to be limited. Unit beds may not be available at times of crisis, and requests for consultation from the leaders of such units often cannot be responded to within an acute time frame. Therefore, outpatient therapists must continue to rely on general units in local hospitals. Thus, in many settings they will continue to face 1) difficulties with staff disbelief in the MPD diagnosis; 2) splitting and burnout of staff as they attempt to work with MPD patients; 3) increased acting-out by other patients in response to the problems that surround the MPD patient; and 4) consequent disruption of the milieu of the unit to which the patient is admitted.

The best approach to resolution of these problems is to coordinate a treatment plan with a general unit staff prior to the MPD patient's hospitalization and to continue this process throughout the admission. This includes providing training and support for the staff as well as contracting and limit setting with the patient. By being proactive, the therapist can improve the prognosis for a successful hospitalization.

Reasons to Hospitalize

The reader must bear in mind that although MPD can reach a gratifying and stable resolution, as demonstrated in the series of MPD patients followed sequentially by Kluft (1986), it is a chronic condition in which crises and regressions may be recurrent despite the skill of the therapist. Although psychiatry's knowledge and skill with MPD has grown, and there are many ways in which the use of a hospital setting can facilitate such patients' recoveries, it is an unfortunate irony that these advances have become available at a moment in history at which the use of inpatient facilities is increasingly curtailed. Therefore, any consideration of the use of hospital treatment must be made with the utmost care, and with an appreciation that a patient's lifetime hospital days may be quite limited and cannot be squandered. The patient should not be hospitalized if an alternative effective treatment is available, and hospitalization should never be undertaken to suit the convenience of concerned others. Having acknowledged these considerations, it is nonetheless all too often the case that alternative settings that are capable of managing the distressed MPD patient effectively are exceedingly rare. The same must be said for the use of the hospital for specific therapeutic interventions. In addition, despite widespread cries to use alternative settings, they are all too often either not available or not able or willing to undertake work with this patient population.

In clinical practice, most MPD patients are hospitalized in the context of a crisis, usually involving danger to self or to others. Nonemergency admissions may be planned to achieve specific clinical objectives that, in the judgment of the clinician, are necessary to advance the patient's treatment but that could not be undertaken on an outpatient basis without subjecting the patient to such a high risk of decompensation that would necessitate hospitalization that patient safety is best served by doing the necessary work in an inpatient setting from the first.

Although crises cannot be predicted, they often can be anticipated. When advance preparation has been carried out between an admitting psychiatrist and a hospital, even a crisis admission need not become an uncontrollable emergency.

Crises of violence.   Crises that bring the MPD patient to the hospital include those that make the patient a danger to him- or herself or to others:

1. Homicidal ideation or acting out toward external individuals or internal alters (which looks like suicide);
2. Suicidal ideation or acting out by one personality or several alters;
3. Violent behavior toward other individuals or their property;
4. Self-mutilation; and
5. Decompensations with flashbacks and memories of traumata that lead to violent behaviors.

Inability to function.   Hospitalization may have to be sought for a patient who cannot function because of the following:

1. Rapid switching;
2. Flashbacks that are temporarily incapacitating;
3. Overwhelming reactions to environmental stimuli; and
4. Overwhelming reactions to a date, an anniversary, or time of year.

Psychological stressors.   Psychological stresses that can bring about hospitalization include the following:

1. The trauma of receiving the MPD diagnosis;
2. A death or another personal loss (the death of an abuser can be particularly traumatic, causing long-dormant concerns to surface);
3. Problems about money, work, friends, or family; and
4. Anniversary reactions.

Prophylaxis.   Hospitalization may be necessary on short notice to prevent a crisis hospitalization when the patient has decompensated further:

1. The patient's safety may be imminently threatened by memories or acting out;
2. Abreactive work with violent alters may mandate the safety of an inpatient milieu with the option of using restraints; and
3. The psychotherapist may perceive that material that could prove too difficult to process in outpatient sessions is about to emerge.

Therapeutic deadlock.   Deadlock in therapy can be an indication for a brief hospital stay and a reevaluation. Therapeutic impasse may be an issue of transference or countertransference; it may be due to a lack of knowledge or experience by the therapist; or it can be caused by a failure of limit setting by the therapist early in outpatient treatment, creating a countertransference issue. On rare occasions, deadlock must be resolved by changing therapists; but more often, all that is needed is a limited amount of time with another therapist who can assess and resolve the impasse. A time-limited intervention by a staff psychiatrist during a brief hospital stay can provide such an occasion. The leverage of the hospital milieu can be simultaneously used to establish limit setting and get outpatient therapy back on track.

Special procedures.   Hospitalization for special procedures may be planned as part of therapeutic strategy:

1. Initiation or adjustment of a medication (e.g., when one drug is withdrawn and a new one started);
2. Preparation of a patient for surgery and dealing with the psychological associations that surgery may have for the patient;
3. Treatment of a medical condition unrelated to MPD in a setting that can respond to the unique issues raised in work with MPD patients;
4. Use of the safety of an inpatient setting to make an initial approach to integration of alters;
5. Use of a quiet room and full leather restraints for abreactive work;
6. Medication-assisted interviews; and
7. A short course of occupational or other special therapy on the hospital unit to get stalled therapy moving again, especially if the patient fears that such movement is likely to initiate violence.

Anticipating the Need for Admission

Even though a significant investment of time and effort is required, therapists should take the steps needed to anticipate rather than respond to the need for an MPD patient to be admitted to a psychiatric unit. The return on investment is twofold: 1) the patient is assured of a more productive inpatient experience, and 2) a cadre of supportive hospital staff is trained for future MPD patient admissions.

The first step in admission planning is confirmation that the outpatient therapist has either direct or surrogate admitting privileges. This is especially important if the outpatient therapist is not a psychiatrist.

A nonpsychiatrist without admitting privileges is unlikely to have any influence on the choice of an inpatient psychiatrist when the patient is admitted in crisis. If the patient is admitted through the hospital's emergency room, he or she is usually assigned to the psychiatrist or psychiatric resident on call, or whoever is next to receive a patient in a rotation system. At best, this psychiatrist will have some training or experience in the treatment of MPD. At worst, the psychiatrist assigned by "luck of the draw" will be a firm nonbeliever in the existence of MPD, will consider the patient a fraud, and will be unlikely to collaborate productively with the outpatient therapist.

Therapists who do not have admitting privileges need to take steps to prevent the "luck of the draw" scenario from occurring. An effective approach is to seek out a local psychiatrist with admitting privileges who will agree to participate in the treatment of MPD patients when they must be hospitalized. Even if the psychiatrist is inexperienced in the treatment of MPD, such an alliance can be valuable if the psychiatrist is willing to consider the legitimacy of the diagnosis.

Cooperation by Therapists

The treating therapist and the admitting psychiatrist can work together to anticipate the requirements of both the patient and the hospital. Hospital policies vary regarding the amount and/or frequency of patient contact permitted an outpatient therapist who is not on staff. When circumstances require that the staff psychiatrist have sole charge of the patient's care, the outpatient therapist can arrange to consult with the staff psychiatrist regularly to assure continuity of care and to communicate with the patient. With the patient's consent, the outpatient therapist may consider having the staff psychiatrist serve as a consultant or cotherapist prior to admission, thereby laying the groundwork for a therapeutic relationship between the patient and the psychiatrist who will provide inpatient care.

Periodic consultation while the patient is hospitalized is important, and at the time of discharge it is especially important with regard to medications, the rationale for their use, and possible side effects. Every therapist (medical or nonmedical) should be familiar with the indications, contraindications, and side effects of all medications taken by his or her patients.

Coordination of Therapist Responsibilities

When hospital policy permits, the best option to assure continuity of care is to arrange in advance for the outpatient therapist to work in some agreed-upon capacity (such as being granted temporary privileges or associate staff privileges) throughout the patient's hospital stay. This permits both the outpatient therapist and the staff psychiatrist to conduct psychotherapy with the hospitalized patient.

Whatever arrangement is made, the outpatient therapist and staff therapist(s) must discuss and coordinate the respective responsibilities they will undertake after the patient's admission:

1. The development of a treatment plan for the patient while he or she is hospitalized;
2. The delineation of each therapist's area of therapeutic endeavor;
3. A division of responsibility for coordinating the treatment plan with nursing and other hospital staff; and
4. An agreement as to how complaints from the patient regarding staff or other patients are to be handled.

With regard to the last item, it is often best to intervene on the patient's behalf only when the therapists are certain they have all relevant, reliable information. If the therapists have doubts about the validity of the complaint, they must refer the patient back to the appropriate staff member for resolution. This may have to be done in a qualified manner, with a cautious ear attuned to the possibility of staff splitting.

Staff Issues

The outpatient therapist can probably assume that the nursing and other hospital staff (including the hospital administrators) have very little understanding of MPD, and that much of what they may know may have come from the popular press and entertainment media. The potential for controversy will be high when an MPD patient is admitted. Staff psychiatrists, with the help of the outpatient therapist, must address and resolve as early as possible the issue of staff belief versus disbelief in the diagnosis. Until this is done, staff training cannot begin in any useful way. If conditions and hospital policies permit, staff training is best initiated prior to the admission of an MPD patient. Arrangements for appropriate staffing patterns also ideally begin prior to an admission.

Staff Training

In a 1984 paper, Putnam and colleagues called attention to the difficulty of making the MPD diagnosis and of gaining support for the diagnosis from professional colleagues. "Like neurosyphilis," they said, "MPD is a chronic illness that may mimic the gamut of psychiatric illnesses, as well as many somatic conditions, especially neurologic, gastrointestinal and cardiac disorders" (p. 172).

MPD patients also are secretive and manipulative, making it even more difficult for untrained staff on a general psychiatric unit to accept an MPD patient's report of his or her history and current symptoms. The fact that the treating psychiatrist appears to accept the patient's report may make matters even worse, until the staff learns that acceptance of the patient's report is qualified with the understanding that it may be flawed in respect to "reality," but it is with the patient's report that one must begin.

Disbelief in the diagnosis may trigger an increase in acting-out by the patient. This is particularly true if the patient feels that a disbelieving staff is affronting not only him or her, but also the therapist with whom the patient has formed a therapeutic alliance. Confronted by disbelief, the patient may flagrantly act out to prove his or her multiplicity, resulting in further disbelief and splitting of the staff between believers and nonbelievers in the diagnosis.

Focusing on Issues That Split a Staff

Given the cooperation of hospital administration, training of staff address the following issues and related topics. The staff psychiatrist and the outpatient therapist, when possible, open discussion and training regarding these issues:

1. Disbelief in the diagnosis;
2. Staff splitting over the diagnosis;
3. Increased acting out by the patient and its effect on staff and other patients;
4. The possibility of general disruption of the unit if other patients become antagonized or co-opted into staff splitting;
5. The probability of burnout in staff who are not properly trained in the handling of MPD patients;
6. The patient's contribution to staff splitting; and
7. Ways of dealing with these problems.

When staff training begins, it focuses on the approaches that facilitate patient acceptance and control. Staff are given information to help them understand and deal with some of the unique features of MPD.

Patient credibility. As MPD patients come to trust staff, they often relate stories of severe abuse that many caring professionals may find unbelievable. A split is likely to occur between those who believe everything related by the patient and those who reject all that is said in disbelief. Once training has started and the staff begins to become more informed on the issues involved in treating an MPD patient, members of the staff may tend to become more hypo- than hypercritical regarding the patient's reports. The experienced therapist must help staff understand that, although it is important to believe and support the MPD diagnosis, objectivity must be maintained. MPD patients are just as capable of lies, distortions, and manipulative behaviors as other patients. In this respect, they are closer to the profile of the borderline patient than to that of the depressed patient.

If more than one MPD patient is hospitalized in the same unit, staff may come to suspect that one patient is copying another in behavior, symptomatology, and recalled history. This suspicion tends to confirm skepticism and disbelief regarding the legitimacy of the diagnosis. However, the mere fact that two or more MPD patients on the unit exhibit similar signs and symptoms does not necessarily mean that one patient is "taking lessons" from the other. Similar presentations may very well be the manifestation by each of the valid signs and symptoms of the severe psychiatric disorder experienced by both. It is curious that one thinks of such "contagion" when two patients with major depressive disorder or schizophrenia do this; it merely is held to confirm the validity of the true diagnosis.

Posttraumatic stress disorder by proxy.　Staff members who become overly empathic with a patient with a complex and painful past open themselves to the possibility of developing posttraumatic stress disorder (PTSD) by proxy (Braun et al. 1987; Olson et al. 1987), especially when the patient abreacts while reporting experiences of severe abuse. Overly empathic staff may try to "make up" for the abuse experienced by the patient (e.g., by granting the patient special favors or special relaxations of unit rules). This can be a sensitive issue on a general psychiatric unit where controversy, staff splitting, and patient jealousies already exist. Feelings of entitlement are frequently seen in patients who have been abused, and this can be magnified in MPD patients, many of whom also have a need to be "special." Exemptions from unit rules should rarely be granted to MPD patients and only for good reason. They must be encouraged to live within unit rules.

Professional equilibrium.　Regular and on-the-spot staff meetings are useful mechanisms for maintaining personal and professional equilibrium. Weekly multidisciplinary staff meetings can help to develop intrastaff support and training. Meetings that can bridge shift changes serve to enhance discussion and exchange of information. In these meetings, staff are able to address and process the emotions that surface in response to patients' reports of severe abuse. Group strategies can be developed for dealing with transference, countertransference, and acting-out. Weekly staff meetings also provide a neutral environment for objectively assessing a patient's therapeutic progress.

　　On-the-spot meetings are called when the therapist has just conducted a heavily emotionally charged and/or abreactive session with staff members present. The session needs to be processed with the staff immediately, no matter how tired everyone may be or how late the hour. It is not in the best interest of the patient or the staff to merely walk away from such a powerfully charged session, leaving all or some of the staff in emotional disarray for dealing with the patient and the rest of the unit. Such meetings are also called to tell staff about such a session if the staff were not present so they will be properly informed and can anticipate problems.

Preparing for discharge. Even before the patient arrives on the unit, staff can attempt to foresee what must occur for the patient to be prepared to leave. Staff can anticipate that some MPD patients may act out and resist discharge, especially at the end of a therapeutically useful hospitalization. They are often reluctant to leave a safe, understanding, and helpful environment where they have had a positive experience and when they face an uncertain reception in the outside world. Sakheim and colleagues (1988) believe that when a hospitalization has extended for months or more, the staff can find it difficult to see the patient become less in need of them as therapy progresses, or, conversely, may be overly glad to see the patient leave. Staff members should discuss their feelings on this issue, reducing the possibility that these feelings may adversely affect their dealings with the patient. On our dissociative disorders unit, we have not seen such problems, probably because of our intensive in-service training efforts and steps taken to develop a strong tradition of mutual staff support.

Staffing Patterns

Given the support of hospital administration, the therapist(s) can seek the assistance of the head nurse and unit director to address the staffing concerns raised by MPD patients. With the assistance of the head nurse, specific nurses may be assigned primary and associate roles for the MPD patient's care. Among the criteria for making such selections are that the primary nurses chosen should have the following:

1. Sufficient general psychiatric experience;
2. The ability to tolerate the material related by the patient;
3. Cognizance of their own feelings and the ability to talk about them;
4. The ability to recognize and speak openly about counter-transference issues that arise from handling the MPD patient; and
5. An interest in working with MPD patients.

Although the primary nurse must have an interest in working with MPD patients, the associate may have less interest, and if objective, may even disbelieve in the diagnosis. By this type of teaming of staff, as the associate nurse learns from the primary nurse, he or she will positively influence other nurses on the unit.

Goals of Hospitalization

The goals of hospitalization should be carefully delineated in a treatment plan that includes a schedule of therapeutic goals to be achieved in finite time periods. Care must be taken as to how the time periods are shared with the patient so as not to put undue pressure on him or her. In my experience, it is usually inadvisable to admit an MPD patient for an open-ended psychiatric hospitalization. Therapeutic goals should include length of stay, and the stay should not extend much longer than planned. Such an approach to inpatient treatment permits goals to be achieved in small steps over defined periods of time. I note that Kluft (1991), though agreeing in general, appears to indicate that this is not a practical approach with the massively decompensated complex MPD patient.

The duration of hospitalization often is predicated upon such issues as the patient's potential for suicide, homicide, or self-mutilation; the severity of abuse in the patient's history; or the difficulty foreseen in unblocking deadlocked therapy.

Hospital stays may be as brief as 3 days or as long as several years. Three to 6 days may be long enough to work through a preplanned special issue, but 4 to 8 weeks may be necessary if there are more difficult diagnostic or therapeutic problems. Patients who require more than 8 weeks of hospitalization often experience significant regression and may need many more weeks or months of additional inpatient treatment to deal with the regression. When hospitalization is for 6 months or longer, the treatment plan may allow the patient to regress in the service of the ego in order to work through specific issues of abuse. Even in a stay of this duration, goals should be set and met and a limit placed on the permissible degree of regression.

Discharge is the end point of the hospitalization, and planning for discharge should begin as soon as the patient is admitted, or (as noted previously) even prior to admission. Within the protocols of the treatment plan, discharge planning continues in discrete steps throughout the hospital stay.

Prior to discharge, it is useful to first evaluate which therapeutic goals have been achieved and to seek the reasons for the failure to achieve goals that have remained unaccomplished. Furthermore, it is advisable, even after achievable goals have been attained, for there to have been a period of continued but less intensive therapy to solidify gains and to assess how the patient will behave as an outpatient. Particular concern should be directed toward appreciating whether the patient will be safe from violence toward self or others and from severe regression.

Discharge planning also includes preparation for outlining new outpatient goals and ways to achieve them. The patient and the outpatient therapist must concur with the goals, especially if the outpatient therapist is not the same person as the staff psychiatrist.

As pointed out by Sakheim and colleagues (1988), before the patient's hospitalization, the hospital staff should assess the availability of outpatient care after discharge. If the original or referring therapist is not able to resume the treatment, and if a new outpatient therapist is not available for one reason or another, and/or if the patient will be discharged into a minimal support system, it may be a mistake to pursue an intensive hospitalization with ambitious goals. The patient's adjustment after discharge under such circumstances could be difficult and cause decompensation. On our Dissociative

Disorders Inpatient Unit, we will not admit a patient who does not have an outpatient therapist who will accept him or her back into therapy after discharge.

Contracting and Limit Setting

Although there must be some flexibility in the therapy of MPD patients, the setting and maintaining of clear, firm limits is mandatory on a unit that undertakes their care. Among the limits to be established is the length of time that staff can spend in one-to-one sessions with an MPD patient.

Patient-staff boundary limits are set to protect both staff and patient. Some degree of openness to patients is useful; but without clearly stated limits, the MPD patient will often try to and succeed in becoming intimately involved with the personal lives of staff. A useful rule of thumb for making personal revelations is "If in doubt, don't."

The therapist is responsible for making contracts with the patient, beginning with a contract for safety. Elsewhere (Braun 1984, 1986) I have described my approach to establishing the safety contract:

> [I ask] the patient to repeat the following phrase without necessarily meaning it, and then ask how the patient would modify it so he or she could live with it: "I will not hurt myself or kill myself, or anyone else external or internal, either accidentally or on purpose at any time." The negotiable points are the duration of the contract and the ability to hurt others as protection from *unprovoked* external attack. If one gets a time-limited contract, it must be renegotiated prior to expiration or this will be perceived as an implicit suggestion to act out. A modification of the time limit might specify "one week or until we talk face-to-face, whichever comes last." This covers the eventuality of an emergency or natural disaster interfering with the next scheduled visit. (1986, p. 12)

To date, this contract has not been broken with regard to violence toward external others or suicide, although patients will frequently tell their therapists that they cannot keep the terms. It has been broken by patients harming, but not killing, themselves. It appears that some self-harm is addictive behavior (Braun 1990) and beyond the ability of the contract to control. Patients report that the contract facilitates their asking for help and reduces the frequency of acts of self-harm.

Suicide Precautions

Medical and nursing staff should be trained to recognize subtle warning signs that the MPD patient may be on the verge of violent behavior. Despite a safety contract, the MPD patient has potential for violence toward self or others. In fact, most are hospitalized because they are actively suicidal or homicidal, or in a phase of therapy that can stimulate violent behavior, usually self-directed.

The treating therapist is medically and ethically bound to advise other staff of any issues that may trigger violence during therapy, and he or she should remind staff when the treatment plan calls for the exploration of volatile issues. When a patient has suicidal ideation, suicide precautions are indicated at an appropriate level of intensity. The following level system has proven useful in units under my direction. Level 1 is the least restrictive level.

Level 1. Fifteen-minute, round-the-clock checks on the patient; no sharp objects accessible to the patient; no straps or other objects by which the patient can hang him- or herself; regular checks for hoarded medications that the patient can use to overdose; monitoring to be sure the patient swallows all oral medications. Room search, clothing checks, and body search with or without cavity search (by a physician) as indicated.

Level 2. All measures listed in Level 1, plus a mandate that the patient must be in public areas during the day.

Level 3. All measures listed in Levels 1 and 2, plus a mandate that the patient must sleep in the hallway in view of staff.

Level 4. Above Level 3, the patient is observed directly, one-to-one, at all times.

At all levels of suicide precaution except Level 4, several patients may be observed by one nurse. This optimizes safety while conserving staff resources and lessening the potential for burnout inherent in placing a substantial proportion of available personnel on such assignments, leaving the remainder overwhelmed.

Patients on suicide precautions, especially those on one-to-one (Level 4) precautions, can come to enjoy the attendant close proximity and interaction with staff. They may seek to stay on precautions to accrue the secondary gains of continued staff attention. This is the main reason for Levels 2 and 3—to reduce the secondary gain. As staff members learn more about MPD patients and their treatment, they also will learn to recognize when a patient's apparent need for suicide precautions has become a desire for continued staff attention. Another reason that it may be difficult to get such patients off suicide precautions is that many MPD patients always have some thoughts of suicide and, in a caricature of honesty, they maintain that they must be *absolutely* truthful and therefore cannot give a 100% ironclad contract for safety.

Titration of Therapy

Discrete, achievable goals for therapy are steps toward the achievement of a comprehensive therapeutic goal. The step-by-step goals and the overall goal are guideposts that help to keep therapy on a rational track.

Throughout the MPD patient's hospitalization, it is best if therapy is coordinated under the overall guidance of the therapist, with the counsel and cooperation of all professionals involved in treatment. Therapy paced under a coordinated approach helps to prevent the inappropriate opening up of additional issues that may be important per se, but that can slow the achievement of the goals of the admission.

The importance of titration is apparent in the outline of a frequently seen treatment plan. A patient with limited insurance coverage is hospitalized. A very specific treatment plan is developed, allowing 3 to 7 days to build rapport and set goals, 3 to 7 days to open up the material, 10 days to 3 weeks to process the material, and 3 days to 1 week to prepare the patient for discharge, including planning for patient safety. This plan is set up for a new patient who is unknown to the admitting psychiatrist. It may be actualized in 4 weeks but might require up to 6 weeks, depending on the material encountered. If the patient is known and there is rapport, similar goals might be accomplished in as little as 2 to 3 weeks. The treatment plan may be successful under the guidance of a single co-ordinating therapist, but uncoordinated approaches by multiple therapists can prevent completion of all steps before insurance coverage ends. If this occurs, the patient will be at substantial risk of decompensation in outpatient therapy, and the progress made during the hospitalization may be lost.

Titration of therapy includes consideration of patient-staff relationships. Healthy, therapeutically appropriate relationships can develop between an MPD patient and hospital staff if the staff are well trained and experienced. MPD patients can expand their circle of trust from the primary therapist to a few staff members on the psychiatric unit; with time, this may extend to other staff members and patients. This expanding trust can be harnessed therapeutically into a support system for the patient. However, without careful therapeutic guidance, the patient can experience dramatically different consequences, because a tenuous alliance with staff may prove inadequate to support the patient's disclosure of traumatic material. A trained, experienced staff member will direct such sensitive encounters into the hands of the primary therapist.

Untrained, poorly trained, or inexperienced staff members can be easily co-opted into inappropriate relationships with patients. Kluft (1984, 1991) noted that hospitalization may encourage the emergence of alters who are afraid, angry, or perplexed at being in the hospital. Alters who are particularly sensitive may identify staff members who are most supportive of the MPD diagnosis and overwhelm them with therapeutically important material and demands for nurture and attention.

Group Therapy

If consistent with the treatment plan, an MPD patient may be assigned to group therapy. Careful joint planning by therapists and nursing staff is required to make group therapy meaningful for the patient. MPD patients often do not work well in ongoing therapy groups that are designed to uncover difficult material through verbalization. Because the uncovering of emotionally charged material should be carefully titrated to limit or prevent regression, patient participation in ongoing process-oriented groups must be optional or specifically ordered by the therapist(s). Also, it is not uncommon for the MPD patient to overwhelm the group with his or her material (e.g., severe sexual abuse [Kluft 1984]).

Task-oriented groups may be useful in blocking regressive behavior as well as providing additional ongoing therapy, because they are goal-oriented and do not rely on the uncovering of difficult material. Attendance at task-oriented groups such as milieu meetings, occupational therapy, art therapy, and goals groups should be mandatory insofar as a given patient can benefit from the experience (Kluft 1984).

Art therapy and occupational therapy are especially useful, because they permit the patient to nonverbally reveal information that may not be accessible verbally. Nonverbal description of abuse can often be tolerated by an MPD patient, whereas verbal "telling" was forbidden by abusers under pain of physical harm or death (Braun 1990).

Participation by the MPD patient in a number of the psychiatric unit's group modalities can significantly decrease the patient's potential for splitting of staff and/or patients. It is also important that the MPD patient cooperate and participate on the unit and *not* be made special.

Conclusions

MPD patients frequently require elective or emergency hospitalizations. Although the obvious choice for such hospital stays is a specialty unit for treatment of MPD/dissociative disorders, that choice is often not available. The patient who cannot be placed on a specialty unit will become a candidate for placement on a general psychiatric unit at a local hospital or a freestanding psychiatric hospital.

The outpatient therapist can be faced by numerous problems when the patient must be hospitalized in a local hospital:

1. The therapist may be a nonpsychiatrist or a psychiatrist without admitting privileges to this particular hospital.
2. The general psychiatric unit staff may have little knowledge or experience in the treatment of MPD, and some or all staff members may be skeptical about the diagnosis.
3. Placement of the patient on a general unit where staff has little experience in treating MPD, and where skepticism about the diagnosis is blatant, will very frequently result in disruption of the unit, polarization of staff, and increased acting out by the MPD patient and by other patients.

Perhaps the worst scenario is the emergency hospitalization of an MPD patient under these circumstances:

1. The outpatient therapist has no privileges.
2. The admitting psychiatrist has no experience in treating MPD and actively disbelieves in the diagnosis.
3. General unit staff have no knowledge or experience in the treatment of MPD.
4. The outpatient therapist is not permitted to coordinate or participate in the inpatient treatment of the patient.

Although the "worst" scenario may not occur, any combination of circumstances that result in less than optimal treatment for the patient must be considered, taken into account, and responded to by the therapist. Aggressive, proactive preparation for hospitalization before it is needed is the therapist's best defense on behalf of the patient.

When the outpatient therapist is a nonpsychiatrist or a psychiatrist without admitting privileges, he or she should find psychiatrists who have admitting privileges, who believe or do not actively disbelieve in the diagnosis of MPD, who will agree to work with the outpatient therapist in treatment of the patient, and who will cooperate with the outpatient therapist in essential training of the general unit staff. Ideally, these steps are all taken in anticipation of the future elective or emergency hospitalization of an MPD patient.

Within the hospital's rules, the outpatient therapist and cooperating staff psychiatrist can work with the administration to arrange for some form of temporary staff privilege for the outpatient therapist, permission to undertake training of the unit staff (to make them better prepared to receive an MPD patient), and permission to work with the psychiatric unit head nurse to arrange appropriate management of the MPD patient.

Staff training is focused on issues such as disbelief in the diagnosis, the prevention of staff splitting over the belief/disbelief controversy especially and many other issues, the variety of ways in which an MPD patient can manipulate and "burn out" staff, and the difficulties that an MPD patient may cause to arise among other patients on the unit.

Staff cooperation regarding coordination of an in-hospital treatment plan for the patient, and in the maintenance of limit setting contracts with the patient is essential. Staff are trained to work with the therapists(s) in the fundamentally important areas of therapy titration and suicide prevention.

When this groundwork has been laid, the outpatient therapist is more assured of a successful hospital stay for the patient on a general psychiatric unit. The therapist will be better prepared to hospitalize the patient electively and will be more confident that the patient can be effectively managed in the event of an emergency hospitalization, thus yielding a more positive experience for all.

References

Braun BG: Uses of hypnosis with multiple personality. Psychiatric Annals 14:34–40, 1984

Braun BG: Issues in the psychotherapy of multiple personality disorder, in Treatment of Multiple Personality Disorder. Edited by Braun BG. Washington, DC, American Psychiatric Press, 1986, pp 1–28

Braun BG: Unusual medication regimens in the treatment of dissociative disorder patients: noradrenergic agents. Dissociation 3:144–150, 1990

Braun BG, Mayton K, Olson J, et al: Post-traumatic stress disorder by proxy. Dissociative Disorders 1987—Proceedings of the Fourth International Conference on Multiple Personality/Dissociative States. Chicago, IL, Rush-Presbyterian-St. Luke's Medical Center, 1987

Kluft RP: Aspects of the treatment of multiple personality disorder. Psychiatric Annals 14(1):51–55, 1984

Kluft RP: The Treatment of Multiple Personality Disorder (MPD): Current Concepts (Directions in Psychiatry, Vol 5, Lesson 24). Edited by Flach FF. New York, Hatherleigh, 1985, pp 1–11

Kluft RP: Personality unification in multiple personality disorder: a follow-up study, in Treatment of Multiple Personality Disorder. Edited by Braun BG. Washington, DC, American Psychiatric Press, 1986, pp 29–60

Kluft RP: The hospital treatment of multiple personality disorder. Psychiatr Clin North Am 14:695–719, 1991

Olson J, Mayton K, Kowal-Ellis N: Secondary post-traumatic stress disorder: therapist response to the horror. Dissociative Disorders 1987—Proceedings of the Fourth International Conference on Multiple Personality/Dissociative States. Chicago, IL, Rush-Presbyterian-St. Luke's Medical Center, 1987

Putnam FW, Loewenstein RJ, Silberman EJ, et al: Multiple personality disorder in a hospital setting. J Clin Psychiatry 45:172–175, 1984

Sakheim DK, Hess EP, Chivas A: General principles for short-term inpatient work with multiple personality disorder patients. Psychotherapy: Theory, Research and Practice 25:117–124, 1988

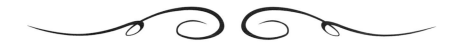

Case Studies in the Treatment of Multiple Personality Disorder: Explorations in the Therapeutic Process

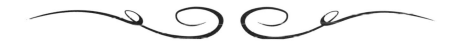

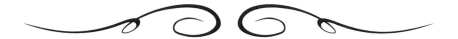

Chapter 9

Dissociation in the Inner City

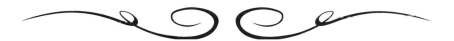

Frank W. Putnam, Jr., M.D.

In July 1986, as part of my interest in the developmental roots of multiple personality disorder (MPD) and other outcomes of child abuse, I began a fellowship in Child Psychiatry at Children's Hospital National Medical Center in Washington, DC. In connection with my training, I became the psychiatric consultant to City Lights, a comprehensive day treatment program developed for black indigent adolescents in the District of Columbia (Tolmach 1985). The program was founded in the aftermath of a lawsuit, *Bobby D. v. Barry,* brought by the Children's Defense Fund against the District of Columbia for its failure to provide a community-based alternative to the institutionalization of disturbed adolescents.

Before City Lights, many disturbed District of Columbia youths were sent to residential treatment facilities as far away as Texas, Massachusetts, and Florida (Tolmach 1985). City Lights has provided a successful alternative for working with disturbed inner-city adolescents. In 1987, it won an award from the American Psychiatric Association for its outstanding program and contributions. This success is due both to the care and dedication of the staff and to the soundness of policy design and administration that provides a supportive environment for students and staff. Tolmach discussed the implementation of the City Lights model in a 1985 article.

The typical City Lights student is a 16-year-old black male who is an adjudicated delinquent with an average of three out-of-home placements (e.g., residential treatment, foster home, group home, psychiatric hospitalization, jail) and who reads at a third-grade level (Tolmach 1985). The majority of students have histories of substance abuse and childhood maltreatment. My role at City Lights was to help the staff assess and manage the psychiatric problems and behavioral disturbances manifested by many students. In addition, I saw several students for individual psychotherapy and/or medication management, and I was a coleader of a therapy group for older adolescents.

Although an occasional student had a diagnosable thought disorder or other psychotic process, most experienced rapid mood shifts, explosive behavior, depression, anxiety, sleep disturbances, and somatic symptoms (Tolmach 1985). Many of the students would meet DSM-III-R (American Psychiatric Association 1987) criteria for posttraumatic stress disorder (PTSD). Panic and phobic symptoms, together with all varieties of school avoidance, were common. Many students had documented learning disabilities, attentional deficits, and episodes of regressed or disorganized behavior. Of course, the high prevalence of substance abuse, primarily phencyclidine (PCP) and crack cocaine, greatly complicated the clinical picture these students presented.

This chapter grows out of my experiences working with the inner-city adolescents who attended the City Lights program. I begin with a brief discussion of the ways in which these teenagers attempt to blot out the frequent trauma in their lives, and I consider the consequences that they experience as a result of their defenses against these traumata. I then illustrate this process with an in-depth presentation of Reginald (a pseudonym), a student with MPD.

It may be difficult for the reader who thinks of MPD in terms of bright, exceptionally verbal, and creative Caucasian women to readjust his or her expectations to accommodate Reginald and his peers at City Lights. Although many in the dissociative disorders field emphasize that these conditions can occur in every ethnic, age, racial, and cultural grouping, and that these factors, along with gender and socioeconomic class, may play an important role in the presentation of dissociative psychopathology, relatively few publications address these considerations (Kluft 1985, 1991). The literature to date has not dissolved the stereotypic gestalt of the most frequently described type of MPD patient.

Escaping

A simplistic but nonetheless useful way to understand much of the behavior that I witnessed at City Lights is that most of these adolescents are almost continually seeking to escape painful stimuli. These stimuli take the form of external events and situations and internal experiences and memories. They have many ways of escaping, but each way exacts a price. By blotting out so much of their world, most have difficulty learning from experience and become extraordinarily difficult to reach and teach. Their avoidance, denial, repression, dissociation, and escape behaviors lead to failures in school and work situations. It also renders them vulnerable to revictimization and substance abuse. Their desperate and often misguided attempts at mastery over frightening or traumatic experiences may lead to violence, incarceration, and death. Within the first months of my tenure at City Lights, I witnessed several students decompensate in a series of rapidly accelerating avoidant behaviors leading to academic and social deterioration, which led inexorably to still further avoidance behaviors, and so on. City Lights attempts to break the suction of this social vortex with multiple and comprehensive interventions. With some troubled teenagers, however, the most dedicated efforts are simply too little and too late.

Why Are They Escaping?

Tolmach (1985) observed that these children fit the description of "the deprived" in the Carnegie Institute's 1979 study of school dropouts (Carnegie Council on Policy Studies in Higher Education 1979). Coming from disorganized families, they experience a combination of poverty, inadequate education, and weak psychological resources. They are surrounded by human and social disaster, high

rates of crime and violence, drug and alcohol addiction, chronic un-
employment, teenage pregnancy, suicide, and physical and mental
illness.

The levels of violence witnessed and experienced by these teenagers are phenomenal. During the period that I consulted at City
Lights, Washington, DC, was undergoing a drug-related crime wave.
There was almost one teenage homicide victim a day. The District of
Columbia was the only jurisdiction in the nation in which homicide
was the leading cause of death from injuries in children (Abramowitz
1989). This violence was happening in the City Lights students' own
neighborhoods and was frequently witnessed by them. Almost
weekly, I heard grisly eyewitness accounts of shootings or stabbings.
In addition, most of the teenagers at City Lights came from disturbed
homes with high levels of domestic violence; furthermore, they lived
in apartments or housing projects where they witnessed their
neighbors' domestic violence. For many, hearing gunfire was a
nightly occurrence. Many were known to have been physically or
sexually abused at some point. Undoubtedly some continued to be
victimized. We suspected that a few periodically were engaged in
prostitution.

Violent nightmares were common among the students and were
often associated with other posttraumatic-like sleep disturbances.
The theme "what you've seen will make you go crazy" pervaded
most of our group therapy sessions. Students often compared themselves to a stereotype of Vietnam veterans driven crazy by witnessing
the horrors of war, or likened surviving on the streets of Washington
to being in wartime Vietnam. Some identified with the aggressors and
openly bragged about the violent acts that they had committed. Many
claimed to own firearms, typically pistols but in some cases auto-
matic weapons. Not infrequently, students would disappear for extended periods because they believed that someone "had a contract
out" on them. In addition to the drug-related homicides, students
faced and witnessed numerous muggings and stickups. Typically
they would know the victim and sometimes they would know the
"stickup boy." These crimes often involved a sadistic element in
which the victim was publicly humiliated in addition to being
robbed, generally being left without pants or shoes.

Beyond the violence and crushing social disaster that surrounds these adolescents, they face many daily threats to their fragile self-esteem. Poverty has deprived them of the easy means to buy the designer-label clothes, shoes, and accessories coveted by American teenagers. When they do manage to acquire name-brand possessions (often at great cost to other needs), their triumph is short-lived. Someone inevitably steals or destroys anything new, valuable, or desirable. They are acutely aware of their educational shortcomings and sense the future implications. They are sensitive to not being in a "regular school" with organized sports and social activities. They resent the therapeutic aspects of the City Lights model, with its implications that there is something wrong with them.

Their self-esteem suffers greatly, in part because they have unrealistic ego-ideals, goals, and standards against which to measure their lot. Television, videos, and movies largely shape their beliefs about life. Most insisted to me that they would become millionaires soon. Dealing drugs, making music videos, and playing professional sports are identified as the fast avenues to the good life. Few want to confront the reality of flipping hamburgers for minimum wage while trying to get the resources together to move into an independent living situation. Collisions between grandiose expectations and grim reality occur daily and usually precipitate escape behaviors, denial, and depression.

Uproar

When adults' criticisms are perceived as threats to their self-esteem, or their requests are experienced as overly taxing to their abilities, these adolescents often simply drown them out. Talking loudly, singing, and rapping are used to overpower any anxiety-provoking request made by the adults at City Lights. Singing and rapping are usually accompanied by explosive sound effects mimicking a synthesizer rhythm section, together with clapping and foot-stomping to the rap beat. As the adult raises his or her voice to be heard, the student escalates his or her performance to match. When a student really gets his or her rap routine under way, it is next to impossible to cut through the din. The rapping may be accompanied by dancing or karatelike movements, which are, of course, also designed to keep people at a distance.

I have found, however, that rapping can be useful in psychotherapy with these teenagers. The rap process, with its focus on rhythm and pressure to rhyme, seems to circumvent to some extent the censorship of charged material in much the same fashion as free association. Although dealing with material in this manner may tax the therapist's patience, relevant psychodynamic material may emerge in this manner. It is even possible to ask questions by phrasing them in rap style.

Hiding

Hiding from the world is second nature for these adolescents. Many avoid tests or other school stresses by staying home, usually remaining in bed. City Light's social workers are infamous for showing up at their homes, getting them out of bed, and escorting them to school. In school, they hide by feigning sleep, covering themselves beneath their coats, pulling hoods or hats over their heads, or hiding behind books. Not uncommonly, a student will spend the entire school day with a coat over his or her head like a tent. Usually the best one can expect in response to one's question is to get some muffled and barely audible responses from beneath. Attempts to look under the coat or otherwise force more direct interaction are strongly resisted; typically, they lead to a behavioral escalation that results in the student's temporary suspension from the program. These overwhelmed adolescents regress into toddlerlike states at times, demonstrating massive regression. On occasion, a student curls up in a corner or on a couch, burying his or her face in a crooked elbow while sucking on a thumb.

Dissociation

Dissociation, manifested by prolonged trancing out or by brief tuning-out episodes, is common. Several of the students have diagnosable dissociative disorders or PTSD with major dissociative features. Spacing-out behaviors in school typically occur when adult authority figures make performance demands on students. When subsequently pressed about the content of the interaction, the students exhibit confusion and memory lapses for the instructions and the expectations.

A depersonalized detachment from their surroundings and from the violence they have witnessed is common. I have been struck repeatedly by the affectless manner in which experienced or witnessed violence is described by students. Out-of-body experiences were often described in the context of violence and trauma. At other times, students would be so detached from the incident itself that they would focus completely on tangential issues. For example, one student was greatly perplexed because a woman that he saw shot four times did not fall down, and he kept asking me how anyone could stand up after being shot four times. He did not react to the assault itself. He would only acknowledge being troubled because what he had witnessed did not match his expectations, derived from movies and television. Another student, describing witnessing an acquaintance being machine-gunned, was upset because the assailant's gun jammed in mid-burst. He seemed to have lost his faith in the potency of machine guns.

Even when no clear diagnosis of MPD can be made in such students, the City Lights staff demonstrate their implicit recognition of a high degree of identity fragmentation and state-dependency in some students' behavior and abilities. For example, staff members often labeled a given student's behavior as belonging to, for example, "the silly Tony" and not representative of "the serious Tony." Students frequently talked about "parts" of themselves and otherwise indicate experiences of self-division.

Reginald: A Case Study

Although I had been aware of his presence for some time, I first formally evaluated Reginald in April 1987, at the request of his case manager at City Lights. She described Reginald as "the most disturbed student" in the program, identifying in particular his rapid mood shifts, explosive behavior, inappropriate and sexualized inter-personal interactions, and disruptive classroom antics. Beyond some records from the District of Columbia Department of Human Services (DHS), there was little background information available on Reginald. At the time of our first contact, Reginald was 17 years old. He was a black male who was a ward of the District and lived in a private group home under a city contract.

The earliest DHS records begin:

> This court appearance is the result of an incident which resulted in the Youth Division of the DC Police Department intervening in a . . . family confrontation. A boyfriend of Mrs. __, Mr. E. S., beat Reginald and verbally or physically interacted with Joseph and Geraldine [two of Reginald's six siblings], forcing all four children to flee to the home of a neighbor. Mrs. __ explains the incident by claiming that Reginald came home from school on October 12, 1982, and asked for money. When she offered him only 50 cents, he became angry, knocked items off the kitchen table, threw rocks at her car hitting it a dozen times, cut her seat covers, and continued to be verbally abusive until dark. At that point, in exasperation, she asked Mr. S. to take a tree branch and whip Reginald. . . .

Most of the remaining records and notes were in the same vein. Reginald's family was broken up after his father was convicted and sentenced to 20 years in Lorton prison for incest with his two daughters. His mother reportedly had sexual relations with her oldest son, Michael, who was subsequently committed to St. Elizabeth's (known as "St. E's" in the District) for uncontrollable temper outbursts. There is also mention of brother-sister incest in the records, although it was not specified which siblings were involved.

Reginald and his siblings became wards of the city and passed into a series of foster and group home placements. Reginald was unable to adjust to one placement after another, living first with a series of foster parents and then, as he grew older and more difficult to manage, in group homes. Judging from the entries in the DHS records, Reginald's situation drew only passing attention. Most of the attention and effort was directed toward the other siblings and his alcoholic mother. By 1986, Reginald was living in a group home. There staff noted, "his progress in the group home has been sporadic in that he has a tendency to experience mood swings and behavior changes."

His first mental health contact was with a psychiatrist who screened him in 1986 as part of his preadmission evaluation to City Lights. Reginald received a diagnosis of adjustment disorder with mixed emotional features. The psychiatrist concluded, "Overall, this seemed a salvageable young man with reasonably good strengths who needs a fair amount of psychoeducational support to make the transition to independent living in the face of hurtful and chaotic family background." On entry into City Lights, Reginald was noted to have "episodes of being disorganized, confused and angry (i.e., not wanting anyone to look at him)." The City Lights clinical director observed, "Although Reginald presents himself as a secure person, underneath he is a youngster with low self-esteem. He will need much support in his process of self-definition."

Because I had been warned that Reginald was violent and potentially dangerous, I arranged to see him first at Children's Hospital, where there was better support and protection. He arrived accompanied by his group home supervisor. In the waiting room I was able to quickly ascertain that he was not dangerous and chose to see him alone. Reginald was a large (6 feet 2 inches, 230 pounds), sloppily dressed black adolescent. He was wearing a faded red canvas jacket, rumpled shirt, dirty pants, and untied running shoes. His overall affect was serious and depressed, although he had a burst of clowning behavior on the way back to my office, tottering around in his untied shoes and waving his hands with a silly grin on his face. His speech was slow. Initially he had difficulty expressing himself and understanding me. Over time we developed an ear for each other's dialects, and communication became easier.

The real shocker came early on in this first session when I asked him to tell me a little bit about himself. What did he like to do for fun? What were his favorite television shows? Did he have any hobbies or play any sports? Reginald looked at me and said something to the effect that there was more than one of him. Unfortunately, he has rarely framed the issue as clearly since. With minimal questioning, he told me that he was really Reginald and Reggie. I was speaking to Reginald, who was serious and tried to do his school work, but Reggie kept getting him into trouble. Reginald was 17 and Reggie was 15. Reggie was angry and wouldn't talk to me directly, but Reginald could relay to me what he thought about my questions.

I was amazed! I had not suspected MPD, though in retrospect all the classic elements were present in his history. I tried to take a standard MPD history, but my efforts met with little success. He admitted to losing time and finding himself in strange places without memory of how he got there, but he was not able to provide clear examples. He called the experience "flicking." He recognized that he would "flick" when he got angry. As my questioning progressed, he expressed increasing misgivings about having revealed these things to me and accused me of plotting to lock him up in a mental hospital or "dope him up" with drugs. I spent a fair amount of time addressing these concerns, which provided a cautionary tale for the future. We agreed to contract about his not harming himself and/or others and his returning to see me later in the week. At City Lights, he was reported to have improved dramatically. Staff at his group home said that he had de-escalated and no longer seemed to be explosive.

My progress notes for the next session begin, "A most unusual session. . . . " Immediately upon entry into the office, Reginald began to pick up the toys lying on the play table and throw them around the room saying, "Whee—this is fun. Let's play with toys. I'm supposed to be crazy, aren't I!" This initial sarcastic stance rapidly evolved, however, into genuine childlike play with the dolls and the toys. In a series of intense play episodes with a family of black dolls and a dollhouse, Reginald reenacted a sequence of gang rapes. First a group of male dolls would gang-rape each of the female dolls, dragging them out of closets and other hiding places and having graphic simultaneous oral, anal, and vaginal sex. Then they would kill each victim by strangulation, saying, "Uhmm, that was good! Let's have another." Eventually the male dolls started to fight over the females and killed off one another. He repeated this scenario three times in a perseverative, stereotypic manner.

He then switched scenarios abruptly and played out a "Night of the Living Dead" theme. He sat on my couch and advanced half a dozen dolls across the cushions toward him as he shot at them with a toy gun. Making classic little-boy sound effects, he would blast a doll down, only to have it get up and continue to advance zombielike toward him. As the dolls converged, he became increasingly anxious, firing wildly as they closed in. Just as he trapped himself, he stopped playing, looked at me angrily, and said, "You're making me do that." When I asked what I was making him do, he said, "Play like a baby." Before I could inquire further, he resumed the play, running the nightmarish theme all over for a second and third time. He then played out yet a third scenario in which a black male doll fought with a much larger baby doll, transformed into a snarling monster. These two figures fought an epic battle across the floor and over the furniture until the black male drew upon his super powers to "zap" the baby doll monster.

Most of the time I sat quietly observing his play. He was clearly aware that I was there, and from time to time he would look over at me as if to make sure that I was still watching. After he finished playing he was able to talk with me in a quite logical fashion. He told me that he was sure that I thought that he was crazy and would have him locked up in "St. E's like his brother Michael." He told me about seeing Michael "all doped up on drugs" when he visited him. He was sure that that was what I was going to do to him. I attempted to reassure him that I did not think that he was crazy but that I did think that some terrible things must have happened to him. He did not acknowledge my speculation.

After seeing Reginald, I spoke with his group home supervisor, who had accompanied him. He said that Reginald was getting into a lot of trouble at home because he kept telling the staff that he hated blacks and wanted to be white. The staff would talk with him about black pride and values, only to have Reginald respond, "all black people are shit." These interchanges would rapidly escalate into shouting matches. Staff were losing patience with him. Some staff members were openly advocating that Reginald be transferred elsewhere on the basis that he did not want to be with black people.

Our next session was in sharp contrast to the previous one. Reginald looked at the toys for a moment and then indicated that there was not going to be any play with toys today. He sat on the couch across the room from me and began to talk in general, vague terms about black-white relations. In an increasingly challenging manner, he spoke about how white men had killed and enslaved people of color around the world. I agreed with him, occasionally illustrating his points with historical examples of my own. Gradually he moved the topic into race relations in the United States. He spoke at length about his fear of traveling in the South and his terror of rednecks and the Ku Klux Klan. Eventually, he began to talk about his own experiences. He vividly described being accosted by police, together with a black friend, in an all-white bar. The police arrested his friend for being under age, but Reginald was able to bluff them into leaving him alone. At the end of the session he asked where I lived. We were able to identify that the issues of my being white and his being black was one of his concerns in the therapy.

Gradually we began to build a fragile therapeutic alliance. For the next several sessions, Reginald talked with me in a serious manner. Although he began one session by coloring childishly with crayons, this rapidly evolved into his drawing detailed maps of Africa and progressed into a further discussion of our black-white differences. One morning, after about 2 months of sessions, the group home staff brought him to my office when he was in a confused and paranoid state. He responded well to simple reorientation and grounding. He had had a nightmare, awakened in terror, and continued to experience intrusive images and affects from the dream. In his nightmare, a zombielike monster named Mr. Mud had broken into his home and killed his sleeping brothers and sisters. He had escaped out a window, but Mr. Mud and his giant black dogs chased him. His train of associations rapidly progressed to his father, whom he described as a stern man. Much later I would learn that his father raised German shepherds and trained them to attack on command.

After the first few sessions, there was no further acknowledgment of alters. He denied ever telling me anything about Reginald and Reggie. He maintained that people called him by one name or other but that he was the same person. I could not elicit alters by direct request, and he refused hypnosis, saying that I was not going to get him under my control. He would then mimic a stage hypnotist, swinging an imaginary watch and saying melodramatically, "You're getting sleepy. You're under my power!" In some sessions, he exhibited shifts in train of thought, affect, and motoric behavior consistent with covert personality switching. Much of the time I just left the issue of MPD alone, choosing to concentrate on developing an alliance, establishing ground rules, and getting some basic contracts in place. Around specific issues, such as contracting, I would sometimes use with good effect the "talking-through" technique developed with MPD patients to address the "other sides" of him (Kluft 1982; Putnam 1989).

Reginald began to talk more about blackout experiences and memory problems, and he began to provide clear examples. In one instance, he found himself standing in the middle of an intersection, shaking his fist at a motorist who was honking back at him. The last thing that he could remember before that moment was walking down a street several blocks away. He blamed these experiences on the people who could make him "flick." He saw this as a power that people held over him. In particular, he blamed the group home staff for making him "flick."

Occasionally there would be sessions that were directly focused on earlier trauma. One such example occurred when Reginald arrived clutching a public library book on raising boxer dogs. He asked me lots of medical questions about dog diseases, particularly heartworm. Finally he showed me a photograph in the book of a dog's heart cut open, revealing a seething mass of worms. He cried as he talked about missing his family's dogs and about how well his father had trained them. This was followed by a covert switch. Then in a trembling, almost incoherent voice, he told me how his father used his dogs to threaten the children if they misbehaved. It was never clear whether or not Reginald or his siblings were actually attacked, but it was obvious that they had lived in an atmosphere of terror and threat.

During this period, we were also able to understand together that a recent major behavioral decompensation had followed his learning that one of his sisters, who was living in another group home, had been raped. However, making this connection did not prevent future crises associated with contacts with his family.

Throughout this period, I met regularly with a range of people involved in Reginald's life, including group home staff, City Lights teachers, DHS administrators, and other professionals. It was manifestly clear from their comments that he had tested the limits of the system. Some wanted him dropped from their programs when he reached the age of 18. In the words of one DHS caseworker, "his next placement will be the shelter for homeless men."

The alters—Reginald, Reggie, and Little Mike (another alter that had been identified)—resurfaced as distinct entities following a pivotal session. He was brought to Children's Hospital on an emergency basis after another nightmare. It was apparent that he was having an extended abreaction that had started the night before. During the preceding night, he had been taken to an emergency room hyperventilating and in panic. He had refused hospitalization and medication. Reginald was discharged back to the group home, where his symptoms waxed and waned all night. By morning, he was confused, agitated, paranoid, and explosively accusing the staff of "messing with [his] mind." They, in turn, were demanding that I hospitalize him immediately or "knock him out" with medication. Instead, we had a highly successful abreactive session.

Interestingly, Reginald and I had begun to try hypnosis in prior sessions. He had remained intrigued with hypnosis and would raise it as an issue from time to time. Finally, he consented to try a few benign trance experiences to test out hypnosis. He was a good subject, easily entering a deepening trance. We had focused on peaceful, safe images that he heightened in intensity and vividness. Now, building on these prior benign trance experiences, he was able to enter trance and visualize the disturbing experiences projected on an imaginary screen. He described being forced to participate in sex with his siblings while his father and his father's friends watched. Out of trance, he cried and cursed bitterly as he talked about being made to have intercourse with his sisters while his father made pornographic movies. In the following session, Reggie identified himself and talked about his anger toward Reginald. Little Mike also appeared and talked about his anger toward "the father."

After these sessions, things seemed to go better for a while. True, Reggie still fooled around at school, but we were making some progress with contracts. Unfortunately, the District of Columbia, responding to a federal court order to reduce overcrowding at Lorton prison, released Reginald's father without having given any warning to the family members. Shortly after his release, he visited Reginald at the group home and tried to get him to leave and "put the family back together again." Reginald refused and was able to tell staff that he did not want to see his father again. A court injunction was obtained against further contact by the father, but this visit set off a chain reaction of events.

Reginald responded to the visit with increased nightmares and abreactions. He began to have two or three major abreactions a week, usually at night. During the days, he missed school, hiding in his room. At times he became paranoid and confused, insisting that people were "messing with his mind" and trying to send him to "St. E's." I started him on clonazepam because of its reported benefit for these symptoms in MPD patients (Loewenstein et al. 1988). It is not clear whether the medication helped. His compliance was poor, and he periodically accused me of trying to drug him. I was able to do some further abreactive work with Little Mike and another alter, Mr. Rage, but these efforts did not succeed in holding things in check. Although I was available by phone at night, some staff disagreed with my approach when he escalated. They preferred to take him to an emergency room with the hope that he would be hospitalized or heavily medicated. On one such night, the psychiatry resident on call committed him to St. E's. Reginald's fear had come true.

Fortunately, Reginald was assigned to a ward run by a psychiatrist experienced with MPD. The ward chief independently made the diagnosis and later described seeing him undergo a classic crisis of rapid switching following admission. Though his treatment team tried from the first to arrange a discharge, Reginald remained at St. E's for 2 months. The group home refused to take Reginald back, and DHS was slow to find an alternative placement. Together with the City Lights staff, I visited Reginald in the hospital weekly and consulted with ward staff by phone. They were receptive to the diagnosis; several team members had worked with other MPD patients. Reginald received only appropriate prn medication and enjoyed a friendly relationship with hospital staff. I was able to negotiate an effective contract with his personality system, and (Little Mike's threats to kick the unit door down notwithstanding) Reginald's behavior was cooperative and nonthreatening.

Eventually he was discharged to a temporary outpatient facility that primarily handled medically ill and geriatric patients. Although not an ideal placement, it provided a domicile from which Reginald was able to return to City Lights. I met with the facility staff and their consulting psychiatrist. Things seemed to go well until Reggie had an altercation over washing his clothes and threatened a staff member with a dinner fork. Reginald was discharged from that facility and transferred on an emergency basis to yet another hastily arranged placement. As luck would have it, the medical director at this new placement had worked with me in the successful management of another difficult MPD patient. We had a good working relationship, and my input was well accepted by the staff.

In therapy, again we seemed to be making some progress. We often played chess, a game that Reginald picked up quickly and played proficiently. Chess is a wonderful metaphor for life and provides a wealth of material that can be worked with in a displaced fashion, as well as sublimating all manner of aggressive impulses. Reginald played the game thoughtfully, setting traps three and four moves ahead. Little Mike blustered at me. He threatened to wipe out all my pieces but usually lost most of his. When he had thoroughly disrupted the board, he would turn it back to Reginald to save something from the mess—and sometimes he did. From time to time, Isaiah, another alter, interrupted the game to sing haunting gospel tunes and talk about making it as a singer.

The chessboard proved to be a useful arena in which to conduct therapy. Within the constraints of the rules of the game, the alters were exploring internal cooperation and communication. It provided a ready source of here-and-now, cause-and-effect examples of how the behavior of one alter affected another. It demonstrated unequivocally their lack of continuity of memory and action, and how some were inheriting situations caused by others. Typically we never finished a game, but we would play to a point at which significant material had been produced to address in therapy. Toward the end, this occurred within a few moves.

Several times over the course of the next year's work in therapy, I would meet an alter with penetrating insight into the personality system's behavior. He could describe how certain triggers (often specific behaviors in others that were reminiscent of his father's) would set off a chained sequence of alters with escalating affects and threatening behavior. He said that once this process got under way, it could not be stopped. Certain alters arranged to activate this sequence by pushing male authority figures such as teachers and group home staff to respond to their provocations. He also indicated that he understood how and why this happened in terms of the internal politics of his personality system, but he would not allow me to be made privy to such information. This alter could and would tell me a lot of what was going on and would work with me in assessing the suitability of contracts and other interventions. As with many inner self-helper(ish)like alters, this personality state was not consistently available.

Reginald adjusted to the new group home satisfactorily and was graduated to an independent living situation. He did well until his new roommate arrived, a newly discharged, heavily medicated schizophrenic man from St. E's. Some strange things happened. Reginald arrived at my office in crisis, and his roommate went AWOL. This typified a pattern for Reginald of bouncing back to the group home repeatedly, after several attempts to manage independent living situations. He needed the structure, interaction, and caring provided by the home. However, the group home was mandated by contract to move him out within a specified length of time. Reginald had already long overstayed his time limit and was stretching thin both tolerance of the staff and official understanding. Staff grew increasingly angry with what they perceived as his failure to use what he had learned to help himself. At some time or other, most staff members tried to get close to Reginald and work with him. Most emerged frustrated by his unwillingness (or inability) to avoid setting up angry, confrontational situations.

In other areas, however, he continued to make some progress. It was clear that he was growing up, dressing more maturely, flirting with women on the way to and from the waiting room and my office, and struggling with what was to become of his life. He explored joining the military, debating the quality of each branch of the service. We talked about various trades, and he fantasized about being a great entertainer. There was a series of girlfriends. These relationships were all intense and short-lived, but they helped raise the question in Reginald's mind of whether he dared to have children. He wanted a son and on occasion spoke to me as if I were a son and he were a father, telling me how the world was and how one has to deal with people. And yet he feared his loss of control and worried that he would do to his son what had been done to him. I tried to help him redirect his parental impulses toward the frightened and needy child parts within him.

From the first, I informed Reginald that I would only be able to see him until the completion of my fellowship, at that time more than 2 years in the future. We picked the termination issue up again in the last year, with a vocal part of his personality system maintaining that he did not want further treatment and in fact did not even want to be seeing me. During the time we were struggling with our termination and the subsequent course of his treatment and schooling, he was having increasing conflict with group home staff around his avoidant behaviors of staying in bed and not attending school. Not coincidentally, he had also begun to seek out his family after a chance encounter with a sister on a city bus. Soon he was visiting his mother, whom he had discovered living only a few blocks away, and was meeting with a sister to discuss their abuse experiences.

After a series of escalating crises, he was temporarily discharged from the group home. In retaliation, he broke into the group home and "borrowed" the home's van for a few hours. Following a week's suspension, during which he lived on the streets, he returned to the group home, but a level of trust had been broken. About 2 weeks later, in a bizarre episode, Reginald developed an extremely high fever and an acute organic brain syndrome. In this delirious state, he brandished a knife and threatened staff members who came too close. He was medically hospitalized for a week. On return to the home, he found himself even more estranged from staff. Shortly thereafter a final blowup occurred, and Reginald once again stole the van. Police charges were filed against him. His story remains unfinished.

Discussion

Clinically, it would appear that there are a spectrum of escape behaviors in the emotionally disturbed inner-city adolescents with whom I worked at City Lights. These behaviors serve as defenses against disturbing memories, affects, and experiences. Although they are somewhat adaptive in the short term, they inevitably lead to maladaptive behavior over the long term, because they block out important information and interfere with these adolescents' ability to learn new information and explore new ways of problem-solving. These adolescents become stuck, perseverative, and increasingly ineffective in coping with the increasing expectations and demands made on them. Some reenact traumatic situations in attempts at mastery, but often these efforts lead to their being revictimized. Most seek additional or more potent forms of escape—often a search that culminates in substance abuse.

Reginald's MPD can be understood as an extreme form of the psychological defenses and escape behaviors manifested by many of the students at City Lights. He was blocking out traumatic memories and affects generated by extensive physical and sexual abuse. The price, however, was a fragmentation of self leading to unstable and discontinuous behavior and the loss of effective self-agency.

Reginald's case illustrates the difficulties encountered in the treatment of inner-city adolescents with major dissociative symptoms. Until the diagnosis of MPD was made, he was seen as manifesting a major behavioral problem that was and would continue to be unresponsive to all interventions. His erratic and explosive behavior led to increasingly restrictive living situations and generated a sense of frustration and despair in those who tried to help him. Reginald was also very much trapped by his situation. He did not have the resources to extricate himself, and he was continually being retraumatized by his environment.

My treatment plan initially focused on trying to stabilize his living and school situations and laying the groundwork for later processing of his traumata. My first concern was nurturing a therapeutic alliance with Reginald as a whole. I did not seek out his alters aggressively during the period when he was attempting to seal over and undo his revelation to me. I was confident that if they were an enduring part of his psychological makeup, they would reappear as a therapeutic alliance developed. I used contracting, even before the alters overtly rejoined the treatment, to control behavior and to structure treatment boundaries. Within the treatment setting, contracts worked well; and although Reginald could become agitated, I never had to face the physical threats and displays of intimidation to which he subjected other authority figures. That may have led to some resentment from others involved in his management who felt that they were bearing the brunt of his pathology.

Hypnotic and abreactive techniques came to play an important role in the treatment but had to be introduced in a gradual fashion. Benign trance experiences served to acquaint Reginald with formal hypnosis and mitigate his fears about loss of control to me (Horevitz 1983; Kluft 1982; Putnam 1989). Spontaneous abreactions were first handled by basic grounding and reorientation and the use of the hypnotically facilitated displacement of traumatic material (screen techniques). Later, a few directed abreactions were attempted using age-regression and affect-bridging techniques to seek out and re-cover suspected traumatic material (Putnam 1989). Altogether, how-ever, probably less than 5% of therapy time was spent on direct abreactive work.

A major element of Reginald's treatment involved providing con-sultation and liaison to the institutions and agencies involved in his care as a ward of the District of Columbia. In many ways, this was more demanding than working directly with Reginald. It is difficult to explain MPD to psychologically naive administrators, group home staff, and teachers, who often labor under the burden of erroneous stereo-types evoked by the media. I found that the best place to begin my efforts to share an understanding of MPD was with his erratic behav-ior. Most people who had worked directly with Reginald shared the experience of finding that he behaved in radically different ways at times. This was often interpreted as oppositional or antisocial behav-ior—"he knows how to behave properly; he just doesn't do it."

I provided an alternative explanation that his inconsistent behav-ior reflected different parts of him that were active in different situations. This alternative explanation was, in fact, congruent with most people's experiences, and they often added details of differences that they had observed in him across different states. I did not emphasize the phenomena of the alters in attempting to explain his behavior; rather, I stressed his different "sides," the ample evidence of amnesias, and his poor continuity of memory. Most staff were responsive to this approach, particularly when I stressed that it was not their responsibility to identify and work with individual personalities, but rather to provide Reginald, in whatever state he was in, with clear, consistent guidelines about expectable behavior.

Interestingly, Reginald never sought to use his diagnosis to evade responsibility, blame his behaviors on alters, or seek special treatment on the basis of being an MPD patient. Instead, he was adamant that there was not anything wrong with him and that other people were externally causing his problems by making him "flick." In the end, however, there was a limit to the patience and understanding of the people and institutions responsible for him. In formulating interventions to be carried out by others at school or in the series of group homes, I stressed contracting, with particular emphasis on consistency and clarity. I recommended that all his contracts be written down and prominently posted and that staff members continually refresh their memories for details of the contract. Particularly during crises, this was ground that I had to go over and over again with the staff, whose patience was quickly exhausted. One of the major difficulties proved to be the inability of group home staffs to carry through their side of jointly negotiated contracts consistently, a shortcoming that seriously undermined the process for all participants. At the same time, many staff members did excellent individual work with Reginald, including abreactive work. Many were from backgrounds similar to Reginald's and could empathize and work in ways that I could not. Still, Reginald remained a master at splitting staff and setting up struggles around him.

I cannot anticipate what the future holds for Reginald, and for untold numbers of youths from similar circumstances. The identification and treatment of dissociative disorders in youngsters like Reginald remains in its infancy, and it will be critical to develop a body of experience and expertise in working with this clinical population.

References

Abramowitz M: Homicide top killer of D.C. children. Washington Post, March 1, 1989, pp B1, B5

American Psychiatric Association: Diagnostic and Statistical Manual of Mental Disorders, 3rd Edition, Revised. Washington, DC, American Psychiatric Association, 1987

Carnegie Council on Policy Studies in Higher Education: Giving youth a better chance. San Francisco, CA, Jossey-Bass, 1979

Horevitz RP: Diagnosis and treatment of multiple disorder: a framework for beginning. Am J Clin Hypn 26:138–145, 1983

Kluft RP: Varieties of hypnotic interventions in the treatment of multiple personality. Am J Clin Hypn 24:230–240, 1982

Kluft RP: The natural history of multiple personality disorder, in Childhood Antecedents of Multiple Personality Disorder. Edited by Kluft RP. Washington, DC, American Psychiatric Press, 1985, pp 197–238

Kluft RP: Clinical presentations of multiple personality disorder. Psychiatr Clin North Am 14:605–629, 1991

Loewenstein RJ, Hornstein N, Farber B: Open trial of Clonazepam in the treatment of posttraumatic stress symptoms in multiple personality disorder. Dissociation 1(3):3–12, 1988

Putnam FW: Diagnosis and Treatment of Multiple Personality Disorder. New York, Guilford, 1989

Tolmach J: "There ain't nobody on my side": a new day treatment program for black urban youth. Journal of Clinical Child Psychology 14:214–219, 1985

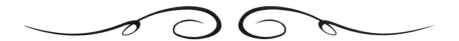

The Deinstitutionalization of Patients With Chronic Multiple Personality Disorder

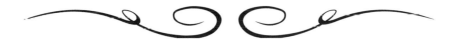

Lucy G. Quimby, Ph.D.
Andy Andrei
Frank W. Putnam, Jr., M.D.

The increasing acceptance and recognition of multiple personality disorder (MPD) is resulting in the more frequent identification of MPD patients in a variety of treatment settings, including chronic care facilities. The confirmation of the diagnosis of MPD in such a setting poses enormous challenges for both the patient and staff. Typically, those who treat chronic mental patients are already overburdened. They have good reason to view as impractical the suggestion that a chronically hospitalized MPD patient could, with appropriate treatment, function adequately as an outpatient.

Our experience has shown that the treatment necessary to effect

Prepared for presentation at the 3rd International Conference on Multiple Personality/Dissociative States, Chicago, IL, September 18–21, 1986.
This chapter is dedicated to the memory of our friend and colleague Christa-Marie Homann, M.D.

such a transition can be provided, resulting both in dramatic clinical improvements in the patient and in substantial economic and administrative benefits for the institution. This chapter is based on the author's collective experiences as consultants and/or therapists with at least five such cases. This experience is illustrated with the discussion of such a case; the identifying details have been altered in the interests of confidentiality.

Jana (a pseudonym), is a young adult who has been almost continuously institutionalized since early adolescence—a period of nearly 15 years. At the beginning of her treatment, Jana was under one-to-one nursing care at a state hospital in the rural northwestern United States. The treatment process will be presented as a series of tasks necessary to successfully transfer a chronically institutionalized MPD inpatient to outpatient status. These tasks include the following:

1. Making the diagnosis in a chronic institutional setting;
2. Acceptance of the diagnosis by the patient, treatment team, ward/milieu staff, and administration;
3. Initiating therapeutic work with the patient as an MPD patient;
4. Working with social services to develop a structure for safe living outside the hospital;
5. Weaning the patient from the hospital; and
6. Maintaining the patient in outpatient treatment.

Making the Diagnosis

MPD has been compared to neurosyphilis in the era before penicillin, in that it may mimic a wide range of psychiatric or somatic disorders (Putnam et al. 1984). There are limited data available on inpatient cases of MPD, but a survey of therapists treating outpatient cases found that the typical patient had averaged 6.8 years from his or her first contact with the mental health system for symptoms referable to MPD until the diagnosis of MPD was actually made (Putnam et al. 1986). The same study found that MPD patients received an average of 3.6 psychiatric diagnoses prior to the diagnosis of

MPD. Although the most common past diagnosis was depression, approximately half of the patients sampled in this survey had received a diagnosis of schizophrenia at some point in their treatment history. It is likely that the typical psychiatric history of chronically hospitalized MPD patients is even more complex. Table 10–1 lists the 19 diagnoses found recorded in Jana's old records.

In outpatient settings, the typical MPD patient presents with a plethora of psychiatric, neurological, and somatic complaints (Putnam et al. 1984). Although many consider amnesia, usually manifest as "time loss" or denial of observed behavior, a universal symptom in MPD (Bliss 1980; Coons 1984; Putnam et al. 1986), patients typically do not report these experiences to clinicians until a therapeutic alliance has been established (Kluft 1987a). Depression is the most commonly reported presenting complaint in MPD patients and is often associated with self-destructive ideation and/or behavior (e.g., suicide attempts or self-mutilation). Extremely rapid shifts in function and behavior are also commonly reported and may be mistaken for the mood swings of affective disorders.

MPD patients usually have multiple somatic complaints with a very high incidence of migrainelike headaches, gastrointestinal disturbances, and unexplained pain (usually abdominal or pelvic). Conversion symptoms and eating disturbances are not uncommon, and at least one-third of MPD patients will describe auditory and/or visual hallucinations. The auditory hallucinations are commonly described as occurring within the head, as opposed to originating in the sur-

Table 10–1. Diagnoses in Jana's records in the 10 years prior to her MPD diagnosis

Question of early schizophrenia	Schizophrenia, acute
Depressive neurosis	Latent schizophrenia
Hysterical neurosis	Adolescent suicidal reaction
Inadequate personality disorder	Reactive depression neurotic
Schizophrenic, chronic undifferentiated type	Borderline personality disorder
	Schizoaffective disorder
Adult situational stress reaction in chronic undifferentiated schizophrenia	Specific learning disturbance
	Hysterical personality disorder
	Temporal lobe epilepsy (supported by electroencephalogram data)
Schizophrenia with catatonic attack	
Depression	Manic depressive, depressed
Borderline schizophrenia	

rounding environment. Schneiderian-like passive influence experiences are common and, together with the hallucinations, may lead to the misdiagnosis of schizophrenia or another psychotic disorder (Kluft 1987b).

In addition to the symptoms described herein, there are a number of behaviors and inpatient-staff dynamics that should lead clinicians to consider the diagnosis of MPD. Most, though not all, MPD patients react in a strong negative fashion to prolonged hospitalization. Typically, hospitalized MPD patients have frequent or almost continuous crises, even after years on an inpatient unit. They do not "burn out" and become compliant with the ward routines as do many chronically hospitalized schizophrenic patients.

Despite their numerous and often bizarre symptoms and behaviors, MPD patients typically have a high degree of relatedness that leads to intensive staff involvement and investment in their treatment. These intense interactions between ward staff and the MPD patient frequently are experienced by some members of the staff as controlling and manipulative and may lead to arguments and staff splitting. Often staff members have very different perceptions of the patient and are unable to reconcile their varying impressions of the patient's behavior, motivation, and needs.

Ward staff may come to recognize the discrete behavioral states manifested by the patient and often give them descriptive names while not recognizing these states as alters. In one case, for example, the staff would describe one patient as being in his "Peacock Mood" when an alter who liked to dress up in flamboyant clothing was in executive control of the patient's behavior. MPD patients may also show rapid regressions in behavior; they can exhibit extreme quasi-infantile behavior when child alters are out. Many staff members will interpret this as manipulative, because it is their perception that the patient appears to move in and out of these regressed states "at will." It should be noted that episodes of behavioral regression are usually more frequent on the night shift. The patient may also deny witnessed behavior and be seen as lying or "sociopathic."

Jana, our case study, is vaguely remembered by one of the staff of her preschool as an abused child who behaved oddly. Her records over the last 15 years document self-abuse and suicide attempts;

eating disorders; substance abuse; auditory, visual, and somatic hallucinations; putting her fist through windows; and reports of "two people inside her head." She also had multiple somatic complaints and many inconsistent allergic responses to foods and medication. She was usually upset and more symptomatic after contact with her family, but at other times she made positive statements about them and asked to see them. Intelligence tests produced scores in the retarded range, recorded in her chart as a probable underestimation of her true intelligence. Presenting symptoms at more than nine hospital admissions have included self-abuse (e.g., cutting and scratching her wrists, setting herself on fire) and suicide attempts (e.g., overdose and wrist slashing) as well as abdominal pain usually diagnosed as a functional bowel syndrome.

Jana's diagnosis of MPD was first suspected by a psychiatric nurse on her ward. However, 4 years passed before MPD was entered in her chart as the definitive diagnosis. During that time the psychiatric nurse and at least one other staff member attempted to treat her multiplicity, but without success. Disagreement over the diagnosis, division among the treatment team, and Jana's refusal of psychotherapy precluded effective treatment. Finally, after a grueling electroencephalogram that showed that much of Jana's seizure activity was without brain-wave correlates, Jana demonstrated powerful abreactive material to a psychiatrist and a student, who were beginning to suspect the true nature of her condition. That experience led the psychiatrist to consult the third author (F.W.P.), who confirmed the diagnosis and, more importantly, made himself available for extended consultation, thus enabling the hospital to organize and implement a treatment plan.

Acceptance of the Diagnosis by the Patient, Treatment Team, Ward/Milieu Staff, and Administration

Reluctance to recognize MPD in a particular patient may have many causes. The power struggles that coalesce around diagnostic disagreements are distractions from the therapeutic goals. An efficient strategy focuses on the task of helping the MPD patient become sufficiently organized for outpatient treatment. Initially, a careful analysis must be made of which individuals' cooperation would be essential for starting the treatment, and of how these individuals might be affected by the diagnosis. This analysis must include all elements of the treatment system. The shorter the initial list of essential participants, the easier it will be to start a process the increasing success of which will generate further support. A similar analysis must be made of the MPD patient's system of personalities.

Factors that may lead both the MPD patient and the hospital staff to oppose the diagnosis include basic skepticism about MPD, reluctance to believe the truth of the MPD patient's memories, dismay at the pain and tumult stirred up by the beginning phases of treatment, and a very chaotic clinical presentation. The chronically hospitalized MPD patient may not resemble the published descriptions or videotapes that show an ordered system with each alter clearly identified and taking turns in speaking or controlling behavior. One novice psychotherapist working with a chronically hospitalized MPD patient described her experience as being more like watching a cat fight under a blanket. It was nearly impossible to make sense out of what could be observed; she knew there was a lot of action, much of it violent, and she put a great deal of effort into trying to get close enough to see what was going on without getting hurt.

With regard to the patient, powerful alters, who may initially be the most defiant and abusive of the body, are important to enlist early on in the treatment. They are likely to be highly motivated to get out of the hospital, and they need to be helped to see the benefits of learning how to keep the body safe. Their abuse of the body and denial of cotenancy with other alters is often an attempt to keep all alters from revealing traumatic memories. Paradoxically, their self-destructive behavior may also be a coded communication about the trauma, reflecting their original predicament of having been abused in an environment in which speaking the truth was dangerous. These alters also fear the emotional pain of sharing their memories with others, both within their own system and with the treatment team. Eventually, they may allow themselves to experience support from both sources. In our experience, the best approach is probably a dogged but low-key insistence that they share a body, that they have to cooperate to maintain its safety, and that they collectively must experience the consequences of any current inappropriate behavior.

On the part of the hospital, successful treatment requires support from the top of the power hierarchy. Given the psychiatric, medical, and legal risks involved and the struggles within the treatment system that will probably erupt before the MPD patient is discharged, the treatment team requires a basic level of support from both the administrative and clinical directors.

The rest of the hospital staff will respond better to a pragmatic focus on the patient's behavior rather than to direct challenges to their own deeply held beliefs (a finding consistent with Kluft 1984, 1991). It is extremely easy to waste energy and incite enmity in power struggles at this point. For example, one therapist involved with Jana's treatment created unnecessary difficulties by self-righteously insisting that unconvinced staff refer to the MPD patient in plural language. Resistive alliances are likely to form between hospital staff and alters. Conflicting endeavors to rescue both the patient and the staff from one another are common. Some staff are reluctant to give up the conviction of "knowing what's best" for a patient whose life they have guarded for many years, often at great personal and professional risk. Others fear the loss of equilibrium in their own personal lives as the patient begins to develop self-knowledge and autonomy. Many of the anticipated benefits of treatment may not be evident during the first year. Several times Jana's therapists discussed the possibility that the resources they had to offer were simply not adequate, and they felt they might have to abandon their efforts. Fortunately, they did not.

In a treatment setting such as a state hospital, where financial and professional resources are overburdened, the prospect of beginning a complex and tumultuous treatment effort may not generate enthusiasm. However, a successful treatment program is likely to be more productive and less expensive in the long run than management of a misdiagnosed MPD patient. Table 10–2 summarizes the financial cost and benefits of diagnosis and treatment of a chronically hospitalized MPD patient and effecting a transition to outpatient status. An initial investment in the intensification of treatment holds the potential of a dramatic reduction in expenditures over the long run of treatment. Although 2 years of Jana's treatment program had not yet brought her to stable outpatient status, she was no longer regarded as a hopelessly chronic patient, her personality system was demonstrating dramatic increases in mutual cooperation and coconsciousness, and both she and her therapists had clearly identified the issues that needed to be addressed in order for her to live successfully outside the hospital.

An important corollary of the acceptance of the diagnosis of MPD is the acknowledgment that the patient was severely traumatized as a child. MPD patients undermine the credibility of their memories in several ways. They describe demonstrable hallucinations and delusions, and they sometimes deny the very abuse they report. Even the alters who remember abuse may recall it in a dreamlike way and may be uncertain of their memories. The severity and unusual nature of the abuse may also lead observers to deny its occurrence. Staff have their own reasons for denying the reality of the MPD patient's mem-

Table 10–2. Weekly costs to a state hospital treating a chronically hospitalized patient with MPD (based on 1986 cost figures)

Service	Prediagnosis	Postdiagnosis in hospital	Postdiagnosis on leave
Basic hospitalization	$862.00	$862.00	0
1:1 specials	$1,779–$2,293	$1,779	0
Diagnostic procedures	+	–	–
Medications	$21	$21	$21
Routine lab work	No charge	No charge	No charge
Psychotherapy			
Mental health worker	0	10 hours/$77	7 hours/$54
Psychologist	0	10 hours/$140	7 hours/$98
Psychiatrist	0	2 hours/$60	.5 hours/$15
Total	$883–$3,176	$1,160–$2,939	$188

ories. If staff know the abusers, the abusers' denials may appear more credible than the patient's often fragmentary memories. If the abusers are family members, staff who are upset by the patient may deny the abuse out of sympathy for the family. It is likely to be traumatic for treatment team members to recognize that such abuse is within the repertoire of human behavior and to bear witness to the MPD patient's display of overwhelming affect as the memory fragments emerge. Additional problems may arise if any treatment team members had been abused as children. It is our experience that they may be more likely to recognize the truth of what the MPD patient remembers, but that the psychological consequences of their participation in treatment may prove distressing.

Initiating Therapeutic Work With the Patient With a Newly Established Diagnosis of MPD

The following concerns are salient in the early phases of treatment.

Trust

Psychotherapy with an MPD patient requires the establishment of a strong therapeutic alliance, based on the MPD patient's recognition that the therapist can provide the external supports necessary to facilitate the MPD patient's own healing processes. The MPD patient needs to experience repeatedly that the therapists can be trusted to respect the truth of memories, to attempt to understand the MPD patient's reality, to be reliably and predictably available without threat of abandonment, to set appropriate limits, and to respect the MPD patient's personal boundaries.

Having learned in childhood that survival depended on learning how to manipulate authority figures to avoid pain, the MPD patient will probably deploy manifold complex strategies to obstruct the course of an inevitably painful treatment. The success of the treatment depends on the MPD patient's learning, through continual reexperiencing in the therapeutic relationship, that these types of manipulations are no longer necessary or helpful.

Contracting

Treatment can be conceptualized as a process of helping the MPD patient to gain more conscious internal control. This requires organization and structure in both the treatment system and the MPD patient's internal system. Contracting is an excellent way to create this structure. A good contract includes concrete descriptions of the behaviors required, the consequences of keeping to the contract, the consequences of breaking the contract, and the length of time the contract is to last (Drye et al. 1973; Thames 1984). A basic contract might read, in part,

> We have decided to work with [therapists] toward developing a New World. We will not physically hurt ourselves or anyone else, now or in the future, inside or outside, accidentally or on purpose, even if we feel like it. We understand that if this contract is broken, the body will be transferred to [locked ward where restraints were used when needed]. This contract must be signed by everyone for themselves; otherwise the signers of the contract will be held responsible for the others and the body. This contract will last through [date].

Contracts serve several purposes. One is to teach the MPD patient about cause and effect in a reasonably benign social context, thus facilitating organization of the internal system. The ability of an MPD patient to experience time in a discontinuous fashion as a way of coping with trauma often leaves the patient confused about the effects of his or her own behavior and even can contribute to the creation of additional traumatic experiences. One of Jana's alters, who had been repeatedly tied down and raped by her father, was left with the body each time the hospital staff put the patient in full bed restraints following other alters' violent behavior.

Another function of the contract is to allow the patient to agree voluntarily to adhere to clear guidelines that everyone can enforce and to define the ways in which the treatment team will hold the

MPD patient collectively responsible for the behavior of the body. This reduces the probability that the patient will experience arbitrary limit setting, which often arouses destructive anger. It also provides support for the ward staff who may also feel angry because of their difficulty in coping with this unpredictable, "special," and sometimes violent patient (Maxmen et al. 1974).

Monthly contracts provided Jana with a fairly frequent reminder of the necessary cooperation. In the beginning, it took several days for the alters to arrange to provide the necessary signatures. The growing list of signatures provided a record of the recruitment of the personality system into treatment. Other issues that call for firm structure include treatment team roles and behavior, time schedules for therapy meetings, guidelines for handling spontaneous abreactions, and the patient's avoidance of further victimization.

Early Treatment Roles

In the absence of general staff expertise in the management of MPD, treatment can be begun by a small psychotherapy team that addresses all issues directly related to the multiplicity. Creating this team may require some administrative and clinical flexibility. Jana's team consisted of the psychiatrist and student who had witnessed the initial convincing abreaction and the psychiatric nurse who had originally suspected the diagnosis. The MPD patient needs to be informed that not everyone will acknowledge the alters' separate identities and that they can use this experience to prepare for life outside the hospital, where they will have to pass as one. Ward staff should be asked to address the patient as the patient requests and to respect the fact that the patient experiences him- or herself as divided (Kluft 1984, 1991). This early organization phase is very difficult. In Jana's case, it required nearly a year's work. Jana's alters were understandably upset by staff members who displayed skepticism about her diagnosis and her memories of abuse. Disagreement among staff members became heated. The general conflict may have lent increased energy to Jana's determination to achieve enough control over her behavior to get out of the hospital. Her subsequent rehospitalizations were on another ward where, as her treatment progressed and she became stronger and better organized, it was easier for more of the ward staff to accept the diagnosis.

_____

Therapy Schedule

Because the only known effective treatment for MPD is intensive psychotherapy (Kluft 1985a, 1991), two or three sessions per week are recommended. In our experience, when abreactive work is being done, one of those sessions may need to last up to 3 hours. Jana's therapists discovered that when they gave in to their urge to spend more time in sessions, both the patient and treatment team became less stable. A balance must be struck with each patient between retrieving memories too fast for emotional processing and assimilation on the one hand and insufficient contact, therapeutic activity, and support on the other.

During Jana's restrictions to the locked ward, one therapist saw her for half an hour daily to boost Jana's morale, allow the alters to ventilate feelings, support cooperation with the contract, and maintain contact while Jana's system "cooled itself off."

_____

Controlling Abreactions

Uncontrolled abreactions present a major dilemma. They often involve self-abuse and other unpredictable, frightening behavior. They frequently follow psychotherapy sessions on traumatic material. Ward staff may respond anxiously by polarizing into one faction advocating increased therapy time and another faction denouncing therapy as the cause of the disturbed behavior. The alters as a group need to develop some capacity to handle minor abreactions on their own and to bring major ones into psychotherapy sessions.

Jana's skill at this improved as alters taught themselves to follow suggestions for increased coconsciousness and practiced trying to see their memories as if on a television screen rather than reliving them. Jana learned to use a tape cassette player with earphones to calm herself and provide protective insulation from her environment. Many of her personalities also agreed on a "password" that would help them to recognize members of the treatment team rather than confusing them with past abusers.

Protection From Abusers

Treatment must include provisions for keeping the patient and the abusers separated. At first, denial of the abuse may obscure the necessity for this. Other agendas, often contradictory, also draw patient and abusers together. The MPD patient may want revenge, support for denial, and confirmation of the reality of the abuse. The abusers may want to silence or disorganize the patient. The patient's family may be expert saboteurs of the most conscientious discharge plans. Effective treatment requires that staff recognize in both word and action the reality of the abuse.

Jana contracted on a monthly basis not to have any contact with her family of origin without the consent of all the alters and the entire treatment team. State laws on reporting of child abuse must be followed while protecting the patient from the possibility of premature and lethally destabilizing interaction with the legal system.

Support for Therapists

Widespread refusal of hospital staff refusal to acknowledge the diagnosis can leave the therapists without the personal and professional supports needed to deal with a Hydra-like constellation of alters. Vulnerable team members may become invested in favored positions as therapists of this special patient and allow themselves to be rendered therapeutically impotent.

In a familiar scenario, the MPD patient says, "If you really cared about me, you'd bend the rules," and then concludes, "You can't be trusted, because you weren't strong enough to adhere to the rules." Each therapist on a novice treatment team should have secure, independent anchors in supervisory and/or personal psychotherapeutic relationships. The highly stressful nature of this work requires that treatment team members also obtain and comply with good medical care for themselves.

Social Service: Resources for Life Outside the Hospital

The MPD diagnosis has important implications for discharge planning. MPD patients differ from other chronically hospitalized patients in their ability to demonstrate dramatic and rapid improvement when they leave the hospital. Active discharge planning should start and continue even when the patient is doing very poorly. This may induce better functioning, especially if the patient is given appropriate responsibility for setting up his or her life situation outside the hospital. The alters should agree that one will be responsible for all interactions with social services and for tasks such as paperwork and apartment hunting. The psychotherapists can encourage that alter to seek consultation and support from other alters. This relieves social services of the confusion of dealing with a variety of alters and allows the alters a protected environment in which to practice the skills that they will need outside the hospital. The discharge plan needs to include six elements: financial support, a place to live, protection from abusive relationships and self-destructive behaviors, a program for development of life skills and/or rehabilitation, a plan for returning to the hospital when necessary, and provisions for ongoing therapy.

Financial support.   Most chronically institutionalized MPD patients meet eligibility requirements for Social Security Disability Insurance (for disabled minors) or Supplemental Security Income. A substantial literature on enabling institutionalized clients to prove their eligibility applies well to this population (Opaku 1988).

The MPD patient often needs help in managing financial resources. Although Jana wanted to receive her Social Security benefits directly, her previous outpatient record showed that she had not paid for rent or food. The hospital arranged to become the "representative payee," having informed Social Security that family members were inappropriate. Jana participated in planning her own budget, which the community support worker used as a focus for life skill development. The hospital's discharge social worker provided the necessary structure through strict controls on Jana's spending.

Jana was allowed more autonomy to decide for herself to request subsidized housing and other assistance programs. Although resistant at first to food stamps, she eventually requested and received her community support worker's help in applying for them as well as fuel and transportation assistance.

Living quarters.   The patient may choose to live alone in an apartment in preference to a halfway house, boarding home, or shared apartment. This arrangement has a number of advantages. It avoids entanglement in the institutional and interpersonal dynamics of a halfway house or boarding home. It offers the alters sufficient privacy to do independent internal group therapy work (Caul 1984). It places responsibility for survival clearly on the patient, thus fostering development of the alters' ability to provide structure and supervision for the system. The nature of federal housing programs makes it most likely that suitable apartments will be located in housing projects for the elderly.

Jana's discharge social worker provided a list of available federally subsidized apartments, from which Jana selected those meeting her criteria for safety. The social worker successfully advocated for her priority admission to a well-managed senior citizens' building.

Protection.   Outside the hospital (as inside), the primary means of protection against abuse by self or others must be contracting. Jana's alters contracted among themselves to prevent substance abuse and regulate sexual activity in a manner that accommodated all their various needs and attitudes. They also maintained their contract to avoid contact with their family of origin. A telephone answering machine with a computer-generated voice provided a means of screening phone calls.

Appropriate responses to abusers' attempts to visit the patient outside the hospital need to be discussed carefully and periodically reviewed with all the alters. The patient may test the therapists by reporting a current abusive interaction and scrutinizing the therapists' response.

Skills for independent living.   MPD patients who have spent most of their teen and adult years in mental institutions and whose childhood environments precluded academic learning and skill development can make excellent use of the same rehabilitation programs typically available to other chronically hospitalized mental patients. Jana's aftercare worker was very impressed by Jana's high level of motivation and her great capacity to improve from a very low initial skill level. Jana needed to learn basic tasks, such as how to comply with her medication schedule, take the bus, count change, read prices in the grocery store, go out for a cup of coffee in a restaurant, and telephone for help in case of emergency. MPD patients with higher skill levels also can benefit from more advanced social and vocational rehabilitation programs. As in the discharge planning program, the MPD patient should designate an alter to represent the group in each program.

The rehabilitation program is a crucial element of the therapy process. It provides opportunities for the MPD patient to develop strong anchors in the here and now and to become desensitized to a wide variety of stimuli that have the potential to elicit traumatic memories and abreactions. It is important that the aftercare worker be flexible and tolerant, possess a ready sense of gentle humor, provide strong positive encouragement, and see the life skills work as complementary to, rather than in competition with, the psychotherapy. The role of the aftercare worker must be clearly defined, and the boundaries of the relationship with the MPD patient firmly specified at the outset (Turkus 1991). Meetings should focus on the practice of skills rather than on the internal processes affecting performance. One 2-hour session per week of direct contact appears sufficient to make good progress. Because the psychotherapy session is likely to disrupt the rest of the patient's day, rehabilitation work can be done more successfully on other days of the week.

Rehospitalization.   Even though the MPD patient may leave the hospital vowing never to reenter "such an awful place," it is important that there be a concrete procedure spelled out for returning to the hospital. Jana and her alters agreed to a contract that specified that in case of any danger to the body, they alone were responsible for going to the hospital, either by taxi or by police ambulance; in addition, they knew that a member of the psychotherapy team would meet with them in the hospital within 24 hours. The contract further stated that if they did not act to protect themselves, they would be left alone to deal with the consequences. When Jana's alters found it difficult to refrain from spending their emergency taxi fare, arrangements were made to keep it for her at the hospital.

Jana's psychotherapists rehearsed with her the procedure they were to follow in case of emergency phone calls. They agreed to gently but firmly remind Jana of the established contract and *get off the phone,* call the ward so that the supervising psychiatrist could be notified if appropriate, and then call one another for support in coping with their own anxieties. These limits will be tested at least once. A vague or uncertain limit that invites testing is more dangerous in the long run than a firm one.

The likelihood of several rehospitalizations and the necessity for continuity of therapeutic relationships may make an extended leave status more efficient than discharge, so that readmission procedures can be avoided. Events likely to provoke rehospitalization include threatened encounters with the abusers, new episodes of abuse (e.g., rape), loss or life changes of therapy team members, and emergence of powerfully disruptive memories, or of violent, self-destructive alters.

Outpatient psychotherapy.   In our experience, the number of sessions can be decreased to two sessions per week, with one of them lasting up to 3 hours to allow time for abreactions (see Chapter 7 for an alternative approach to abreactive work). The psychotherapy needs to deal with various issues:

1. Helping the alters to live cooperatively;
2. Developing the interpersonal skills and orientation to present reality necessary to live independently;
3. Developing alternatives to denial and dissociation;
4. Recovering and abreacting traumatic memories; and
5. Working through the material that is uncovered.

Because MPD patients are so dependent on their psychotherapy relationships for both support and anchoring in the present, continuity of care is extremely important. It is preferable that the same therapist should follow the MPD patient in and out of the hospital, at least until the MPD patient has a stable outside support system.

_____

Making the Transition:
Weaning the Patient From the Hospital

Moving out of the hospital requires developing coping skills and control in the internal system. During this phase the treatment team should continue to be available for support while maintaining the boundaries and limits that permit the MPD patient more autonomous functioning. Heightened anxiety in both the MPD patient and the treatment team can make this transition arduous and lead to behaviors in either or both that complicate the process.

Preparation.   Ideally, the weaning process should begin while the patient is still in the hospital. After moving out, one or more of the personalities will have to be responsible for maintaining the safety of the body. For at least a week before the move, the MPD patient should begin to assume this responsibility by choosing to go to a locked ward or even be placed in restraints if alters threaten damage. At this point, the patient's verbal assurance should also be sufficient to permit leaving the locked ward or restraints. This exercise transfers control to the MPD patient and can strengthen the position of the caretaking personalities, as well as reassuring anxious staff that the MPD patient's internal system has the capacity to keep the body safe.

The treatment team should outline for the MPD patient in concrete detail the support system available. These supports should include the option of moving out gradually—for example, spending either days or nights out at first, then working up from 2-hour absences to week-long leaves. Therapists and ward staff should be available for well-structured telephone contacts. A reasonable plan would be to allow up to 20 minutes per day total (shared by all alters) per psychotherapist, at hours convenient to the therapists, with the clear understanding that calls may be used for brief questions, reassurance, and reality grounding, but not for work that belongs in the therapy session. During other hours, or when the therapist cannot be reached, the patient may call the ward to talk to staff, with the same constraints on time and content.

Pitfalls.   If the staff remains split over the diagnosis and the psychotherapy team isolated, certain pitfalls are nearly inescapable. The therapists' anxiety is likely to be acute as they watch their mercurial and potentially self-destructive patient leave the confines of the hospital. This anxiety is easily compounded by anticipation of anger and blame from staff members who did not accept the diagnosis, should the patient become self-destructive or otherwise fail to prosper. If many of the ward staff are still vehemently resisting the diagnosis, it will be difficult for them to support or relieve the therapists as providers of telephone or other support. The therapists may be caught in the impossible position of feeling responsible to the rest of the staff for the welfare of a potentially very demanding patient whose risky behavior they cannot control. They may also fear that contacts with openly skeptical staff will trigger self-destructive behavior in the patient.

In addition to the pressures created by staff splitting, there are other dangers for the treating therapists. After the patient moves out of the hospital, the greater privacy of the relationship between patient and therapists leaves the therapists vulnerable to seductive alters, misperceptions arising out of abreactive realities, and hospital gossip about the nature of the relationship between the patient and the opposite-sex therapist. Because of their anxieties, the therapists may make frequent lengthy telephone calls to the patient or make personal rescue visits to the patient's apartment. In the long run, these interventions are destabilizing to the patient and professionally dangerous to the therapist. Finally, visions of postsuicide lawsuits may lurk menacingly in the minds of those clinically responsible for the patient.

Support and trust.   To maintain effectiveness, the psychotherapy team needs to have developed a level of interpersonal trust sufficient to allow them to continue to remain available to the patient while taking the structured risks necessary for the progress of treatment. The inevitable presence of risk must be openly acknowledged, and the therapists' anxiety recognized as a normal (if uncomfortable) response. It sometimes appears as though MPD patients communicate their emotional predicaments to their therapists by inducing feelings in the therapists that mirror the MPD patient's own feelings. The therapists' responses then become a model for the MPD patient to emulate. An anxious or fearful MPD patient induces anxiety or fear in the therapy team and watches to see how the team members handle it. The therapists should take reasonable steps to protect themselves and their professional lives but resist the temptation to try to avoid their own anxiety by attempting to control the MPD patient. It is a mistake to accept the challenge of keeping the MPD patient alive, in or out of the hospital. A more viable goal is to offer the MPD patient consistently repeated opportunities to choose life (Kluft 1985b).

Communication among team members, respect for one another's positions, and consensus behind clinical decision making and therapeutic structure are essential ingredients for team members' emotional, clinical, and legal support in complex situations. Good record-keeping is essential. The documentation of clinical interventions, their rationale, and the patient's responses are an important element of this support. Team members also need to be able to trust one another's adherence to the structure and boundaries of the therapy.

Hospital policies and routines and the presence of other staff provide some role definition and structure for the therapy process in the hospital. The meaning of the therapeutic relationship and its boundaries and an explicit clarification of the difference between a "friend" and a "therapist" need to be redefined and restated in both words and behavior, both before and after the MPD patient moves out. Useful guidelines include the following:

1. The psychotherapists will not visit the MPD patient's apartment;
2. Opposite-sex hospital staff members will not enter the MPD patient's apartment unless accompanied by another staff member of the same sex as the MPD patient;
3. Therapists and other staff will not telephone the MPD patient;
4. Crises are to be handled by returning to the hospital, if necessary, rather than telephoning the therapists.

The therapists can expect these boundaries to be tested both subtly and strenuously. Consistent gentle firmness can enable both the MPD patient and the therapists to experience that benign structure facilitates trust and productive work.

Maintaining the Patient Out of the Hospital

Building secure community support systems and gaining independence from the hospital can be a long, slow process lasting 18 months or more. A variety of obstacles must be overcome. The patient may lack any experience of living independently and feel so different from "normal" people that even living among them seems impossible. Alters may compete and argue with one another so that everyday tasks such as getting dressed in the morning become complicated and drawn-out events. The MPD patient may experience voices and even sensations reminiscent of physical punishment that shed doubt on the possibility of successful independent living. The process of choosing attainable life goals and working toward them may be unknown to the patient. Finally, the patient may with good reason fear to be the victim of or even the perpetrator of further abuse, making chronic hospitalization appear preferable to reentering society.

Three elements are required for a successful outpatient treatment plan: the availability of rehospitalization when needed, the continuity of outpatient psychotherapy and social support services, and the development of an outside support system (Turkus 1991).

Availability of rehospitalization. Rehospitalizations are of two kinds. One is a relatively brief (1 day to 6 weeks) return to a secure environment, necessitated by environmental events that the MPD patient does not have the resources to handle independently. Examples of such events are threatened encounters with former abusers; new abuse, violence, or threats of violence; physical illness; and loss or threatened loss of a psychotherapist. Optimally, the MPD patient takes the initiative to return to the hospital when needed. Sometimes this does not happen, and the MPD patient is taken to the emergency room after an overdose or is rescued from serious mishap before being returned to the hospital.

These rehospitalizations should be kept as brief as possible. The problem in the patient's environment needs to be identified, and the patient helped to work out successful coping strategies. If the contracts have been adhered to, appropriate recognition and appreciation are indicated. If contracts have been broken, the therapists should find out why the MPD patient did not conform to the agreement. Then the therapist should restate the importance of the contracts and help the MPD patient to find the resources necessary to adhere to the next set of contracts. As soon as new contracts are created that satisfy both the MPD patient and the therapy team, the MPD patient should be allowed to leave the hospital. If the hospitalization has lasted for more than a couple of days, a gradual increase in time out of the hospital over several days or a week may be appropriate.

The second type of rehospitalization is necessitated by the emergence of traumatic memories that the MPD patient is not yet strong enough to face without the support of the structured hospital environment. This type of rehospitalization is likely to be of longer duration, especially if treatment is being conducted by a novice therapy team. Several factors make this type of hospitalization more complex:

1. The memory material may arouse powerful responses, such as guilt, anger, or grief, which both the MPD patient and the psychotherapy team avoid dealing with openly, so that the MPD patient's dissociative defenses are not challenged adequately.
2. Once the dissociative defenses are given up, the MPD patient has to develop new ways of coping with both self and world.
3. Retrieval of powerful memories may change the structure and organization of the constellation of alters, so that there is, in effect, a new ball game to be figured out, with different players, some ardently suicidal.
4. When both the MPD patient and the ward staff begin to better understand the nature of the MPD patient's problems, the ward staff become more curious and sympathetic. Unless they respect professional boundaries, their attempts to participate in the psychotherapy can obstruct progress with a maze of distractions.

In her first year after leaving the hospital, Jana spent 32 weeks in her apartment and 20 in the hospital. She had two brief rehospitalizations precipitated by external stresses in the first 4 months, a period of 4½ months out of the hospital, and then a longer rehospitalization for memory-related work.

Continuity of Outpatient Psychotherapy and Social Support Services

Together, the psychotherapy and rehabilitation programs can provide the trustworthy structure necessary for the MPD patient to continue to develop internal order, awareness, and controls. Familiarity with the MPD patient over time allows the psychotherapists, aftercare, and rehabilitation workers to develop appropriately increasing expectations. They can reflect back to the MPD patient the progress achieved. The patient's experience of progress over time can be a potent incentive.

If the patient's outside living situation has been satisfactory, its continued availability during rehospitalizations can be an important inducement for the patient to recover effective functioning. Jana's apartment was the realization of one of her strongest dreams. Visits to it while hospitalized often inspired the "caretaking committee of alters" to work on whatever had to be done to get out of the hospital again.

Development of an outside support system.   The initiative for developing a support system outside the hospital will probably have to come from the treatment team, who should communicate the expectation that the MPD patient will become an autonomously functioning member of the community. An early treatment goal should be helping the MPD patient to formulate life goals outside the hospital. The MPD patient may need to be taught how to develop and use short-term and intermediate goals. Ways to begin development of an outside support system include the following:

1. Beginning to use a primary care physician outside the hospital and filling prescriptions at a nonhospital pharmacy;

2. Entering an education or training program outside the mental health system;
3. Participating in community social organizations, including ones for former mental patients;
4. Spending time with friends outside the hospital; and
5. Finding part-time employment.

Conclusions

As increasing numbers of previously unrecognized MPD patients are identified in chronic care facilities, their appropriate rehabilitation and deinstitutionalization will become a growing concern. Their outpatient management offers the hope of a new life to individual patients and the prospect of significant economic benefits to the state system in which they are found. Attention to the issues discussed in this chapter may facilitate such transitions.

References

Bliss EL: Multiple personalities: a report of 14 cases with implications for schizophrenia and hysteria. Arch Gen Psychiatry 37:1388–1397, 1980

Caul D: Group and videotape techniques for multiple personality disorder. Psychiatric Annals 7:51–68, 1984

Coons PM: The differential diagnosis of multiple personality. Psychiatr Clin North Am 7:51–68, 1984

Drye RC, Goulding RL, Goulding ME: No-suicide decisions: patient monitoring of suicidal risk. Am J Psychiatry 130:171–174, 1973

Kluft RP: The treatment of multiple personality disorder. Psychiatric Annals 14:51–55, 1984

Kluft RP: The Treatment of Multiple Personality Disorder (MPD): Current Concepts (Directions in Psychiatry, Vol 5, Lesson 24). Edited by Flach FF. New York, Hatherleigh, 1985a, pp 1–11

Kluft RP: Presentation (untitled) at the Introductory Workshop, Second International Conference on Multiple Personality/Dissociative States, Chicago, IL, October 24, 1985b

Kluft RP: Making the Diagnosis of Multiple Personality Disorder in Diagnostics and Psychopathology. Edited by Flach FF. New York, Norton, 1987a, pp 207–225

Kluft RP: First rank symptoms as a diagnostic clue to multiple personality disorder. Am J Psychiatry 144:293–298, 1987b

Kluft RP: Hospital treatment of multiple personality disorder: an overview. Psychiatr Clin North Am 14:695–719, 1991

Maxmen JS, Tucker GJ, LeBow M: Rational Hospital Psychiatry: The Reactive Environment. New York, Brunner/Mazel, 1974

Opaku S: The psychiatrist and the Social Security Disability and Supplemental Security Income programs. Hosp Community Psychiatry 39:879–883, 1988

Putnam FW, Loewenstein RJ, Silberman EK, et al: Multiple personality disorder in a hospital setting. J Clin Psychiatry 45:175–178, 1984

Putnam FW, Guroff JJ, Silberman EK, et al: The clinical phenomenology of multiple personality disorder: review of 100 recent cases. J Clin Psychiatry 47:285–293, 1986

Thames LH: Limit setting and behavior contracting with the client with MPD. Paper presented at the 1st International Conference on Multiple Personality/Dissociative States, Chicago, IL, September 22, 1984

Turkus J: Psychotherapy and case management for multiple personality disorder: synthesis for continuity of care. Psychiatr Clin North Am 14:649–660, 1991

Chapter 11

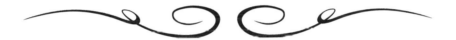

The Use of Amytal Interviews in the Treatment of an Exceptionally Complex Case of Multiple Personality Disorder

Robert A. deVito, M.D.

Throughout my career, I have had a penchant for working with people whose problems have been characterized as diverse, complex, mysterious, and sometimes impossible. Diagnostically, these problems have ranged from adjustment disorders with mixed emotional features to schizophrenic disorders and rare and "unclassifiable" disorders such as *koro* and the Capgras syndrome. Early on in such endeavors, I became interested in dissociative disorders and particularly, multiple personality disorder (MPD), but it wasn't until 1969 that I had the opportunity to diagnose and treat my first case.

At that time—and, I must admit, due in large measure to Gregory Peck's movie portrayal of a psychiatrist in *Captain Newman, M.D.*—I had begun using Amytal (amobarbital) narcosis as an adjunct in the diagnosis and treatment of posttraumatic stress disorder (PTSD), conversion disorders, and dissociative disorders, with significant success. In those instances in which both hypnosis and Amytal were used to induce a state of deep relaxation, MPD patients experienced Amytal as bringing about a more profound narcosis and, hence, a state in which alters could emerge with greater ease. Thus, over the years, I have utilized Amytal more frequently than hypnosis, even though Amytal interviews tend to be more time-consuming and more easily done in inpatient rather than outpatient settings.

To illustrate the strengths and weaknesses of the Amytal interview, I have chosen to share my clinical experience with Nora (a pseudonym), a young woman with whom I continue to work on an intensive basis. I first met Nora in October 1985 on a 35-bed closed general psychiatry inpatient unit at a university hospital medical center. She had been referred to me for a second opinion by a colleague who had diagnosed her as having atypical bipolar disorder, unresponsive to all pharmacologic regimens to date. These regimens had included 1) lithium alone, 2) lithium and chlorpromazine, 3) lithium and thiothixene, 4) lithium and haloperidol, and 5) trifluoperazine alone.

As I discussed the reason for the referral with my colleague in more depth, it became clear that she (my colleague) did not want a second opinion after all. Instead, she wanted me to take over as primary therapist. My colleague had become extremely frustrated with Nora because of Nora's irascibility, rebelliousness, and failure to comply with any and all treatment plans, no matter how sensitively or creatively they had been conceived. It turned out that, in addition to Nora's Axis I diagnosis of atypical bipolar disorder, she had been viewed as having an Axis II diagnosis of borderline personality disorder. Its hallmarks were impulsivity, unpredictability, self-mutilative behavior, overvaluation and devaluation of others (including the unit's staff), identity confusion, and chronic feelings of emptiness. Beyond this, she had exhausted her commercial insurance coverage for inpatient psychiatric care and had applied for medical assistance. In a fit of incredibly clear thinking bordering on autochthonous ideation, I thanked my colleague and accepted the referral sight unseen, giving as my reasons that the patient would be challenging and that she could potentially benefit from being in an educationally stimulating environment. Beyond this, I had the gut feeling that Nora had been misdiagnosed and that, as a consequence, she had not yet been exposed to a potentially therapeutic treatment strategy.

My first encounter with Nora proved to be a riveting experience for both of us. A tall, slender, redheaded woman with pale green eyes, Nora had a striking physical presence. She eyed me with mixed suspiciousness and derision, letting me know that I was simply another in a "long line of shrinks" who would undoubtedly brand her as "crazy," certify her to a state mental hospital, and "feed [her] to the sharks." I told her that her view of the situation made some sense to me, because her records had indicated that before me, she had had 24 therapists in 10 years. These therapists included 14 psychiatrists, 6 psychologists, and 4 social workers, who had collectively evaluated her to have had 15 different psychiatric disorders ranging from catatonic schizophrenia to dysthymia; they had seen fit to certify her to state mental hospitals on 6 different occasions. Although she was only 22 when she first met me, she had already received mental health services in 4 different states. Orphaned at birth, she had lived in 8 different foster homes before being adopted at age 10 by a childless couple who raised her in a far suburb of Chicago.

In our first session, Nora did her best to impress me that she was not only symptom-free but characterologically healthy. It was clear that she was tired of being in psychiatric units, public and private, and that she simply wanted to return to living alone in her suburban apartment in an effort to bring some semblance of "normality" into her life. She had never been married or pregnant, or employed for more than 3 months at a time. She had hoped that since she had been admitted to our psychiatric unit on a "voluntary" basis, I would agree with her and give her an opportunity to have a fresh start.

Despite her efforts to appear as mentally healthy as possible, three of Nora's statements caught my attention:

1. On at least four occasions, she had used the word "we" when she could easily have said "I."
2. When I asked her if she had ever had the experience of discovering clothing in her closet for which she could not account or of noticing entries in her checkbook that she did not remember

making, she hesitated and looked surprised and momentarily bewildered before answering "no."

3. On five different occasions, she had lost track of what either she or I had been saying, asking me to repeat what had just been said.

The intrainterview amnesia had little diagnostic significance by itself; but in the context of a history of multiple psychiatric hospitalizations and a plethora of therapists, in a person with a spectrum of psychiatric diagnoses, it raised the question of a primary dissociative disorder as the principal clinical condition (Kluft 1987). Nora was to tell me later that she was so "freaked out" by some of my questions that she had thought I had the power to read her mind, yet she "knew" in this first encounter that I would "be the person to really help her."

Nora's first hospital stay lasted 10 days. It included a blend of biological and psychological evaluations and resulted in her being diagnosed as having a mixed bipolar disorder with melancholic and dissociative features, requiring a mood regulator, Lithobid (lithium) and a noradrenergic antidepressant, Norpramin (desipramine). These medications were selected on the basis of ongoing clinical observations, entries by Nora in her own "mood journal," and psychoendocrine testing that revealed an abnormal dexamethasone suppression test (DST) and a normal thyrotropin stimulation test (TST) and serum prolactin test (SPT). Both Nora and the psychiatric staff noted that her moods would "cycle" several times a day, covering a range from "deep despondency" to hyperthymia punctuated by episodic tearfulness. Though at times her short-term memory was poor, at other times Nora displayed a particularly astute memory and was capable of remembering events with richness, detail, and accuracy. On two occasions while on the psychiatric inpatient unit, Nora experienced minor fugue states, during which she would find herself in the rooms of other patients, completely confused as to how she got there. When she first regained awareness of her surroundings, she was disoriented as to time, place, person, and situation, as well as amnesic for what had occurred. Despite these events, she asked that she be permitted to be discharged after 10 days in order to return to her apartment, obtain a job, and begin seeing me for outpatient psychotherapy.

In the ensuing 9 months, Nora managed to maintain her apartment while working as a waitress in a posh suburban restaurant. However, in the spring of 1986 she began to experience increasing episodes of "lost time," both at home and on the job. On one occasion during a holiday weekend, she found herself at a roadside bar in Wisconsin, totally at a loss to explain how she had gotten there. Later, she discovered a road map in the glove compartment of her car that revealed a "route" penned in red from her home to Milwaukee, Wisconsin. She did not recall outlining the route, nor did she remember knowing anybody in Milwaukee. To her further dismay, she found in her purse the names, addresses, and phone numbers of two men from the Milwaukee area who were total strangers to her.

Given the intensity and frequency of her "lost time" episodes (not to mention the embarrassing situations in which she had begun to find herself), Nora agreed to a voluntary hospital stay to better understand what was happening to her and to learn to regain control of her life. She was thus admitted for a second time on July 16, 1986, and placed on "elopement precautions" to alert the staff of her rapidly changing mental status.

During my first inpatient individual session with Nora, she appeared to experience a cascade of quick and facile changes, too numerous to identify clearly. She seemed to be experiencing what I have described as "dissociative panic" (deVito 1984). One could sense an overwhelming fear deep within her. The personality transformations were so rapid that they disguised a dominant mood state or major psychological issue within any single alter. Speaking very firmly but quietly, I tried to acknowledge her distress, without mentioning anything about a possible diagnosis of MPD. I did not confront her with the possibility of seclusion, leather restraints, electroconvulsive therapy, certification, and ultimate commitment to another psychiatric facility, or anything that I anticipated her alters would perceive as threatening. Rather, I let what was happening "happen," and I tried to remember and to document as much of it as I could. I suggested that she keep an "experience" journal similar to the "mood" journal that she had kept during her first psychiatric hospitalization, a journal with dates and times of disremembered experiences and signatures of those who were undergoing the experiences. It did not appear at first that she understood me, but later I was to learn that "the system did."

It was during this admission that I first suggested the possible use of Amytal narcosis as an alternative to hypnosis in helping Nora better access perceptions, feelings, thoughts, and behaviors (my version of Bennett Braun's 1988 BASK System). She had already described an aversion to hypnosis, but she did not seem totally at ease with Amytal narcosis either. I gave her two journal articles to read on the subject. The first described a single case study of the Amytal-facilitated treatment of MPD (Hall et al. 1978); the second offered a more general description of its uses in an emergency room setting (Perry and Jacobs 1982).

By the next day, Nora decided to try this treatment intervention on two conditions: first, that the interview be audiotaped for review during psychotherapy sessions; and second, that if probing produced too much anxiety, dysphoria, or dissociation, her request to halt the proceedings would be honored. I agreed that both requests were reasonable and informed her that they in fact were part of the routine procedure for Amytal narcosis. All patients undergoing this procedure are given the option of having their interviews either audiotaped or videotaped or, for that matter, the right of declining to have them recorded. From a medicolegal standpoint, the taped interview material belongs to the patient and can be used for educational or other purposes only with the patient's fully informed, written consent. For the first and all subsequent interviews, we obtained two written consents: consent to do the interview and consent to have the interview audiotaped.

Initial orders were as follows:

1. Patient reclining in bed in a semidarkened room
2. Nothing by mouth as of midnight of the previous day
3. All medical materials relating to the interview to be on the unit as of 8:00 A.M. of the interview day
4. Amytal: Three (3) 250-mg vials
5. Three (3) 10-cc syringes with three (3) 1-inch 18-gauge needles

6. Three (3) 1-inch 22-gauge needles with intracatheter setups
7. One intravenous (IV) stand with an extension, arm board, and tourniquet
8. 1,000 cc 5% dextrose in water

It was explained to Nora that intracatheter setups would be used in lieu of scalp vein or butterfly needles because of the tendency of patients with traumatic histories to thrash about once under the influence of Amytal. On the day of her first Amytal narcosis, Nora was extremely anxious. Just prior to the introduction of the intravenous intracatheter, she demanded to check the 5% distilled water bag as well as each syringe to make certain that all were free of air bubbles. Despite our reassurances, she seemed to be reexperiencing a series of traumatic events and was under the misperception that she would be given a lethal bolus of air intravenously. Within moments, her veins seemed to collapse, making it impossible for us to start her intravenous line. However, when I acknowledged the existence of "presences" within her who seemed able to control her autonomic nervous system, her veins filled, making intravenous entry possible.

In the course of the first Amytal interview with Nora, which was witnessed by a psychiatric resident and a medical student, four alters emerged, confirming the diagnosis of MPD. Two of the four were children—Nora Ann, age 7, and Molly, age 8. Both alters reported memories of a satanic cult group with whom Nora was seemingly involved between ages 7 and 8, while she lived in foster homes in Nebraska. (The reader may wish to consult Ganaway 1989 and Kluft 1989 for a discussion of the issues raised by such allegations. Also, Lanning 1991, Putnam 1991, Sakheim and Devine 1992, Jones 1991, and Young and colleagues 1991 provide a variety of opinions about these phenomena and their veracity.) However, in the clinical context, I elected to meet Nora "where she was at."

Nora Ann recalled vivid scenes of ritualistic sacrifices in which both children and adolescents died following some kind of injections; Molly described similar rituals in which individuals in black hooded robes had to drink something in golden cups that tasted "awful." These "child" alters spoke in childlike voices, expressing intense fear and helplessness. Their emergences were spontaneous and occurred when the Amytal dose was between 175 and 230 mg. Before each alter surfaced, Nora experienced an intense left frontotemporal headache of sudden onset and brief duration. The headache would disappear with the emergence of either Nora Ann or Molly, but it reappeared as an equally intense right frontotemporal headache with the reappearance of Nora. Headaches are such common phenomena in work with MPD patients that I have developed the terms "entrance" and "exit" headaches, with entrance headaches signifying the imminent emergence of alters and exit headaches reflecting their disappearance. It is my view that MPD headaches are vascular in nature. This is suggested by regional cerebral blood flow studies that demonstrate numerous cerebral perfusion abnormalities in individuals with MPD, including distinct contrasting abnormalities between host personalities and their alters (deVito et al. 1985).

With a dose of Amytal between 300 mg and 575 mg, two extremely angry alters emerged, neither of whom would offer a name or a physical description to facilitate her identification. One told us (the psychiatric resident, medical student, and me) to "get lost," because further probing could prove dangerous to our health. When I noted that, as threatening as that statement may have sounded, it also sounded "like fear," the alter left, and Nora reemerged with a pounding occipital headache. I gave her the option to listen to the voice of this angry alter to see if she could recognize it. This provided Nora with an opportunity to acquaint herself with a very unfamiliar part of herself. She indicated that she had heard that voice before on at least two occasions; each time it had exhorted her to jump out of a moving automobile. On both occasions she had resisted the pressure, but she was left deeply shaken by the experience. She had come to think that she might be "crazy," that perhaps some of those psychotic diagnoses she had received were "right on the button." Despite this, there was something else, some other force or voice within her telling her to "hang on."

At the level of 500 mg of Amytal a second angry alter surfaced, even more rageful than the first. It was difficult to determine the gender of the alter, because the voice seemed deep and raspy. "It" asked what I wanted, and when I suggested that I wanted to know more about "it," it replied: "None of your business. She's mine.

They're all mine." At that point, "it" faded and within about 40 seconds, Nora "returned" once again, this time with a violent occipitotemporal-retro-ocular headache. Gradually the headache dulled and Nora was able to reorient herself as to place, person, and situation. When this segment of tape was replayed, Nora claimed not to recognize the voice, but she did appear to be viscerally shaken by it. She demonstrated the abrupt appearance of a left-sided piloerection. The skin on her left arm and left leg seemed cooler than that of her right upper and lower extremities. Nora could not offer any insight about these phenomena. She seemed to be fully alert at the level of 600 mg of Amytal but suddenly switched yet again for just a few seconds before apparently falling unconscious. Within 2 minutes, Nora emerged again, completely alert but totally amnesic for what had just happened. At this juncture we concluded the first Amytal interview.

I encountered similar phenomena during many Amytal interviews. Varying levels of alertness among different alters on the same "dose" level of Amytal were quite common. These phenomena may reflect regional cerebral differences in blood flow across the personalities, but as of yet no methodologically sound study has definitively established such a correlation.

In the 5 years following her second hospital stay in our inpatient unit, Nora underwent a course of intensive, psychodynamically oriented psychotherapy, averaging 2 1½-hour sessions per week on an outpatient basis and 2 50-minute sessions per day when she was an inpatient. These sessions were augmented by 66 Amytal interviews, all in inpatient settings, and by 24 hypnotherapy sessions, all in outpatient settings. On two occasions I combined the use of Amytal and hypnosis to approach two specific conflict areas. Between 1985 and the present, Nora has had a total of 9 psychiatric hospitalizations ranging in duration from 10 days to 3 months. Her Amytal usage per session has averaged 640 mg, with a range of 450–900 mg. We do no more than two Amytal interviews per week, and we process both with conventional therapy sessions and sessions for audiotape review.

Nora's psychotherapy, Amytal interviews, and hypnotherapy were augmented by the following:

1. Her writings in her "experience" journal;
2. The "milieu" observations and therapeutic interventions of the inpatient unit's treatment staff;
3. Ongoing communication with Nora's adoptive parents, with her permission and most often with her active participation; and
4. The periodic use of a multiple personality map documenting identifying data and other important information about the birth personality and every alter, fragment, and special-purpose fragment (Braun 1986).

In the course of this treatment, it has emerged that Nora has most likely been dissociating since her earliest years and that several overlapping systems of dissociated elements developed within her, each organized and dominated by an oppositional alter, as listed in Table 11–1.

The systems identified in Table 11–1 were discovered in the order in which they are numbered, a reflection of the phenomenon of "layering" (Kluft 1984, 1986). Some alters play a role in all four systems.

Including the presenting or birth personality, Nora; the four dominant oppositionals; and the 122 alters, fragments, and special-purpose fragments, a total of 127 personality elements were documented. It is of interest that there was a 128th personality, known as "The Timeless One," a female alter who claimed to be separate and distinct from Nora and from all of the major dissociative systems within Nora. She saw herself as both ageless and timeless and as having been present in Nora's life from before the time of her birth. She emerged only when Nora showered because of her attraction to the feeling of water spraying on her skin. I became aware of her presence through writings in Nora's experience journal, done just after showers had been taken. Her existence was confirmed with the help of a female psychiatric resident who arranged to interview her immediately after Nora had showered. The resident described this alter as soft-spoken but articulate, intelligent, mysterious, and quite knowledgeable about Nora. She offered no name, no age, and no self-description, except to say that she would always be there "in some form." She was neutral to the other alters and she predicted that a unification of all personalities would eventually take place. A final fusion of these alters occurred on August 17, 1989, after working through several issues, themes, and feelings that preoccupied System #4. Since the final fusion, we have not "heard" from "The Timeless One" or from any other alter, even on direct invitation or hypnotic inquiry.

Perhaps "The Timeless One" is best understood as a memory trace personality, a concept first described by Cornelia Wilbur. I have come to regard alters, regardless of their function and elaborateness, as being analogous to living memories of a hidden past—memory

Table 11–1. Nora's systems of dissociated elements

System #1:	Claire and 27 alters foster mother #3 introject	Established to cope with feelings of pathological jealousy toward various foster parents, siblings, and peers
System #2:	Asudem (Medusa spelled backwards) and 22 alters satanic cult "queen" introject	Developed to ensure survival while coping with feelings stimulated by exposure to ritualized satanic cult abuse, including human and animal sacrifice, burials, torture, beatings, brainwashing, sexual abuse, and programmed intimidation
System #3:	Nathan and 43 alters foster father #3 introject	Designed to maintain survival while dealing with feelings triggered by early childhood trauma that occurred in foster homes #3, #5, and #7, involving foster mothers #3 and #7 and foster fathers #3 and #5. These feelings include rage, helplessness, fearfulness, humiliation, guilt, shame, and confusion and anxiety over gender and sexuality.
System #4:	Marsha and 30 alters biological mother introject (maternal imago)	Created to cope with personal losses and their impacts on her emerging self-representations and her dissociative defenses. These losses included her biological twin sister, multiple foster parents, and a fetus that was aborted in the fourth month of gestation. In the context of these losses, the feelings that were ignited included profound sadness, guilt, futility, aloneness, deep anger, and self-abnegation.

banks initially inaccessible to the presenting personality, but increasingly accessible with psychotherapy. One might construe a memory trace personality as a form of partial dissociation—an internalized, depersonalized self, aware of a sequential series of events but not necessarily aware of the feelings that those events evoked. If they are aware of such feelings, they may not be able to communicate those feelings directly.

Since August 1989, Nora has steadily developed an increasingly strong sense of self, with enhanced self-esteem and self-confidence. She now has a new apartment, a new job, and a new car. Her relationship with her adoptive parents is becoming more mutually satisfying and reciprocal. She has begun to attend self-help groups aimed at enhancing her socialization skills. In psychotherapy, she has been dealing with a concatenation of feelings, perceptions, and cognitions previously hidden in the layered alter systems. In so doing, she has been experiencing a series of PTSD symptoms, particularly flashbacks of childhood abuse experiences (Ross et al. 1989; Spiegel 1984); but thus far, she has been up to the challenge of facing the feelings connected with these traumatic events without dissociating again. She has gained insight into her role in the genesis and development of her dissociative disorder and has come to value the impact of psychotherapy on her personal growth.

Conclusions

To summarize the strengths and weaknesses of Amytal narcosis as an adjunct in the treatment of MPD, it can be a very useful alternative to hypnosis. Some patients who have experienced both believe that Amytal is more efficacious than hypnosis in breaking through resistances. On the other hand, it is more time-consuming and more labor-intensive than hypnosis. Though I have found it to be medically safe, it is possible that one could accidentally induce a respiratory depression by infusing Amytal too rapidly. The mechanism is its direct activation of chloride channel iontophoresis, with resultant hyperpolarization of brain stem medullary respiratory centers.

One other danger is that the more frequent the Amytal narcosis, the greater the possibility for the development of barbiturate dependence and abuse. Thus far, I have encountered two MPD patients who have admitted to having alters who enjoyed "getting high" on the Amytal. In both instances, when the problem was recognized and acknowledged, it ceased to be an issue of contention.

Finally, study of the effects of Amytal-facilitated interviews on regional cerebral blood flow may provide scientists with new insights into the biological underpinnings of dissociative disorders. Because Amytal interviews have both clinical utility and research potential, I would strongly advocate their continuing use and study in this burgeoning field.

References

Braun BG: Introduction, in Treatment of Multiple Personality Disorder. Edited by Braun BG. Washington, DC, American Psychiatric Press, 1986, pp xi xxi

Braun BG: The BASK (behavior, affect, sensation, knowledge) model of dissociation. Dissociation 1(1):4–23, 1988

deVito RA: Explorations into the phenomenology, etiology, and treatment of multiple personality disorder, in Dissociative Disorders 1984—Proceedings of the First International Conference on Multiple Personality/Dissociative States. Edited by Braun BG. Chicago, IL, Rush University, 1984, p 2

deVito RA, Braun BG, Karesh S, et al: Regional cerebral blood flow studies in MPD, in Dissociative Disorders 1985—Proceedings of the Second International Conference on Multiple Personality/Dissociative States. Edited by Braun BG. Chicago, IL, Rush University, 1985, p 84

Ganaway GK: Historical truth versus narrative truth: clarifying the role of exogenous trauma in the etiology of multiple personality disorder and its variants. Dissociation 2:205–220, 1989

Hall RCW, LeCann AF, Schoolar JC: Amobarbital treatment of multiple personality. J Nerv Ment Dis 166:666–670, 1978

Jones DPH: Commentary: ritualism and child sexual abuse. Child Abuse Negl 15:163–170, 1991

Kluft RP: Treatment of multiple personality disorder: a study of 33 cases. Psychiatr Clin North Am 7:9–29, 1984

Kluft RP: Personality unification in multiple personality disorder: a follow-up study, in Treatment of Multiple Personality Disorder. Edited by Braun BG. Washington, DC, American Psychiatric Press, 1986, pp 29–60

Kluft RP: Making the diagnosis of multiple personality disorder, in Diagnostics and Psychopathology. Edited by Flach FF. New York, WW Norton, 1987, pp 207–225

Kluft RP: Reflections on allegation of ritual abuse (editorial). Dissociation 2:191–193, 1989

Lanning KV: Commentary: ritual abuse: a law enforcement view or perspective. Child Abuse Negl 15:171–174, 1991

Perry JC, Jacobs D: Overview: clinical applications of the amytal interview in psychiatric emergency settings. Am J Psychiatry 139:552–558, 1982

Putnam FW: Commentary: the satanic ritual abuse controversy. Child Abuse Negl 15:175–180, 1991

Ross CA, Heber S, Norton GR, et al: The dissociative disorders interview schedule: a structured interview. Dissociation 2:169–189, 1989

Sakheim DK, Devine SE (eds): Out of Darkness: Exploring Satanism and Ritual Abuse. New York, Lexington, 1992

Spiegel D: Multiple personality as a post-traumatic stress disorder. Psychiatr Clin North Am 7:101–110, 1984

Young WC, Sachs RG, Braun BG, et al: Patients reporting ritual abuse in childhood: a clinical syndrome. Child Abuse Negl 15:181–190, 1991

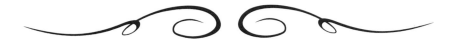

Observations on the Role of Transitional Objects and Transitional Phenomena in Patients With Multiple Personality Disorder

David Fink, M.D.

D. W. Winnicott described the transitional object as the first "not me" object (Winnicott 1971). In his view, the transitional object arises at a time when self and other are not clearly differentiated. It occupies a unique intermediate area of experience, which facilitates the child's gradual process of separation from the mother, and nascent self- and object definition. Winnicott describes this realm of experience: "The intermediate area to which I am referring is the area that is allowed to the infant between primary creativity and objective perception based on reality testing" (1971, p. 11). The transitional object, then, is not a part of the symbiotic hallucination of the infant-mother, nor is it a separate, external part of reality perceptions. The transitional object is both at the same time. It is the magical imbuing of a material possession with the comforting qualities

241

of the mother. By means of this creative use of illusion, the child begins to gradually negotiate separation from the parent and consolidate the distinctions between inside and outside, dream and reality, and self and other (Deri 1978).

It has been my observation that many patients with multiple personality disorder (MPD) possess and have remained deeply attached to transitional objects. What is more, many of the feelings and the patterns of interrelatedness described with their transitional objects are similar to the way these patients describe and experience their relationship with certain of their alters. In this regard, it is my contention that certain alters serve a transitional function.

Winnicott (1971) alludes to possible pathological disturbances that may occur during and disrupt the transitional object phase. He states, "An infant may be so disturbed in emotional development that the transitional state cannot be enjoyed, or the sequence of object use is broken. The sequence may nevertheless be maintained in a hidden way" (p. 5). Marmer (1980) describes how alters can represent transitional objects that are forced inward, and states that the exigencies of severe trauma may not allow the use of external transitional objects. It is the hidden continuation of this transitional process that is at times a fundamental aspect of the process of creation and pathological persistence of alter states.

In this chapter, I review several cases of MPD in which alters were observed to function in a transitional way. I illustrate how these personality states occupy the intermediate area of experience between "me" and "not me" that Winnicott describes, and how they serve a transitional object function by maintaining a stabilizing self object bond that assuages the difficulties of traumatically engendered separation and loss.

Alters can be formed based on representations of either the self or the other, although their connection to their point of origin may become quite disguised. Both types of personalities can serve a transitional function. When the alter is based on an object, the individual's subjective experience of that alter is a strong sense of the other's presence. Regardless of whether this is a positive or negative representation of the other, this type of alter serves to preserve the threatened attachment.

When alters are based on a representation of the self, they function as transitional objects to the extent that they provide a link to aspects of the self that are experienced as more soothing, coherent, capable under certain circumstances, or whole. In many instances these alters are split-off self states that are adaptive versions of the self used to survive specific abuse. These self-based alters are held in relation to the primary personality in much the way a transitional object is held by the child; like the transitional object, the alternate version of the self serves a stabilizing function.

In general, then, in addition to the more familiar appreciation of alters as dissociated posttraumatic defensive organizations, these same alter states contain the unresolved relationship to the ambivalently held object. Particularly in those cases in which the dynamic interaction between the primary personality and the alters is persistent and represents a primary preoccupation for the patient, the stabilizing functions of the alters must be explored. Although alters may obviously persist as an indication of incompletely worked through traumata, they may also persist because they play an essential homeostatic function in the form of a transitional object.

The Case of Melissa

Melissa was a 32-year-old single woman from a small factory town who was admitted to the hospital for treatment of nearly continuous dissociative episodes and incessant uncontrolled switching among alter states. She was the sixth of seven children born to a working-class Catholic family. After Melissa's birth, her mother experienced a postpartum depression. During her next pregnancy, which occurred when Melissa was two, complications necessitated the mother being away from home and in the hospital for weeks at a time. When Melissa was five, her mother again experienced a serious depression and made a suicide attempt. Not only was her mother unstable and unavailable, but her father was by Melissa's report a rigid, angry, and authoritarian man. He was verbally and physically threatening and abusive. Melissa reported genital contact with her father from the age of four, with digital penetration. She also described her father's preoccupation with cleansing her. He frequently maintained that she was dirty and "required" his scrubbing her genitals in order for her to be clean.

Melissa's development of an inner world of alters dates from about the age of two, with her persistent sense of a baby for whom she would care. Over the years a total of six alters came into being. Each had a specific age and a set of well-defined characteristics. The alters ranged in age from 2 to 14. Melissa reported the persistence of dialogues within her head among these "others" and "between the others and [her]self."

For each alter, Melissa had a stuffed animal that bore the name of that alter. By her report, her acquisitions of the stuffed animals all chronologically followed (in most cases by years) her sense of the internal presence of the alters. She was conscientiously concerned with the well-being of her stuffed animals. They were regularly cared for and nurtured; she would hold and rock and talk to each of them. She described ongoing dialogues with each stuffed animal, dialogues that corresponded to her dialogues with the alter of the same name. She would describe in detail the concerns of each, such as "L. doesn't like to be rolled on her back" or "S. is so frightened that she can't move and can only look out from blackened eyes." Both the alters and their externalized representations in the stuffed animals were for Melissa the repositories of dissociated memories. Each represented a view of herself as a young girl; each related a particular set of traumatic memories with well-defined sets of responses to trauma, including fear, despair, catatonic immobility, and the wish to flee from harm. Each also contained a set of visual and somatic memories.

As in most cases of MPD, Melissa's alters were part of an overall dissociative response to physical and sexual abuse. In addition to their adaptive role in the face of acute trauma, Melissa's alters served an additional stabilizing function. Melissa received essential comfort from the presence of the alters. The personalities were fantasy-based constructions of herself that, during development, she had used to manage her mother's absences and her father's violence. As highly adaptive views of herself, the alters were experienced by Melissa as more powerful or capable then she. With the unavailability of external, reality-based sources of protection and soothing, Melissa attempted to comfort herself by means of a splitting of the ego and the formation of alters. These split-off aspects of herself were then experienced, and relied upon, as transitional objects in an effort to maintain her psychological equilibrium. Melissa's reliance on her alters in this way is consistent with Marmer's (1980) view that traumatic circumstances inhibit normal outward expression of transitional objects and supports the notion that some alters are transitional objects that have been driven inward.

The Case of Beatrice

In addition to easing the pain of separation, transitional objects play a role in the development of an increasingly reality-based construction of self and others, as observed by Winnicott (1971). Beatrice's use of transitional objects demonstrates both of these developmental functions.

Beatrice, a 35-year-old writer with MPD, was hospitalized because of sustained dissociative episodes. After these spells she had found herself mutilated inexplicably. A host of voices in her head dominated her thoughts, and she was overwhelmed by the conflicting directives and commands that were constantly being voiced. A complex system of alters was defined in the course of her assessment.

During the course of treatment, several central dynamic themes became clear. The first was Beatrice's terror of being "seen." To identify herself—to be "seen" in a physical or psychological sense—was to be exposed to a great risk of destruction. Her abusers had threatened to kill her if she spoke of what had occurred. Consequently, she feared that any revelation she made in treatment would be considered a betrayal of her instructions. Her highly complex system of alters was designated to maintain secrecy, hiddenness, and invisibility.

In the early months of therapy, each time an alter would emerge, spontaneously or at my request, Beatrice would feel that this had occurred at the risk of her annihilation. After such emergences, she would frequently hear voices in her head threatening her for revealing herself. Not infrequently, she would experience an intense revisitation of traumatic flashbacks, which she would interpret as a punishment for her wrongdoing. In the early months of treatment, an alter's contact with me would be followed by its disappearance. In Beatrice's world, these alters had been "banished" and further access to her or myself would, for a time, be declined. Despite Beatrice's enormous distress and determined motivation for treatment, she found herself initially unable to directly and openly engage in the psychotherapy.

A number of symbolic interactions that relied on the use of transitional objects came to play an important role at this time during the psychotherapy. In this regard, Beatrice used a number of transitional objects to concretely express her struggles between her wish to reveal and explore her traumatic experiences and her terror of being destroyed if she were to do so. Over time we came to understand how she was using these transitional objects in her effort to define herself, myself, and our relationship to one another.

Several examples will illustrate the nature of these transitional phenomena. Early in our work, Beatrice pointed out a complex arrangement of glass beads on her desk. She indicated that in the arrangement there was always a fixed triad of beads that was in a shifting relation to a configuration of some 20 or 30 other beads. Beatrice revealed that the triad of beads was a representation of me and that the ever-changing larger grouping of beads depicted herself. She pointed out how the bead representation of herself was in continuous flux, whereas the representation of me was constant. Furthermore, she indicated how the bead representation of myself was in a shifting physical spatial relation to the larger grouping. Each day the arrangement of beads on her desk would be different. Sometimes the two groupings would be in close proximity to one another, but on other days they would be separated by a great distance. Sometimes no beads were to be found at all.

Beatrice's beads served as transitional objects in several respects. First, as we studied the bead representation of herself, we discovered that individual beads within the organization were identified as representations of important individuals from her past. She referred to several of the beads as dybbuks, or dead souls. These beads were literally a part of her effort to hold onto and maintain a sense of connectedness to individuals she had lost.

Other subsets of beads within the bead representation of herself were identified as representations of known alters. These alters were representations of divergent views of herself. Although they varied widely in terms of their particular presentations (i.e., many were views of a young girl, whereas others were powerful male alters, etc.), they all fundamentally represented the dynamic interplay between Beatrice and an abusive other. On the one hand, these representations of herself represented versions of Beatrice as an individual who could successfully remain connected to an abusive but essential other. They were created in an effort to sustain the literal relationship between herself and her abusers. They allowed her to maintain her object bond by dint of a recreation of the self. On the other hand, however, they reflected the extreme inaccessibility of the other as a stabilizing force. Because of the profound disturbance of the stabilizing interpersonal bond, she resorted to using split-off aspects of her self for this purpose. Many of the alters represented powerful, comforting, protective, or whole versions of herself on whom she then relied. In this regard, these alters functioned as transitional objects.

As I noted previously, in addition to the complex bead representation of herself, Beatrice had identified three beads that were a representation of me. This triad of beads was a stable and reliable presence. Between sessions, Beatrice would change the organization of the beads, and in this process the relation of this triad to the larger grouping would change. Beatrice used the bead representation of me as a transitional object that helped her to symbolically hold onto a sense of myself while I was away, and also negotiated a tolerable relation between us representationally for when we would again be together.

In the sixth month of therapy, Beatrice introduced a doll that she had made. The doll was in fact only the head of a doll made of rags and paper. She had one eye, long strands of hair painted blood red, and a neck. The doll was introduced with a name familiar to both of us as that of one of her alters. Beatrice related to this doll intimately. She treated her lovingly and respectfully. She spent much time holding her, soothing her, and listening to her. Initially this figure was a comfort to Beatrice, someone who could ease her pervasive terror and panic. At night she would frequently sleep with the doll in her arms. At times she would withdraw from the doll in fright, saying "She was telling me things I could not bear." Beatrice clearly recognized the doll as a thing, but not just a thing. She was a doll but was also experienced as a separate, important other. A true transitional object, the doll was "neither external object nor powerful wishful hallucination; it was both at the same time" (Deri 1978, p. 51).

In time a second figure was created. The second doll possessed a different set of qualities but served a similar stabilizing role for Beatrice. As with the first figure, the second was based on a known alter. Both of these figures took on an increasingly important role in the therapy and were experienced by Beatrice in much the same way that she experienced alters. Both these figures and the alters carried on dialogues with her, provided her with information, and served an essential role in her emotional homeostasis. These two dolls were created at a time in the therapy when Beatrice was almost continuously flooded with traumatic memories and desperately struggling to find a source of comfort or relief from their almost continuous onslaught. In the world of her alters, she had become able to identify a number of "protective" alters that could help her get through times of crisis. The dolls became tangible representations of two of these alters. The alters (and subsequently the dolls) functioned as transitional objects for Beatrice as they allowed her to feel a connection to a sense of the presence of a comforting other.

Beatrice's relationship to the transitional objects and their parallel representation as alters reflects the similarity in psychological function carried out by these tangible and intrapsychic representations. In the course of her psychotherapy, it was an indication of therapeutic progress that the transitional object role played by the alters could be gradually reexternalized and come into view in the intermediate space of the psychotherapy.

Discussion

The persistent use of transitional objects for Melissa and Beatrice and the associations between their transitional objects and their alters allow for a number of observations about the significance of transitional phenomena for these two individuals with MPD. In addition, such use provides an opportunity to explore the relationship between transitional objects, dissociative disorders, and those forms of psychopathology that arise subsequent to experiences of sustained abuse. The normal developmental role of transitional objects is to help the child negotiate separation from the mother and to make the fundamental distinctions between "me" and "not me," inside and outside, fantasy and reality. The developmental phase of transitional objects and transitional phenomena is the time when, under favorable conditions, the child comes to terms with the impingements of reality into his or her world and gradually relinquishes omnipotent fantasy for reality-based perception. When abuse intervenes, it undermines the child's ability to define physical, psychical, and interpersonal boundaries and blurs the growing distinction between inside and outside and between self and other. Abuse impinges on the child's efforts to relinquish a primary reliance on fantasy and develop more reality-based perceptions and relatedness.

In the event of such trauma, the bond between the child and the other is radically ruptured. Under these circumstances, the persistence of a transitional object represents the child's effort to sustain a fantasy connection with the other. In MPD, the most extreme sequela of such abuse, the persistence of transitional objects and/or the creation of alters serve a similar dynamic function in that they represent the individual's wish to sustain object relatedness.

As Winnicott (1971) writes, "Just before loss (i.e., the child's relinquishing of his [or her] transitional object) we can sometimes see the exaggeration of the use of a transitional object as a part of denial that there is a threat to its becoming meaningless" (p. 5). In normal development, this loss of meaning in the particular transitional object is tolerated, because its meaning becomes generalized and "diffused . . . spread out over the whole cultural field" (Winnicott 1971, p. 5). Under the pathological conditions of severe abuse, however, this process of generalization can be inhibited, and the transitional object that was initially created to serve as a temporary bridge to the other during absence becomes a necessary substitute for the other in toto. It no longer serves a temporary or transitional function but, in Greenacre's (1971) words, takes on a fetishistic quality and becomes an emotional "patch." The very real experience of the loss of meaning of the object as a result of physical, sexual, or psychological trauma necessitates the persistent reliance on a substitute in the form of a transitional object or an alter.

Although the existence of alters and the persistence of transitional objects implies the "fetishistic" need described by Greenacre (1971), the degree of fixation is variable. In the case of Melissa, the possibility of separation from or loss of the stuffed animals and, similarly, the possibility of integration of her alters filled her with overwhelming anxiety. She mounted unyielding resistance to preserve her autistic world of alters and clearly indicated that any steps toward integration (which for her meant intolerable separation) had to be rebuffed out of her fear that she could not survive without her created "objects." Melissa's alters protected her from the terror of separation and the associated sense of loss of identity and "dissolution." Her primary allegiance was ultimately to her alters rather than to reality-based relatedness with external others.

In contrast to Melissa, Beatrice was able to move beyond this fetishistic reliance on alters to a true transitional phase during the course of therapy. For Beatrice, this progress was seen in her movement from the protective hiddenness of her alters and their inner world of relatedness, to their revelation and subsequent tangible representation in the form of beads and dolls. This was understood by Beatrice as movement from an internal object relatedness (with its primary reliance on fantasy) to a phase of transitional experience, and subsequently to a more reality-based object relatedness in the transference relationship.

For Beatrice, the use of transitional objects was a way of bringing her experience into the intermediate space where both she and I could view it together. It was a tentative, exploratory attempt at interpersonal relatedness. In the bead play, our proximity to one another was tested in representational form, and I was ultimately included, in bead form, as one of her transitional objects. Beatrice began to increasingly use this transitional representation of myself as a stabilizing source. Gradually, the transitional objects gave way to a more complex object use in the transferential relationship. For her, therapy was the process of giving up the primacy of the self-contained relationships to the alters in favor of interpersonal relatedness in the world.

This therapeutic process very much resembled the "gradual loss of meaning" seen with transitional objects. For Beatrice, the primary importance of certain alters was relinquished as the issues of the transitional phase were worked through in psychotherapy.

References

Deri S: Transitional phenomena: vicissitudes of symbolization and creativity, in Between Reality and Fantasy: Transitional Objects and Phenomena. Edited by Grolnick S. New York, Jason Aronson, 1978, pp 43–60

Greenacre P: The fetish and the transitional object, the transitional object and the fetish: with special reference to the role of illusion. Emotional Growth 1:315–334, 1971

Marmer SS: Psychoanalysis of multiple personality disorder. Int J Psychoanal 61:439–459, 1980

Winnicott DW: Playing And Reality. New York, Basic Books, 1971, pp 1–26

Chapter 13

Play Therapy With Children With Multiple Personality Disorder

Polly Paul McMahon, Ph.D.
Joen Fagan, Ph.D.

Children with multiple personality disorder (MPD) have experienced some form of trauma so severe, intense, or prolonged that the development of two or more dissociated parts to reduce pain and dispel intolerable awareness was seized upon as a means of psychological survival. The sequelae of the trauma may be manifested in a variety of ways, including extreme fear, anger, aggression, withdrawal, or rejection of contact. However, the child with MPD (Kluft 1984, 1985) or incipient MPD (Fagan and McMahon 1984) may first present a carefree and friendly demeanor to the clinician and deny any problems whatever. No matter what the presentation, the treatment of a child with a dissociative disorder has to be predicated on trust. The child may offer information designed to please, to hide from, to test, or to drive the therapist away. In response, the therapist must find a way to build rapport and connect with a deeply wounded youngster. This chapter is based on the authors' assessment of approximately 60 children with dissociative disorders, and one author's (P.P.M.) therapeutic work with 30 such children, half of whom met diagnostic criteria for MPD, and half (with less fully developed signs and phenomena) who would be more appropriately described as having incipient MPD, which would be classified as Dissociative Disorder Not Otherwise Specified (DDNOS).

Gaining entry into the heart of the child with MPD is not an easy task. Play therapy, because it speaks the universal language of childhood and lets the therapist function in a role that avoids authority and judgment, provides an ideal route of access. Play therapy brings adult and child together where hopes as well as painful struggles can be explored. It also provides sufficient distance and space so that defenses can be respected as well. By its very nature, play therapy is tailored for the individual child. The child who behaves aggressively receives something different from the shy or withdrawn child (even if it is the same child showing very different behaviors within and between sessions).

Although therapy must be individually structured for each child, there are some standard guidelines in treatment. The mnemonic *LOVING* helps describe our conceptualization of the tasks of therapy. A somewhat different effort to outline treatment was developed by Kluft (1986a).

> L—Lend an ear—Develop trust.
> O—Outside support—Get help.
> V—Value and find all parts of the system.
> I—Intensify friends in the system—Develop alliances.
> N—Negotiate and release pain.
> G—Go for it! Integrate.

Lend an Ear—Develop Trust

The first stage of listening and gaining trust may take a few sessions or many months. The initial friendliness shown by many MPD children often proves to be what they perceive as a necessary disguise. Life events have given them ample reason to adopt a cooperative appearance, as a defense rather than as an invitation to closeness. Other therapy tasks may proceed while trust is still being established, and trust may develop at variable rates for different parts of the system. In our experience, the question of determining when trust has been established is an intuitive one.

For the angry or hostile child, trust can be developed by permitting a safe and effective means of allowing the expression of anger. Allowing the child to make noise, hit appropriate objects, and have free release of emotions while preventing harm to property or the therapist is essential. Initial efforts to facilitate the release of anger should not be confused with the process of expressing anger in the course of abreaction, which comes much later. The therapist must show the child that anger is accepted and welcomed and the therapist is not afraid of such volatile outbursts. At other times, the angry child may desire no openly interactive contact with the therapist. Simply acknowledging the anger and respecting the silence may be sufficient:

> It's okay if you don't want to talk today. Sometimes if I'm angry, I don't want to talk, so I know how that feels. Or maybe you are not really angry, but just want to be quiet.

Sometimes identifying with the emotion, and allowing it to be experienced secondhand with a toy or a game can be useful:

> Sometimes when I have feelings stuffed inside, I like a small room where I can just feel safe and then say and do anything I want. Other times, I like to move around a lot and sometimes make pictures about how I feel. Maybe you would like to do one of those things?

For the younger child, the therapist might say:

> The great big Mr. Green Frog has been very mad at Mr. Bear all this week. They have had a hard week together. Maybe you can understand how they feel. Let me show you what's been happening. . . .

For the very withdrawn child, building trust may require more therapist initiative, but such efforts must proceed with care so as not to trespass prematurely into the child's space or across the child's emotional boundaries. The first few sessions can well be spent with the therapist using puppets, art, and movement, and sometimes by giving a one-person show. The newer electronic talking toys can be a useful part of the therapeutic armamentarium, especially for children younger than age eight. Some of the toys will repeat words said by the child or therapist; others will tell stories or read poetry that can then be acted out, perhaps by therapist and child together. By these means, information about the course of therapy can be given gently, and it may be possible to gather some of the child's history:

> The children you have seen in this doll house had a life something like your own. The little boy couldn't stay anymore with his mommy and daddy. They were fighting all the time and sometimes they would hurt him. See these marks that he has? I think that they are like the marks that you had before you had all those stitches. Now you just have a scar, but this little boy is still bleeding. Maybe he needs stitches too. . . . So he had to leave his mommy and was in this new home. He felt very sad and angry because strange people were around him all the time. There were even police officers. Can you show me what you think happens next and tell me more about how he might be feeling?
>
> One day he visited a lady who had an office in a house with lots of trees around it. He saw her so he could learn more about feelings. He had lots of different feelings and they were all confused inside. He saw some toys and art supplies just like the ones here. Show me what you think he needs to learn. . . .

Gradually, slowly, personal feelings can be touched. One way of approaching feelings initially may be by making a list of feeling words. Or feelings may be identified through toys and other situations that are nonthreatening. Then different toys can be associated with different feelings, and different situations related. A number of books and games are available that help children label and express emotions. After the child develops a vocabulary for feelings and learns to relate them to different situations and people, he or she may then be willing to relate feelings to moods and experiences. For example, the child may demonstrate through role-playing the feelings a small animal or child has when crossing a street for the first time. Gradually, situations that directly affect the child are confronted:

Can you remember how you felt the first time you came to foster care? Please tell me what that was like. I think it might be sad, angry, and hurting all mixed together. . . .

The child could then be offered toys and art materials for expression, as appropriate for his or her age and interests.

Outside Support—Get Help

Finding support systems within the child's immediate environment is a step that must be accomplished while trust is being developed. Communication must be maintained with all important persons in the child's world, including caseworkers, foster home providers, schoolteachers, and court service workers. Not only parents and stepparents must be kept informed to prevent sabotage of the therapy, but also important friends and relatives. All can be helpful, and it is important that the therapist ensure that they not feel ignored. An alliance with these external therapeutic support networks is most important and should be made as soon as the diagnosis looks probable, and even before the child's major issues are clearly identified.

Contact with important adults will enable the therapist to acquire additional background information and obtain valuable behavioral observations from other people, who may have different perceptions of the child. Communication must be initiated by the therapist, who also encourages helpers to call on a regular basis. Because people may perceive the child and the goals of treatment differently, distrust among the therapeutic network is a likely occurrence. In our experience, keeping communication current among all the "people resources" is necessary for successful therapy. Obviously, it is essential that the therapist be aware of any potential plans or changes that might upset a child or require a large adjustment, such as an operation, a change of schools, a move from one home to another, and so on. These may sound like obvious recommendations; but all too often major changes are made, such as by a casework agency, without contacting the therapist.

An absolutely essential part of assessing resources is evaluating the likelihood that the child is still being abused. If the reports of others and/or the therapist's best judgment suggests that abuse is ongoing, this must be ended before the next stages of therapy can be initiated. The therapist is mandated to report child abuse and suspected child abuse and must fulfill his or her legal obligations. Until the child's safety is absolutely assured, dissociative defenses against the abuse must not be altered or removed. Therapy is often initiated only after the child has been placed in a safe setting, often by his or her removal from the abusing home. If so, the issues associated with separating from family and moving into a new home must be addressed before treating the elements created by the abuse. If the child who will be returned to an abusive family seeks therapy, the focus again must be on eliminating the abuse. Defusing family violence by providing family nurturance, releasing individual feelings and fears, supporting limit setting, finding crisis resources, and negotiating disciplinary actions are essential. Obviously this aspect of treatment may require many months before formal treatment of the child even begins.

In addition to the external support, every child should ideally have at least three personal support resources. Preferably, these are actual people; but if necessary, they may be animals, inanimate objects, or some part of nature. These can be identified by the therapist by simply saying:

> Name three people who are important and care about you. . . . Do you have any animals in your home right now that you love and who love you? . . . I would like to meet some of the special toy friends you have at home. Would you bring them in?
>
> Outside my window in my backyard you can see a big tree. Trees are so fine for touching and they are strong too. Sometimes it can feel good to just go outside and touch a tree. Do you have a tree at your house?

Other resources to help develop internal support include a variety of cognitive and affective games such as those described by Gardner (1975). These include board games designed to identify feelings, ideas, and values, and the creation of stories conveying lessons that can help the child develop badly needed coping resources.

Value and Find All Parts of the System

After trust and diagnosis are established and external resources are assessed and made as supportive and healthy as possible (or weak links contained), the journey into the child's inner world can begin. Until this point, play therapy has been mainly a means of gaining trust, getting acquainted, and establishing boundaries. Although certain boundary situations are universal, some are unique to each therapist-child dyad, simply because people are different. Some therapists tolerate more freedom, responsiveness, and messiness than others; children vary in how much direct intervention they can tolerate, the firmness of the limits they require, and how much freedom they need. Sensitive attention to limit setting, tact and ingenuity in determining how the child can best be approached, and the capacity to understand and to listen without words being spoken are all important ingredients of communication with children.

With the initial assessment accomplished, the therapist is aware of the healthy as well as the problematic elements in the child's personality. With these assets and liabilities in mind, the diagnosis should be explained to the child. Usually he or she has long been aware of having separate selves. In our experience, often these selves are related to imaginary playmates and aspects of self experienced as the "good" child, the "bad" child, and the "hurt" child. With the child's help, a list of all the different parts should be made, together with their characteristics. Fantasy games may serve to define the ones that are known more clearly as well as to discover others. For example, Tommy may be the part of the child who can feel anger and Sally is the one who feels sadness. However, in fantasy or play, it is discovered that Tommy can only be angry at certain people and Sally must act happy when circumstances are stressful. A new solution needs to be discovered to broaden the scope of the emotions. Sometimes the child creates another personality pattern, or seeks help from an animal, an aspect of nature, or the playroom toys to help develop a new and more adaptive response. Mr. Green Frog or Mr. Bear may help Tommy become more broadly angry, whereas a cave (either a fantasy cave or one created from a table and blankets) may provide protection for Sally until she can experience her sadness fully.

Communication with family and teachers about their observations of different personality patterns or sudden changes in behavior is helpful, allowing amplification of the list and the description of personalities to others. The different personality patterns and changes should first be described using behavioral terms. This is less threatening to family and teachers than giving names:

> Johnny shows only a cheerful side in school, but he gets extremely upset when he plays with peers on the playground. Teachers describe him as a very different child when these two circumstances are compared. Likewise, he is often angry and hard to control at home; then sometimes he may suddenly seem as if he is a stranger and not part of the family situation at all. These are the main differences noticed between school and home, and apparently the family and teachers do not see the same child. Suppose we describe the children observed at school as Johnny A and B and the child at home as Johnny C and D. Later we may have more information regarding these changes, and Johnny himself may find he has names for them.

Although the tools previously mentioned may still be utilized, the focus now moves toward greater internal exploration. Guided imagery, hypnosis, and fantasy games are valued tools to help develop communication with the child's internal world. Gardner and Olness (1981) provide an excellent resource on child hypnosis. Quite frequently, a deep trance is not needed for a child who is in a safe place and for whom the secrets and trauma are quite fresh.

A valuable step is for the therapist to plan and prepare the child for the next session at the end of each session. Sometimes, of course, the actual agenda may change because of external events such as illness, a change in family life, or some important everyday occurrence that needs attention. Whenever the external support system changes, this also requires exploration, because the child's absolute safety must always be assured. More extensive exploration of the different elements should not be attempted again until the security of external support networks is assured as much as possible.

When initially introducing fantasy techniques, the creation of a special sanctuary or "safe place" inside can make later opening of painful material less traumatic. The sanctuary is a place where the child can find inner safety and protection to diminish the pain of memories or current experiences. As part of developing the sanctuary, the child's inner self-helper or guide needs to be located and an alliance established among the child, the therapist, and the guide. The guide will then be available to understand what is happening and to give direction when the therapist and child are lost. The fantasy may be introduced by the therapist as follows:

> Tell me about some places where you were really happy. [The child relates some places.] Now tell me about what made these places so happy. Did you feel safe in those places? Were there any other people there? When did you last visit these places?

After these experiences are discussed at some length, the therapist, at the appropriate time, begins a fantasy trip by saying:

> Now let's see if you can find some of these places within your mind even though you may physically still stay in the playroom. Take a long deep breath and let's go back until you can find that safe place that you told me about.

In this way, the place of known security is reexperienced. Next, the therapist can proceed with guided imagery to a forest or a seashore that the child has not perhaps yet experienced, which will be used to begin the process of entering the sanctuary. Finally, the child can be led by guided imagery to the setting; then a doorway or a tree stump or some other symbol can be described that will allow the child to find his or her own special sanctuary. Some children choose gardens or places with animals; others may find familiar places such as a room or comfort with a special person. Often children may define a sanctuary as a closed space such as a room or a comfortable lap, in contrast to adults, who may choose a place without narrow boundaries such as the seashore or a mountain top. Whatever the sanctuary, the child should explore and experience it as fully as possible, including both its contents and sensory elements. The therapist should emphasize that the child can use this sanctuary whenever it is needed and especially whenever a situation is very frightening. The child can learn from this that safety and quiet are available within him or her, even when old memories become terrifying.

The creation of the sanctuary and the development of fantasy skills may take from two to six or eight sessions. Some children may require more tangible creations. Children younger than age four may need a sanctuary, concretely designed, using stuffed toys, dolls, or sand tray objects. Imagery of the tangible safe place can be encouraged by saying, "Now close your eyes, take a deep breath, and see how this happy safe place looks and feels!" Feelings should be attached to the words and the idea given that this special place will stay snug inside forever and ever.

The guide is identified in much the same way:

> Now let's visit the sanctuary. We'll take our special big blue bird [or whatever setting or transport object the child may have created] and fly deep inside until we see the sanctuary while I count one, two, three. Now tell me about the sanctuary today. [The child tells about the experience at the sanctuary.] Now today there is someone you have not recognized before. This is a marvelous, marvelous guide like we have talked about. [Up to this time the idea of a guide and special people have been explored. As needed, this may be accomplished by tangible play.] This guide may be a familiar person, a friendly animal, or even just colors. Keep breathing and feel everything and tell me what you are experiencing.

Sometimes children will see unicorns, Jesus, rainbows, teddy bears, dolphins, or dogs. Other guides have been identified, but those noted here have occurred at least twice. The guide should be accepted and an alliance clearly obtained. It is essential that a commitment be gotten from the guide to protect the child and the sanctuary. It is quite possible that a harmful part of the child's personality may provide a false guide, and requiring this commitment can prevent trauma within the sacred space.

The learning of fantasy and imagery skills comes naturally to children. They usually begin imaginary play before age three and identify quite easily with this kind of thinking. Establishing the sanctuary and the guide underlines the importance of protective elements and furthers the process of trust. The guide and sanctuary will also be resources the child can use whenever external events or therapy itself become overwhelming. Visiting the sanctuary and guide can be part of beginning and ending every therapy session. Children are delighted by safe rituals and routine. Establishing this visit as a beginning and an ending process provides a safe continuity.

Assuming that the child has been prepared and outside supports have been functioning well, the deeper level may be addressed. The next step, that of exploring the different elements, can now begin. The therapist may say:

> Now, get down on the mat and breathe deeply. We are going into the magic space capsule that takes us deep inside and far away from the playroom. Breathe very deeply, because we need lots of oxygen for this journey. We will stop and visit with the unicorn guide in the sanctuary along the way. [The child is led into the familiar imagery.] Now, going on beyond the sanctuary we are going to visit Mark, who came along when you were a little baby about one year old. Let's see if we can find Mark. We know what Mark is like, so let's see if you can see him in your mind right now. Breathe deeper now, and when I count, we will find out what Mark is like. One, two, three. . . .

Meeting every element that the child has awareness of can be accomplished in this way. Perhaps some elements are aware of others not yet known by the child's most usual personality. Typically, the personality system of the child with MPD is not nearly as complex as that of an adult (Kluft 1985). However, children can be seductive with simplicity, and the therapist should never assume that information is easily gained or complete without thorough investigation.

As each element (or personality) is identified, it should be valued, even if it is hostile toward the therapist:

Well, John, I understand you don't like big people very much. You have had the important job of protecting Sandy from big people who were bad. We are not going to take this job away, because we don't want Sandy to get hurt either. But we may need you to do some other kinds of different things. You are very important, and we are glad to have you.

As elements are identified and contact is made, some may fight the therapist or each other, and some may be cooperative. One element may be unaware of others, but often many of the different elements are coconscious in children, and permission for them to express themselves is usually well received. Sometimes elements may be mute but still able to communicate through art, movement, or the creation of special playroom scenes.

It is most wise, as always, that the therapist not move too quickly. After the elements are identified, they can be named, described in words, have their pictures drawn, and talk and share through play and art. An important part of this process is making sure that each part is identified as having valuable functions and shown how to be helpful as well as destructive. In our experience, such naming and describing practices are quite helpful. (For another perspective, see Kluft 1986a, who does not advocate all of these interventions.)

Intensify Friends in the System—Develop Alliances

This step is an extension of valuing every part of the system. It begins with understanding the history of each element. At this point, an alliance is gained with each part of the personality and a plan of treatment is developed and communicated. Each of the elements has an official duty and a reason or reasons (based on fear, trauma, or providing some kind of protection) as to why that element must continue its existence. An alliance among the elements can be encouraged only after communication and an alliance has been created between the elements and the therapist. It is especially important to note the presence of destructive parts of the personality.

Although it was initially believed (Kluft 1985) that children did not identify internal persecutors frequently, one of us (P.P.M.) has found an element represented as an internalized abusive adult in half of a sample of 30 dissociative children. This often reveals itself when the system begins experiencing strength and the overall health of the child has improved. The child may then become more aggressive and abusive toward other children and even adults, as well as toward him- or herself. This can be initially dealt with by forming a peace contract with the internalized aggressor and, as soon as possible thereafter, releasing the pain that created the aggressive element in the first place. It is essential that the aggressive element realizes that although a different job description may be needed, its existence certainly can continue. Children seem frightened of being banished from the world; any threat that a part of them may no longer exist can be terrifying. There is still a great fear of trusting and sharing secrets, and punishment may be demanded by the internal system when such "sinful behavior" occurs.

Especially with children younger than age 10, active play therapy can be very effectively paired with fantasy work. Clearly defining the different experiences, behaviors, and conflicts that each element encounters can become a very involving process. The child may take the part of the element, or it may be represented by dolls or other toys; sometimes they may use artwork or tell stories with a tape recorder. Children older than 10 often can internalize the feelings and images entirely and may be less interested in a more concrete or externalized approach. On the other hand, play therapy techniques may be useful for adults, especially those who are handling issues coming from very early childhood experience.

Once these steps have been accomplished, then the reexperiencing and abreaction of traumatic events can begin.

Negotiate and Release Pain

The release of severe traumatic events is started by negotiation as to how the process will occur. For many children, abreaction may occur through doll play, stuffed animals, or puppets. Other children may make elaborate structures in a sand tray. Each element has a story, and that story must be fully reexperienced. Although the experience often is associated with intense emotional release, this is not always the case. Not all of the elements may have experienced severe trauma, and their purpose may have been to perform specific tasks, such as schoolwork.

The reexperiencing and releasing of traumatic materials may be completed over several sessions. While this is happening, the family and others who provide external support need to be alerted for possible regression. Sometimes the primary caretaker, who is seen as a nurturing resource, can be part of this release. For example, an abreactive experience may be started by saying:

> This time we will take the space capsule and go into the very hard places that we have talked about where Cleo has been very frightened. Cleo protects the rest of the children and is the only one who knows so much fear. Now everybody can know this fear so Cleo won't have to carry it alone. I know this can be a scary thing, but this time your new mamma and I will be with you. You also have all your friends and your teachers outside this playroom pulling hard for you. Okay, so are you ready? This is a very brave journey. We will also take all our other animals [stuffed toys, etc.] with us on this journey. Is there anybody else we should make sure is in this room with us, even if they cannot really be here? [The child may ask for a deceased but loved relative, such as a grandparent, or a pet. A photograph or a picture may be added if the visual imagery is not sufficient by itself.] As always, we will stop by the sacred sanctuary and visit with our spirit guide before we go so deeply. Okay, breathe a great big deep breath and we will go backward to the times when you were so small and frightened and alone. . . .

Sometimes an elaborate format is required for the abreactive journey. Once the stage is set, it is unwise for the experience to be delayed. This can either create too much anxiety in the child or establish excessive distance between preparation and experience. The child may need some kind of transitional object, such as a special stone or toy, that will "help him or her stay strong" from one appointment to the next. During abreactive work, it is usually helpful to have the appointments close together. However, sometimes the child may need more space between one intense abreaction and the next, especially if there is considerable real life stress. Certainly external events must always be taken into consideration. If the child is being treated on an outpatient basis, as is usually the case, the child's experience within the community, including school, friends, activities, and holidays, must always be recognized. The internal experience frequently attains primary importance, but it can be intensified more effectively if other events are not competing for the child's attention and energy.

The different personality elements may reexperience and release the trauma one at a time or combine experiences. The next step, that of integration, may follow such abreactive release. More often, two or more of the elements may merge. However, in our experience, true final integration does not occur until all the abreactive work has been completed and all the elements then can be joined together in an integration ritual.

Go for It! Integrate

Integration can happen quietly, but children usually appreciate a ceremony or ritual even if the elements have integrated smoothly and without dramatic external manifestations.

Kluft (1986b) writes beautifully about integration rituals. It is essential that the integration be accomplished in both a tangible and concrete manner and on an abstract level as well so the child is assured that it actually has occurred on many levels of consciousness. Following are some examples of integration rituals that have been effective with children:

> A bridge or wall is created or visualized in fantasy and one by one the different personality elements cross over from one side to another and join hands. . . .
> The process can be accomplished by climbing up a mountain to the top, crossing over a lake or other body of water, and sometimes

by joining one star with another and forming a great sun. . . .

A doll can be chosen to represent the "new" child and the different elements can give symbolic gifts to represent their continuing characteristics. The therapist can join the elements into each other with a hug.

The common theme of integration rituals is that as the different elements are united and merged, they become one strong individual. For older children, this may be primarily a symbolic process; but the younger child may require a specific and tangible focus such as a doll, poster, or picture that symbolizes the integration. After integration is completed, the work is still far from finished. The child may experience frustration as he or she becomes more fully aware of misbehavior and its consequences. He or she may need to get used to being more emotional, responsive, and joyful. Observations made by teachers, family, and associated caregivers will be of value. Follow-up with outside support is also important, directed toward maintaining communication with all the caregivers and helping the family and child cope with normal developmental issues, many of which may have been sidestepped. Now is the time for the therapist to focus on family therapy, primarily for the parents; but at times there also are indications including work with the child and his or her friends. Individual sessions from time to time are still strongly encouraged, because the strong relationship that has existed between the therapist and child will continue to be a very important factor in the child's continuing growth.

Initially, it was believed that the therapy process with children with MPD could be achieved in a relatively short time, especially compared with adults (Kluft 1984, 1985). Although the time may be much shorter than is necessary for therapy for adult MPD patients, in our experience the length of preparation time and follow-up care, combined with other parts of the therapeutic process, may extend over several months and on occasion may require as long as 2 or 3 years. If the child arrives at therapy with an intact family network and supportive external environment, the work will be much easier. Also, if the child has become fragmented because of a specific extrafamily trauma rather than an extensive history of abuse, the therapy time can be shortened. In any event, it is best that the therapist not rush the process, work within the child's pace, keep all elements within the child's internal world well informed, and also involve and encourage support systems in the external world.

A Case Study: Cassie

Six-year-old Cassie looks out with enormous chocolate eyes holding fear-filled knowledge that new places and people can bring harm. She has been in foster care for 2 months. The foster mother reports many problems. Cassie hoards food and seems to have no awareness when her tummy is full. She hides dirty underwear all about the bedroom in the same places where she hides the food. She forgets events that have just occurred. One moment she laughs happily; the next she lapses into a frigid silence. She is a strange child, smiling while she is being punished and denying events when evidence is clear that they occurred. There is no known physical reason for Cassie's strange behavior; she is healthy and seldom physically ill. She seems to have average intelligence, although sometimes she cannot answer very simple questions. Her school performance fluctuates daily and even hourly.

The agency caseworker reports that little is known about Cassie's early development and nothing about pregnancy, delivery, and the first important days of life. Her mother abandoned her early, leaving Cassie unattended for days at a time. She stayed with her maternal grandparents for periods of time; then her mother would return and reclaim her for a while. When Cassie was almost two, a baby brother was born. He was prized by the grandparents and nurtured by them, although his mother cared for him no better than she had Cassie. The grandparents wavered in their ability to help with Cassie. They were old and tired; the demands of the children were overwhelming to them. More and more frequently, the children would be returned to the mother, who would often leave for another town, sometimes taking the children with her and sometimes abandoning them.

When Cassie was three, she was found wandering the streets

searching for food. She would climb into garbage bins and spend the night. Agencies attempted intervention by working with the mother and grandparents, but nothing could be done to keep the mother stable and the children fed and clean. The grandparents were exhausted and finally ended all involvement; the mother and her two small children moved to another state. When Cassie searched the house for food, she was beaten and left for days at a time in a locked room. At four, she became a child of the streets. Finally, by the time she was six and home-based intervention had repeatedly failed, Cassie and her brother were placed in foster care.

The foster parents were dedicated and energetic. They cared for children lovingly and efficiently. The mother, a full-time homemaker, was the primary caretaker. The father was firm and somewhat distant, but quite supportive of the children. Cassie and her brother were dressed beautifully, looking like children from a fashion magazine. The brother adjusted well and everyone loved him, but Cassie was perceived as a strange child from the beginning. Within a month of foster placement, the behaviors that had been merely strange became frankly bizarre. Her occasionally glazed look became a strange, silent solitude lasting for several hours at a time. She would eat until she began vomiting and immediately beg for more food. She claimed that it was another child who hid the underwear, took the excessive food, stole and threw away toys that belonged to other children, and wet the bed. On other occasions she denied these events completely. Her behavior was becoming intolerable to the foster parents.

Finally, the caseworker asked one of us (P.P.M.) to see Cassie for therapy, and we began to work. I also spent time with her foster mother and contacted her teacher. The diagnosis of incipient multiplicity (Fagan and McMahon 1984) was confirmed when radical shifts in behavior were noted hour by hour, and data about the very different presentations Cassie made among different surroundings were collected systematically. Everyone saw Cassie differently. She was one child at home, another at school, and someone else around strangers.

For the first few weeks of therapy, Cassie seldom spoke except to answer "Yes ma'am" and "No ma'am." As therapy continued over those first few months, Cassie began playing more easily with the playroom toys. She especially enjoyed playing with the puppets and drawing. This was the initial state of trust; although her comfort level in the playroom increased, she still interacted little with me.

While trust was developing, the teacher, the foster mother, and the caseworker were all interviewed. The caseworker needed support to accept that, in this case, long-term foster placement would be needed; prospective adoptive parents would not consider Cassie after reviewing her history and current behavior. The foster mother needed a place where she could express her frustrations to someone who could believe that the "silent beauty" could also be a "holy terror." The teacher needed help in understanding why this child was so strange and silent. Eventually, as problems became more pronounced, Cassie received half-day special education services for children with severe emotional problems.

Meanwhile, in therapy, Cassie became more interactive. Feelings were identified, and she acted out events that occurred at home and during the school day with puppets and dolls. She showed her version of the day, and then I showed her how people may see the same incident differently. However, she often perceived this as blaming and withdrew into solitary play, avoiding interaction. I learned again that when a child is so withdrawn, confrontation at any level must be attempted only after trust is gained, and trust develops at the child's own pace. With Cassie, this came very slowly.

After a month's regrouping, Cassie used different puppets and acted out her history. She remembered much that had happened but showed no overt affect. Therefore, we talked about feelings. We played games about feelings; we chose puppets and dolls and let them have different feelings. Some feelings were happy, some were sad, and some were very frightened. Cassie said she never had experienced some of these feelings; she never felt fear and she was never angry. "But, all little children are angry," I said, "and they are scared too. So maybe some of these dolls can feel those things for you." A hurdle was crossed. Cassie began letting the different dolls express feelings that she could not do herself, becoming more animated and making faces of anger and sadness. She was able to create situations that the dolls might experience, such as being frightened when attending school for the first time, but it was clear that Cassie had not experienced these feelings herself.

Now work began to deepen and we started to find the different parts within her system. We talked about different feelings people have within themselves. Cassie had been aware that people saw her as good and bad, very sweet and very naughty. Ever so slowly, she began letting the dolls and puppets act out events that she actually experienced in her life. A white puppet in a doctor's uniform was called "Doc." Doc was always around, helping the other puppets continue the story. One important story was about a little doll hiding during the night in a garbage can. Cassie realized that this doll was very frightened, leading to her learning how different dolls could hold some of the feelings that she had experienced.

Cassie was now able to close her eyes and think about different feelings even though they were still only experienced by the dolls. Now it was time for the creation of the sanctuary, using the dolls and playroom toys. Her choice was the beach with sand, and the sand box and the small miniature toys were used to make a beach with a happy house and many animals. No children were ever lonely, and there was always plenty of food at this beach. Hot dogs were especially enjoyed by Cassie and all the animals and dolls. When memories were painful, Cassie returned to the beach remembering the sand smells, the taste of hot dogs, and the sounds of ocean surf.

We had begun to integrate affective work with actual remembering of experiences. Cassie herself began experiencing those feelings that the different dolls were holding, and she could show some affect. She was still role-playing feelings, but the first step had been made. It was never Cassie who was sad, but Amy or Bessie. Cassie did not get frightened, but Rick could be, and Tommy could be very naughty. This was the beginning of identifying dolls who had experiences and could be connected with experiences that Cassie had endured.

The mystery of the past and its relationship to the present became more vivid. Cassie began recognizing and acknowledging her history. The emotions connected with events could be experienced through the dolls, who showed a variety of different feelings.

We had begun our second year of therapy. Cassie's behavior at school was no longer that of the silent child, but at times she was simply obnoxious. There was more similarity between her behavior at school and at home, and the foster mother was relieved because people now believed her. In therapy we talked about which of the different dolls should attend school. Lisa was always a sweet doll and did well when Cassie took her to school and let Lisa sit on her lap. Sometimes, however, she hid Lisa in her desk; this was when she became sassy to the teachers, stole from the other children, or made sexual advances to boys.

I had started talking with all the dolls, who were given names and told why they were special. Their histories were discovered—some of them had spent many nights in garbage cans, and one ate over and over until she threw up. There were seven main dolls and puppets, although several of these had some special friends who I suspected were also part of Cassie's system. Some of the dolls (like Lisa, the one in charge when Cassie met new people) had a very happy family and never had any sad things happen to them. Doc was identified as the internal self-helper, usually sitting high on a shelf watching. Doc always knew the right things and was always the helper of children, but sometimes even Doc could not get them out of garbage cans or feed them when they were hungry. Doc helped the other dolls care for each other.

This point in therapy was critical. Different elements had been identified and given names, and Cassie was aware of how they were related to her even though the elements still existed separately, with their own histories. There was more awareness that different feelings can be expressed, and Cassie showed more consistently disruptive behaviors, requiring patience from all the support people. This necessitated my making phone calls or even visiting with them.

We began reliving the trauma each of the doll children had endured. I began, mistakenly, with the youngest of the children, who was just a baby. Cassie was able to close her eyes, enter into a fantasy game, and feel the same experiences that Cindy (the baby) had felt when tossed around, covered with dirt, and very hungry. Cassie wanted to feed Cindy and then let me know when she wanted to be fed like that! She let herself be rocked and held; the foster mother participated also in this during some of the therapy sessions. When the feelings of being the small infant Cindy got too sad, Cassie could remember the safe beach place.

However, as Cassie experienced the pain of early infancy, this influenced her behavior at home and school as well. Cindy assumed too much control, and as a result, control over bowel and bladder control were lost, solid food was rejected, and crying continued for hours. The children ridiculed her for urinating in the classroom, and we "realized" that a tiny baby should not attend school. Very quickly we found the oldest child, Big Bruce, who was 13 and whose job it was to protect the small children. Big Bruce could handle school, but he had not yet dealt with the problems related to his need to be so strong. Cassie became somewhat of a bully at school, but this was better than her behaving as a regressed infant.

Cassie's foster mother had been able to overcome her irritation and find patience as the system became more stable. She agreed to bathe Cindy, feed her baby food at home, and give her extra cuddling. After 3 weeks the baby had been healed enough so that Cassie could cry and be angry, and there was a clear relationship between affect and remembered experiences. Other children then let us know that they were also wanting their turn in treatment, and one by one they emerged and told their stories.

The stories were revealed one by one. Sometimes they were filled with grief and profound despair (e.g., Emily's wanting a mamma and giving up crying when no one appeared). Big Bruce was large and angry because he was always the fighter. At other times, elements presented themselves as if they could only laugh and play. The children began to act with one another; behaviors learned by one child were not totally forgotten by the others. The children would leave messages for each other by sandcastles on the beach during fantasy play and in the sandbox at the playroom. The children were finally helping each other.

Some of the older children were integrated with little fanfare or notice. They simply shared their stories, reexperienced the pain, and ceased to be separate. The environment by this time was providing adequate support, so the initial reason for splitting was no longer necessary. Nonetheless, four of the children remained separate. The smallest baby, Big Bruce the bully, the very good child, and the toddler looking for a home needed to achieve acceptance of one another before integration could be completed.

Several weeks of sessions passed while communication among the elements increased. They gave each other presents, shared food, and realized they could fare better together than separately. The baby liked bananas, whereas Big Bruce wanted beer; they compromised on a banana milkshake. One element loved soft lullabies, another hard rock. A time for both could be arranged, and a mutual acceptance established. An increasing appreciation for one another was developed. There was more consistency now than ever in daily functioning and between cognition and affect. The final four children were represented by a sweet doll, a small baby, a monster man from the sandbox, and a cuddly teddy bear. Each child had a special offering of a picture, a toy, or a special memory. They shared what they liked and found difficult about each other, but mostly this was a time of high positive regard. The formal integration ritual was actually almost anticlimactic. All the treasures were placed in the middle of the circle and the symbolic children held hands and formed a solemn pact:

> We are Mr. Teddy Bear and Little Baby Girl, Big Bad Bully Boy and Crying Black-Haired Child. We hold our hands and close our eyes. We come closer with each breath. We are no longer shattered like broken glass. We become one and I'm Cassie, I'm Cassie, I'm Cassie. I need family and friends. I need love and protection. I need school and playgrounds. I need to know Cassie.

Despite the integration, Cassie's therapy was by no means complete. Rather than several elements acting separately without warning, there now was a single disturbed child who, as she said, needed to know Cassie. Cassie was no longer a wary, fear-filled child, but one capable and fully aware of joy and mischief. The enormous chocolate eyes were filled every day with more knowledge, and Cassie grew stronger.

Now 5 years have passed since Cassie began her treatment. She continues to function with special educational support in a school setting for emotionally disturbed children. She never became a star student, but her destructive and disruptive behaviors have ceased. As she improved, she received more support from her teachers and her friends. She continues to show satisfactory progress and apparently has made a stable adjustment.

Carrie became more lovable and was able to do much better in foster care. She did so well that her foster family adopted her. Recently the family relocated to a new community, where Cassie and her family and friends still struggle, but indeed survive.

Cassie is an example of the type of child who exhibits severe dissociative symptoms, but who might never be considered by many clinicians to fulfill diagnostic criteria for MPD. Instead, she might be considered to have DDNOS and/or to demonstrate the clinical picture of incipient MPD (Fagan and McMahon 1984).

Her case was chosen as an illustration because she represents a type of child who could be encountered frequently by therapists who consult with agencies that serve high-risk children (traumatized children, survivors of abuse, foster children, etc.). Cassie's behavior is not a florid example of childhood MPD. She is, however, an example of a child who is split into many parts and has at times become dull and lifeless and at other times uncontrollable while preserving her most creative and precious potential.

References

Fagan J, McMahon PP: Incipient multiple personality in children. J Nerv Ment Dis 172:26–36, 1984

Gardner GG, Olness K: Hypnosis and Hypnotherapy with Children. New York, Grune & Stratton, 1981

Gardner RA: Psychotherapeutic Approaches to the Resistant Child. New York, Jason Aronson, 1975

Kluft RP: Multiple personality in childhood. Psychiatr Clin North Am 7:121–134, 1984

Kluft RP: Childhood multiple personality disorder, in Childhood Antecedents of Multiple Personality Disorder. Edited by Kluft RP. Washington, DC, American Psychiatric Press, 1985, pp 167–196

Kluft RP: Treating children who have multiple personality disorder, in Treatment of Multiple Personality Disorder. Edited by Braun BG. Washington, DC, American Psychiatric Press, 1986a, pp 79–105

Kluft RP: The place and role of fusion rituals in treating multiple personality. Newsletter of the American Society of Clinical Hypnosis 26:4–5, 1986b

Chapter 14

Ego-State Therapy in the Treatment of Dissociative Disorders

Helen H. Watkins, M.A.
John G. Watkins, Ph.D.

Ego-state theory holds that humans develop their personalities through the process of integration, a putting together, and differentiation, a taking apart. Integration consists of a regrouping of experiential elements to allow us to develop generalizations and evolve higher-level concepts. Thus, a child learns that horses, dogs, and cats all belong to the category animals. Differentiation helps the child distinguish between those animals that are dangerous and those that are not, or between those individuals who care for the child and those who may be hostile. Both processes are originally adaptive. They increase the likelihood of survival and facilitate coping with an increasingly complex world (Watkins and Watkins 1991).

Most psychological processes lie on a continuum. Over certain portions of this continuum they are adaptive and facilitate life and growth; at others, usually when excessive, they become maladaptive and may impair the individual's adjustment. For example, mild anxiety may stimulate an individual to solve a personal problem, but severe anxiety may prove crippling. This holds for integration, the unifying function, and differentiation, the separating function. At one portion of the continuum, differentiation helps us make finer discriminations and can be quite adaptive. However, an excess of differentiation is less adaptive, and as it intensifies, it becomes increasingly maladaptive. In its extreme form, it is so different from its more moderate forms that we no longer call it differentiation. It is now better understood as dissociation and may involve the segmentation of the mind into ego states, extreme forms of which may lead to the development of multiple personality disorder (MPD).

Paul Federn (1952), an associate of Freud, apparently first coined the term "ego states" to describe personality segments. However, he made no attempt to develop any model of therapy on this concept. We have adapted Federn's observations and theories regarding ego states and have included them in a novel model of therapy. In our theory and therapy (Watkins 1984), we define an ego state as an organized system of behavior and experience whose elements are bound together by some common principle but that is separated from other such states by boundaries that are more or less permeable. Such a definition includes both true cases of multiple personalities and those less rigidly separated personality segments that lie in the middle of the differentiation-dissociation continuum and that may be more "integrated" and hence more adaptive.

In working with research subjects under hypnosis, we have found that individuals who show no sign of mental illness may nonetheless manifest segmented divisions in their personalities that may act like "covert" multiple personalities. However, the boundaries that separate them from other such states are more permeable and are not necessarily maladaptive. These parts often have awareness for one another but retain their individual senses of identity. They are "integrated" in the same sense that Montana and Idaho are "integrated" within a larger "federal" jurisdiction. We have also noted that these entities ("covert" ego states) seem to represent the same class of phenomena as the "hidden observers" reported by Hilgard (1977); see also Watkins and Watkins (1979–1980).

In MPD, on the other hand, the dissociated parts exist near the extreme end of the differentiation-dissociation continuum. There are often rigid, impermeable boundaries between the ego states, which permit little communication between them; they often posess no awareness of one another. Sometimes it seems as if these ego states live behind locked doors, oblivious to the needs or feelings of other aspects of the mind. The first personalities to be formed are the result of an extreme and excessive use of the separating function, mobilized in the face of tremendous childhood stress. Thereafter, the mind may make further such divisions under various circumstances.

Ego-State Therapy

Ego-state therapy uses group and family therapy techniques to resolve conflicts between the various ego states, which in this model are understood to constitute a "family of self" within a single individual. Its techniques are applicable to both treatment of diagnosable MPD (in which ego states are overt and can emerge spontaneously) and to other behavioral and neurotic disorders (in which symptoms result from clashes between "covert" ego states, whose differences usually become manifest only under hypnosis [Watkins 1992]).

In treating patients with classic MPD, we help them progress down the continuum toward increasing integration and lesser dissociation—hence, toward levels where the remaining degree of differentiation among the personality segments cease to be maladaptive. The personalities of some of our increasingly integrated MPD patients express their situation in this manner: "We are still here, but we are no longer separate persons. We are now parts of her, and we work together." Because we find ego states in control subjects, from the perspective of ego-state therapy it seems both unnecessary (and perhaps not even adaptive) to attempt the elimination of these states through "fusion." Personalities in control subjects are integrated but not fused. Efforts to totally eliminate all boundaries between personality segments increase resistance. Ego states (or part-persons) may at times join other parts or even voluntarily leave (such as a fragment may in a true MPD patient). However, to enforce the need for the fusion of all parts may be viewed by the patient as the therapist's attempt to push the personalities toward nonexistence or death. One alter expressed her apprehensions quite graphically: "You aren't going to make a goulash out of us, are you?" The struggle for life is strong in part-persons as well as in whole persons.

It is our impression that undertaking therapy from this perspective makes the task of the therapist become easier. Because the goal is a harmonious cooperation of the various ego states with a "federal" jurisdiction of the whole personality, there is less likelihood of encountering massive and entrenched resistances by alters invested in retaining their own separateness.

We appreciate that this perspective is at odds with a prevailing point of view in the dissociative disorders field, which favors a definition and a pursuit of integration as that concept is discussed by many of the contributors to this book, and as explored in depth in Chapter 6 (i.e., the personalities becoming a single entity). We also appreciate that many of the clinicians whose work is illustrated in this book may be treating primarily patients with severe MPD and not those who manifest only covert ego states—hence, those who are not diagnosed as having MPD.

Our clinical cases range from severely disturbed multiples to those patients in the intermediate range of the differentiation-dissociation continuum. Our clinical work with both neurotic patients and patients with true MPD, plus our research studies with non-mentally ill volunteer subjects, indicate that non-mentally ill individuals are not "fused" into single entities, but frequently manifest covert segmentation under hypnosis. Successfully treated MPD patients, who show all overt evidences of "integration," may under hypnosis reveal their former alters as continuing covert existence, but now adaptive and with flexible boundaries—such as those we find in college students who are research volunteers.

Ego-State Therapy: The Case of Mikale

The following case study demonstrates the application of ego-state therapy techniques in resolving the conflicts of a patient who had both neurotic symptoms and dissociation bordering on overt multiple personality. The ego states were integrated into a cooperative whole. The illustrative materials are excerpted from tape recordings of the sessions and are discussed from the perspective of the therapist (H.H.W.)

Session I

A perky 22-year-old blond student plopped herself into the recliner in my office and said, "I had the shock of my life the other day when I found out from the nurse at the Health Service that not everyone has voices in their head. Is that true? I've always heard three voices—two that argue and a third that decides what to do depending on who wins the argument!"

Thus began my first session with Mikale, an attractive-looking college senior scheduled to graduate soon. She had been seen at the University Health Service for over a year with little or no improvement in her insomnia and depression. When she casually mentioned voices in her head to the nurse, she had been referred to the consulting psychiatrist, who in turn had sent her to me.

An effervescent young woman, casually dressed in blue jeans and sweatshirt, Mikale began to relate the story of her life. "Dad was an alcoholic but stayed dry when I was in high school. I remember he used to yell and threaten, especially at Mother. They would fight, and she'd throw things. It was scary." Mikale's mother rarely listened to her and did not believe what Mikale related about mistreatment she endured. "I tried to tell her when I was around 8 or 9 that my uncle sexually abused me, but she said I was a liar." Mikale played the role of the good little girl, never expressing anger. She felt very unloved. In recent flashbacks she had experienced herself as being young and vulnerable. A strange man was hurting her in the basement. She remembered telling her mother and hearing her say, "Oh, it's just your imagination. There's nobody in the basement." By the 7th grade, Mikale had developed severe gastritis: "the doctor told me I almost had an ulcer." Her mother told her that at age 2½ she had come close to death with a kidney infection.

I inquired about the voices in her head and Mikale said,

Well, there's a kind of mother figure who says, "you're making it all up; you're a failure; you can't do anything right." Then there's a mad but hurt, feisty little girl who cries or argues with the mother part. Then there's a kind of silent center who listens to the two argue and decides on a course of action, depending on who seems to be winning the fight. When I'm real tired I can also hear a man's voice, yelling and screaming. That voice is kind of muffled, but it's scary anyway.

Our first session ended, leaving me to consider what I could do about these various voices. There was communication between the states and no evidence of complete amnestic barriers between them. In the ego-state model, these findings allowed me to eliminate the possibility of a true multiple personality diagnosis. I appreciate that others might not agree with this line of reasoning. However, there was no doubt about the presence of dissociated states in Mikale's personality structure.

Session II

At the beginning of Session II, Mikale mentioned that she had a pesky, intermittent rash on her thighs and buttocks "that just won't go away, even with medical treatment." This statement, seemingly out of context, sounded like a coded message of some importance. I hypnotized Mikale and asked for a part of her "who knows about the rash." She spontaneously regressed to age 4 in the basement of her family home. "There's a bad man, and he grabs me and my bottom hurts!" I decided to rescue her. "I'm not going to let that bad man hurt you any more. I'll take you upstairs and you wait while I get rid of him." She felt relieved. Upon my "return upstairs," she confided in me, "my name is Misha." I then asked (with her permission) for an internal volunteer to come and take care of Misha. The voice of an adult female age 19, called Mike, agreed to take care of Misha. In a later session I learned Mike was the previously mentioned "silent" center. After arousal from hypnosis, Mikale developed a severe headache. I asked her to close her eyes and concentrate on the headache. A different voice then came out. It sounded like the voice of a stern mother figure who said, "She's made it all up!" I convinced this mother part that the experience was a valid one, and the headache went away.*

Session III

Excitedly, Mikale began Session III with "The rash is all gone!" But now, again seemingly out of context, she told me she was afraid of strong, gusty winds. I took this as another hint, a coded communication I needed to explore. Working within the ego-state model, I hypnotized her and asked to speak with a part who could tell me about her fear of the wind. Out came the voice of Mike frantically shouting, "I promised to take care of her, but I can't find her!" I replied: "I think we can find her in the wind." I asked for Misha directly. She emerged crying, "Nobody's coming and it's dark! The wind's blowing, I'm holding on to a tree. Mommy said I was bad. Daddy's coming home. I'm afraid to tell him why Mommy put me out here. Now he's taking me inside and puts me in the sleeping bag." "How old are you, Misha?" "I'm three." I comforted the sobbing Misha and reassured her that she was not a bad little girl. Then I asked Mike to pick her up and take her away where she will be safe. "Some place, Mike, where she will never be afraid of the wind again." Mike agreed. The purpose of this therapeutic maneuver was to abreact fear, to relieve guilt, and to arrange a reassuring, more favorable "internal outcome."

---

*Many clinicians unfamiliar with clinical hypnoanalysis might take issue with such a direct and active intrusion of myself into the spontaneous reliving of a traumatic experience. Clinical hypnoanalysis differs from psychoanalysis in many respects, and one of these is the importance accorded to providing a corrective emotional experience within the medium of trance. Clinical hypnoanalysts often actively attempt to assuage the pain of the traumatic past in the course of their interventions. They perceive such efforts as invaluable tools to enhance rapport, build healthier object relationships, modify pathological internalized object relationships, and provide a greater sense of safety and security while dealing with difficult material. In the case of Mikale, her description of her own mother's refusal to listen or to become involved suggested a clear model for introducing these beneficial interventions into the treatment (i.e., assuming the stance of an empathic and deeply concerned maternal figure).

Session IV

During Session IV Mikale reported she had felt no discomfort when the wind blew during the week. Now she began to tell me about her allergies, which seemed to have started at the age of 16. Again, taking note of her implicit cue, I hypnotized her and asked "for a part that knows about the allergies." A stern, motherish voice declared, "I did it!" The "allergies" were designed to punish her for "being too uppity with her sister" who was 11 months younger. "I decided to teach her a lesson," the stern part stated. It became clear that this mother ego state was an introjection of Mikale's actual mother. I interviewed this ego state, and was told that she was "born" shortly after the patient's birth.

> Th: Do you know what your purpose is if you were there at the beginning?
> Pt (Mother): I was there to protect her and to keep her safe and make sure she follows the rules.
> Th: What happened at the time you came on the scene to protect her?
> Pt (Mother): Well, there was this big shock when she was born, and she started to cry, which is probably understandable, but we can't have that.
> Th: Oh, how come?
> Pt (Mother): Because Mother said not to. She tried to keep us quiet, and so I took over that function.

Here is the apparent beginning of the introjection of Mikale's mother (in the sense of initiating a separate ego state). At some level she interpreted (if such an intellectual term is appropriate) the behavior of her mother in shushing her as a command to be quiet. The ego state's function was essentially protective. In urging Mikale to follow the rules perceived to be decreed by mother, this ego state attempted to maximize the probability that she will be accepted by the external mother.

> Th: Are you the one who says she's making it all up?
> Pt (Mother, in a haughty manner): Well, I really think she is. She's

creating it to get attention. She did something wrong, and she deserved it.

Th: She didn't make up that rash and the experience in the basement. That really happened.

Pt (Mother): I don't know about that, but I still think she made it all up, and the rash was just a symptom of her overly active imagination.

Th: You talk just like her mother, don't you? You must believe everything her mother said.

Pt (Mother): Mother says she's always right. If she's an adult she must know; so therefore, Mother must be right.

Th: I see. So if she's an adult, and you say she's always right, then you must be a little girl.

Those ego states that are more or less based on parental figures are constructed from the child's perceptions of the parents. Hence, they are really rather childlike states in their attitudes and thoughts, even though they act and speak in the roles of the perceived adults. Mikale's maternal introject reminds me of a little girl playing "dress-up" in her mother's clothes and trying to mimic her voice.

The purpose of ego-state therapy is not to attack the existence of apparently unconstructive states (such as this mother introject), but rather to change their internal "behavior" toward the patient without disturbing their protective functions, which may be far from obvious. The internal behaviors, which can consist of put-downs and criticism, enforce conformity to rules heard in childhood. Their goals are to ensure that she will be accepted by the "world," the child's original world being mother. The therapeutic goal is to change the attitude of such ego states toward the whole personality and to the other ego states to a more positive and constructive stance. Assuming that the motive of the mother ego state's behavior is protective, I convinced it that punishment was not a useful way to teach in the present, even though Mikale's actual mother may have done so. I also pointed out that if protection was her function, then she must love Mikale and have her best interests at heart. Initially, her internal behavior toward the patient was not loving. However, ridding the body of the allergies would be both protective and loving.

Ego states and multiple personality alters can sometimes say that they initiate destructive physical processes, which they claim are punishments for specific forbidden behaviors, but they then find they are unable to stop the process. When considering that my reframing of the situation was possibly legitimate, she expressed genuine concern that she might not be able to influence the allergies: "Right now, it's part of her body chemistry; I'm not sure I can turn it off." Nonetheless, she agreed to try.

Session V

At the beginning of Session V Mikale told me the outside mother had visited her, whereupon the allergies worsened. I hypnotized her and asked for the "inside mother." She emerged, and in her typical strained voice, asserted that she was tying to decrease the allergies but seemed unable to do so.

> Th: It isn't like you to lose control, is it?
> Pt (Mother): No, and I don't understand why. I don't understand how she on the outside could have more effect than I do on the inside. It just doesn't make sense, but it wasn't me doing it. I wish I knew what happened.

Thinking that one of the other ego states might shed some light on this mystery, I asked for Misha but suggested that the "inside mother" listen in. Misha's pipey little voice, bubbling with energy, burst forth:

> Pt (Misha): I'm here! I'm here!
> Th: Misha, do you know anything about these allergies?
> Pt (Misha): No, but you said something about guilt the last time, and that fits. Mommy always told me I was a bad girl and I should feel guilty and I would, but I didn't like it. It made my tummy hurt.

That comment made me think of Mikale's ulcer medication in the seventh grade, but I wanted to pursue the allergy problem. Because Misha denied any direct knowledge of the exacerbation of the allergies, I told her she could go wherever she wanted to go. Before leaving to play, Misha thanked me for rescuing her from the man in the basement and losing the rash and her fear of the wind, because, she said, "I feel much better now."

Still in the hypnotic state and in response to my query about the allergies, Mike, with a calm, adult-sounding voice, came forth. Mike explained that the inside mother was acting differently as a result of the therapeutic intervention, "and I was afraid that if things changed they're going to get worse. At least with them being the same, I know how to deal with that."

Apparently change is unpredictable and therefore confusing, not only to the total personality but also to the ego states. An analogy to family systems seems appropriate. When one member of a family changes, the others are also affected and may be disturbed. The balance is disrupted; the rules change. This principle is also exemplified by the internal psychological family, as shown here.

I gave Mike evidence that change can be good in that Mike helped me rescue Misha from the basement. Misha was now more carefree and happy but still not out of control. I appealed to Mike to trust the therapeutic process, to expect rather than fear the gradual changes occurring in all three of them. I told Mike that the inside mother was listening, and I invited Mike to listen while I spoke to "mother" again, thus diminishing barriers between them. I explained Mike's confusion to the inside mother and told her that Mike did not know what to do. When she softened her control over Misha, when Misha became more carefree, and when the allergies began to abate even though they were supposed to be physical manifestations of guilt, Mike became perplexed.

> Th: She got kind of confused as to what the rules were, that is, when you feel guilty, you're supposed to have an allergy.
>
> Pt (Mother): And I wasn't creating the allergies any more. But the guilt was still there, so the allergies had to be there. So Mike let them in. That makes sense.

Underlying ego states, regardless of their perceived roles, are subject to childlike and magical thinking, because they usually were created in childhood. Their thinking is literal and concrete.

The inside mother revealed that she and Misha were beginning to cooperate instead of argue. She understood that Mike felt she was left out with no function. With that comment I countered, "But maybe she (Mike) needs a function." All ego states want a purpose within that internal family. In order to effect a compromise, I brought all three ego states together to dialogue. Misha suggested that Mike could take over her thinking function so that she would be free to have fun and play. Mike was delighted at this arrangement and agreed to "stop letting the allergies in." The three ego states reached a compromise that met the needs of each, thus reducing the rigidity of the boundaries that kept them separate and moving them closer to the integration of their behaviors.

After arousal from hypnosis, I checked on the permeability of the boundaries between Mikale's main personality and the ego states:

> Th: What do you remember?
> Pt: That's weird, they're all talking—all three of them. Sometimes I wish I could just turn my eyes around and see what's going on.

Session VI

By this session I was prepared for a cue as to how to proceed. My anticipation was rewarded. The allergies were improving and Mikale was happy to have found relief, but she was disturbed about something else. She felt "shut out" when her fiancé entertained himself on his computer. Taking that clue, I hypnotized her and asked for the part that felt "shut out." Out came Mike:

> Pt (Mike): I've always been shut out. Misha and Mother always have fought, I never had anything to do with. I'm alone most of the time now. I don't like it.
> Th: Tell me about the first time you felt shut out.
> Pt (Mike): (Pause) We were little, probably real little. We were crawling but not walking. Mommy was fat, and she just started not paying attention to me . . . us. And the inside mother said, "Oh, you must have done something wrong; that's how come she's ignoring

you." She was talking to Misha even then.

Th: How old was Mikale when you were born?

Pt (Mike): I wasn't there at the beginning. I was there later. I guess I kind of came in before she was crawling, but about that age, when she started investigating things. I was there, and I was busy because I was helping her to figure out what all those things were.

Th: Is that why you came?

Pt (Mike): I think so, yeah. But then Mom started ignoring all of us, and Misha was the only one who could get attention, not that it always worked. There was a new baby when we were 11 months old. And she wanted that one. She didn't want us.

Th: How do you know that?

Pt (Mike): We felt it.

Th: I understand. Your purpose in coming, then, was to help her investigate her world. You didn't come because of any trauma at that time.

Pt (Mike): No. But things got worse and worse. I kept trying to help her explore, but like with the stranger and Mom not believing us, and instead of my being there, I think things just kind of got split, and they went either to Misha or to the "mother," and I didn't have anything. Before that there had been a kind of slow split, because the inside mother got attention because she was always prim and proper when she was in control. Everybody thought that was real cute . . . "look how well behaved she is." And Misha got attention by being clever and pretty. Nobody wanted me, a kid who asked questions.

Hence this curious, intellectual side of Mikale felt left out even to the present day at the university, because the mother ego state directed Mike's activities and took credit for the resultant academic achievement.

Pt (Mike): I get the good grades, but I don't get any credit for that. It's just expected of me. "Mother" just nags at me and tells me what to do. It's like, "okay, you're on; we don't need you any more; you're off."

Apparently Mikale was nagged to study at home but not given praise for her accomplishments. I pointed out to Mike the importance of her intellectual work and that she deserved credit for her efforts.

I called for a "conference" among Misha, Mike, and "Mother." Not enough days had elapsed since the last session for Misha to give her thinking function to Mike, but she was more than willing to do so. In that way Mike would feel important, and "Mother" felt good in shifting to a more nurturing, protective attitude, giving positive reinforcement to Mike. Misha could then devote her time to play.

> Th: I think that's fine that you play.
> Pt (Misha): So do I. But the big person, the outside one, she doesn't know how to play. The minute she starts to play, she feels guilty. I try to tell her that she doesn't have to feel guilty.

It was clear Misha no longer retained the guilt she once felt as the "bad girl."

In ego-state therapy, we think of the various entities possessing contents, such as thoughts, feelings, experiences, memories, and so on. During our internal therapeutic diplomacy, it is possible for them to give these psychological items over to other alters. For example, an ego state or alter originally created as a repository for unacceptable rage and hate can be induced to "give this garbage back" to the primary personality from which it had become dissociated. As affects can be interchanged, so also can perceptions, memories, and behaviors. With a good "therapeutic self" (Watkins 1978), the therapist can often induce a dissociated state to return to the original self those contents that the original had split off. Through acceptance and ego-strengthening, the primary ego state can reclaim the disowned feelings, such as rage, and release them through abreactive expression.

Ego states originate through normal differentiation of function, introjection of significant others, and severe trauma. Because hypnosis is a form of dissociation, it is logical that those individuals who are more toward the dissociation end of the differentiation-dissociation continuum will be more hypnotizable than those at the lower end of this scale, and that they may benefit from therapeutic interventions that make use of their hypnotizability. Furthermore, ego states will be formed and accessed much more easily with patients at the upper end of this continuum. The positive correlations among dissociation, ego-state formation, and hypnotizability are evident, especially in those who have MPD.

Session VII

Mikale's allergies were better, except for one tree in bloom that was bothering her. Mikale was surprised to hear so little noise in her head; no one seemed to be arguing. She reported that Mike was practicing thinking, and "Mother" was trying not to scold. Misha had a temper tantrum during the week, stomping her feet. I used hypnosis and asked for anyone who wanted to talk to me first. By the smile and giggle I could tell it was Misha:

> Th: I understand you had a temper tantrum.
> Pt (Misha): That was fun! I have something to tell you, though. I forgot what it was. She told me to tell you something.
> Th: Who told you to tell me?
> Pt (Misha): The big part.
> Th: "Mother?"
> Pt (Misha): No, not "Mother." The whole thing.
> Th: Oh, the main personality.
> Pt (Misha): Yeah.

Misha's comment reveals an interesting perception of herself as an aspect of Mikale rather than as actually separate. Later on, in speaking with "Mother," she commented:

> Pt (Mother): Oh, I know what the main part wanted to tell you. She wanted one of us to tell you that she hasn't been hearing us as much. She knows what we're thinking, but she doesn't hear us.

Obviously, the walls of dissociation were breaking down, and cooperation was taking the place of competition. However, Mike raised a concern.

> Pt (Mike): This is something all three of us are kind of worried about. Sometimes listening to people talk about integration, it sounds like we're all going to become one, and we don't want that. Now that

the roles are changing it's kind of nice to have three there to kind of jump in and out of.

I reassured Mike that our goal was a happy internal family, wherein all parts were important with different functions but with the unity of being a family. In speaking with Mike about the main personality, Mikale, she shared her perceptions:

> Pt (Mike): Her function? Ah, I guess she's all of us, you know. She can take the input from all of us, and she's the part that has to function with the outside world. We don't, except when Misha's throwing a temper tantrum, or I'm taking a test, or "Mother's" now being the reassuring friend type. That's the only time we really have contact with the outside world. She's the only one that deals with reality.
>
> Th: And she's the one who has to decide when it's appropriate, for example, for Misha to come out and when it's not appropriate—like a dispatcher.
>
> Pt (Mike): Yeah, that's right.

I also wanted to find out how the ego states perceived themselves physically, "within the brain." They all agreed that "Mother is on the left side near the back of top, Misha is on the right side, and Mike is in the middle toward the front." This was Mikale's inner landscape.

Session VIII

Mikale reported that the previous night she felt edgy. She heard within her head the words "I'm gonna die" and "Poor little girl." The three parts did not seem to know what was going on, but her associations led to a hospitalization at the age of 2½ when she had had a kidney infection. Using hypnosis, I brought her back to the hospital scene. Misha came out to complain of pain but also to remark "I'm not supposed to remember." I asked for any part that says she's not supposed to remember:

> Pt (Who?): *I* say she's not supposed to remember. I'm not even supposed to be here!
>
> Th: Who are you?

Pt (?): I'm before.

Th: Well, she's in the hospital and you're there, is that right? And you tell me you're not supposed to be here, or she's not supposed to remember. I'm a little confused. What are you there for?

Pt (?): I don't know why she's still here. She should have been dead! It's not logical. Something went wrong. When she was supposed to die, which was supposed to have been about 2 or 3 days ago, I was supposed to take her up. I was there to escort her, but she didn't die, and now I'm stuck here, and she's not supposed to remember me!

Th: Oh, I see. That's why you wouldn't let me take her back to remember everything, huh?

Pt (?): She can't go back any farther than this, because she can't remember what I told her. I told her she was gonna die, not to be afraid, that she would have no pain and that she would be loved all the time.

She identified herself as a kind of spirit guide, who was afraid that if Mikale found out that death would be beautiful, Mikale might consider suicide. In fact, as a teenager Mikale had thought about suicide but had made no actual attempts.

Th: Let's talk about what the advantage might be in going back there and having her reexperience this. Do you see any advantage to it?

Pt (Spirit Guide): I guess the main advantage now is that it's so close. All the work she's done and the remembering and the getting everybody straightened out and the dealing with her parents and the whole bit, that's so close that if she doesn't go back and remember, it's gonna get her sometimes, and she probably will still hear that voice, because I can't erase that.

Th: What voice can't you erase?

Pt (Spirit Guide): The feeling she got—it wasn't really a voice—that "I'm gonna die." I can't erase that now.

Th: I see. Well, I'll let you decide. You are from before, and you have more wisdom than I do.

Pt (Spirit Guide): (Sigh) It's a tough one to call. I mean, do I break the rules and give her some peace of mind, or do I leave that uneasy feeling and follow the rules. This isn't in the program. Well, I guess a lot of people who "die on the operating table," see the light, and then come back and remember. So I guess it must be all right.

I asked the spirit guide to remove the memory block. Misha was able to remember in detail what happened: the kidney infection, a high fever, hospitalization, her heart stopping and restarting, nurses giving her shots and saying "poor little girl," the fever not going down, hurting, feeling scared, and a voice saying, "It's all right; it's going to be over soon; we're going to go some place where you're always loved and taken care of." Then a doctor came in and lowered her into what she recalled as a tub of ice. The fever subsided.

> Pt (Misha, still under hypnosis): And that voice becomes frantic and tries to erase my memory of what it said and my memory of being hot and sick up to the point where my fever is down and I'm back in bed again. The voice kind of dies and goes away. It's like a tiny spot in the back of my head at the bottom. It's gone, and there's just the three of us again.
>
> Th: Now you know what came the other day when you thought about "I'm gonna die" and "poor little girl"—what this was all about. And now you understand it, and you don't need to be edgy and afraid and scared about it anymore. Okay?
>
> Pt: (Nods agreement)

Session IX

By this session, everything seemed at peace and Mikale was "feeling great." Therefore, I decided to ask her about an internal male voice she reported she sometimes heard when she was fatigued or when other people were fighting (which reminded her of her parents fighting). The words of that voice were not clear, she explained. It was as if they were heard through a wall or floor. She recalled that when her parents fought at night in the living room, she was upstairs in bed.

I attempted to induce hypnosis with a hand levitation induction, but Mikale's hand wouldn't move. Instead, the patient opened her eyes, and Misha, in a pouting voice, objected to remembering:

Pt (Misha): I don't wanna remember. I'm supposed to have fun; and that's not fun.

I explained that we needed to do something about that internal voice; otherwise Mikale would always be afraid of anger. With more explanation, Misha finally agreed to remember; she promised "not to sit on the hand again." I repeated the hypnotic induction, suggesting that she "go to wherever that loud male voice is." She regressed to age three. Misha was in bed upstairs listening to her parents "yelling and screaming and throwing things." I suggested we go downstairs and confront the parents.

Pt (Misha): I don't know. They might hurt me.

Th: Well, they're not going to hurt you because I'm here now.

Pt (Misha): Promise?

Th: Promise. Now, one of the things that I could do if you want me to: I could go in there and you could just stand behind me, or beside me, and I could hold your hand, and tell them what I think of this. Would you like that better?

Pt (Misha): They're pretty big.

Th: Well, I'm a lot bigger than they are, and I'm going to make sure they don't hurt you. And any time you want to interrupt and say what you want to say, that's O.K. All right?

We find that a close relationship with a "strong" therapist often enables child ego states to confront threatening parent figures and permits a safe abreactive release.

I confronted the parents with their unruly behavior and how they had caused a voice in her head to yell and scare her. Then Misha warmed up to the task and chimed in:

Pt (Misha): It's not fair you guys beat on me and holler and scream at me. And I'm not doing anything! I'm just trying to be a good little kid. I don't know what I'm doing wrong, because all you do you tell me I'm not supposed to cry and spank me, but you don't tell me what to do besides cry when you guys yell and scream and throw things. It's not fair!

We took turns confronting the parents until she saw them sitting down, surprised at this onslaught. She began to feel the full force of her power and sent the parents to their room to solve their problems without fighting. Misha felt strong and relieved.

Session X

Mikale noticed tension building up the evening after the last session. She had a dream that night. She was flying in a church trying to release something but could not. I hypnotized her and brought her back to that evening again. We revivified the event and built up the tension. This time the internal mother objected to the patient's feeling angry: "It's not proper for young ladies to get angry; besides it's destructive." I convinced her there were ways to express anger that are not destructive, and that releasing anger from the past is to let go of psychosomatic symptoms like headaches, tight shoulders, and gastritis. I suggested that she could "fly away with that anger of the past and feel good and free." With the reassurance that the anger wouldn't hurt anyone, the mother ego state agreed to let her return to the parents fighting in the living room. This time the patient's confrontation was more vociferous. Still more anger was released. She reported that the male voice was gone: "It's more like a memory of a memory."

Session XI

After the last session Mikale felt agitated. She released her agitation by beating on her fiancé with a harmless foam bat, an arrangement he had accepted playfully. Thereafter her tight shoulders felt more relaxed, her headaches went away, and she slept soundly at night. It also felt good to use the bat on her fantasized parents. I hypnotized her to find out which ego state was using the foam bat. Out came Misha. She had had a lot of fun with the bat. She described the satisfaction of beating up the outside mother in fantasy, even though the fiance was the physical target. In addition she told me:

Pt (Misha): We have dreams. She doesn't remember in the morning, but I do. I've been playing in the water a lot. Mom never liked that. I smashed in the potty. We splash in the puddle and we squirt the flowers with the hose—you're supposed to water them at the base. And I fly sometimes. I like to buzz people, and they run away. It's great fun.

Th: How did the internal mother feel about this?

Pt (Misha): Some of the time she's O.K. Once in a while some of that guilt creeps in with "you shouldn't be thinking those types of things, Misha; that's not the proper thing," and then I start beating on her. And then most of the time she understands. She starts mellowing out my frustrations, and it's O.K. for me to be an obnoxious little brat, because I'm real little. I'm only three or four. And so then she lays off.

Th: Does Mike have any thoughts about any of this that you are aware of?

Pt (Misha): She feels good about it, because the body feels good after all this. The stress and tension leaves. The allergies are gone, except when we run into smoke or cats and dogs. I think we're really allergic to those. Everything else is gone. I know it sounds really strange, but the more I beat on Mom, the bigger I get. So when I'm done with Mom, I'll be big enough to start beating on Dad. He's easy to yell at, but harder to beat up. He was nicer than Mom.

In talking with the internal mother ego state, I thanked her for her cooperation and for exercising her protective function by making certain the patient used a foam bat, which wouldn't hurt her hands. "Mother" perceived that she and Misha were no longer polarized but moving closer together, yet they were still happy to be separate. Mike revealed that she was now feeding information into both "Mother" and Misha so that they understood each other better, "and I'm not the deciding factor; I'm helping make the decisions." Mike continued:

Pt (Mike): The way we communicate among each other has changed. We talk to each other, and so she probably doesn't hear us because the dynamics are different. We're not projecting ourselves out trying to make decisions. We're working together to reach a consensus.

Session XII

We knew this session would be our last. Mikale had graduated and was moving out of state to be married, and I was leaving on a trip. We spent the hour in clarification and review. She no longer heard voices in her head. Instead Mikale experienced a Misha-type voice when she played, a Mike-type voice when serious, and a nurturing mother voice when playing with a neighbor's child. Wistfully, she ended the therapy with a smile, "I know it's been good for me, but I kind of miss those voices sometimes."

Ego-state therapy can bring many surprises to the therapist. Because part-persons are likely to be childlike states, it is worthwhile for the therapist to empathize with childlike patterns of thought that are literal and concrete. To begin this type of therapy, the therapist needs to discover whether an ego state can be accessed by means of hypnosis. To minimize the possibility of producing an artifact, the following approach is suggested: "I'd like to talk to the part that [mention known feeling, attitude, etc.]; but if there is no such separate part, that's just fine." Such words give reassurance that the patient need not produce what may not be there.

Not every ego-state case is as clearly delineated, cooperative, and charming as the case of Mikale proved to be. Two months after the end of our work together, I received a note from her telling me she was happy and symptom-free.

References

Federn P: Ego Psychology and the Psychoses. Edited by Weiss E. New York, Basic Books, 1952

Hilgard ER: Divided Consciousness: Multiple Controls in Human Thought and Action. New York, Wiley, 1977

Watkins H: Ego-state theory and therapy, in Encyclopedia of Psychology. Edited by Corsini RJ. New York, WIley, 1984, pp 420–421

Watkins JG: Hypnoanalytic Techniques: The Practice of Clinical Hypnosis, Vol 2. New York, Irvington, 1992

Watkins JG, Watkins HH: Ego states and hidden observers. Journal of Altered States of Consciousness 5:3–18, 1979–1980

Watkins JG, Watkins HH: Hypnosis and ego-state therapy, in Innovations in Clinical Practice: A Source Book, Vol 10. Edited by Keller P, Heyman S. Sarasota, FL, Professional Resource Exchange, 1991, pp 23–37

Chapter 15

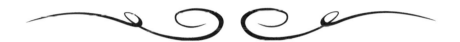

Use of Sand Trays in the Beginning Treatment of a Patient With Dissociative Disorder

Roberta G. Sachs, Ph.D.

The past decade and a half has witnessed a renewed interest in the concept of dissociation (e.g., Braun 1984; Hilgard 1977; Schacter 1987; Spiegel and Spiegel 1978) and the rediscovery of dissociative syndromes (e.g., Braun and Sachs 1985; Kluft 1985). In the laboratory setting, researchers have been using hypnosis to study how information that is inaccessible to conscious recollection under some conditions can become accessible under other conditions (e.g., Hilgard 1977). Clinical observers have witnessed similar phenomena in patients with various dissociative syndromes. For example, in patients with multiple personality disorder (MPD), a particular personality state may know information that is consciously inaccessible to another personality state. Both the research and clinical examples illustrate how memories can become dissociated from deliberate conscious recollection. However, dissociated memories can still affect a person's behavior without that person's being aware of their

influence (Braun 1984; Kluft 1987; Schacter 1987), often with dis-
maying results.

Investigators and clinicians working with normal subjects and dissociative disorder patients have been exploring a variety of techniques for bringing previously inaccessible memories back to
conscious awareness. The purpose of my discussion here is to illustrate the clinical use of sand trays for uncovering dissociated material.
First, I offer a brief historical review of the sand tray techniques.
Second, I illustrate the use of sand trays with materials from the
treatment of a patient with dissociative disorder, supplemented by
the patient's retrospective verbal reports about her state of mind during the time of her experiences with the sand tray technique.

The reader must bear in mind that this discussion of the sand
tray technique with dissociative disorder patients is more a report of
work in progress than a definitive statement. It describes my first use
of this approach, in response to a patient's spontaneous initiation
of it. At this point in time, I have used this technique with many
more patients, and I am confident that the sand tray is a powerful
clinical technique. But I am still trying to discern whether it has
particular indications and contraindications, and I cannot objectively compare its efficacy to that of the more traditional nonverbal psychotherapies. It also remains to be established how to best
achieve a constructive synergy among this and other therapeutic
modalities.

A Brief Historical Review of
the Sand Tray Technique

The use of sand trays may have its beginnings in the ancient rituals
of primitive tribes who drew protective circles on the ground as a
symbolic act. However, the first person to seriously write about the
therapeutic use of sand play was the Swiss psychoanalyst C. G. Jung.
Deeply affected by his break with Freud, Jung went to the shores of
Lake Zurich, where he had spent many happy times as a child.
Along the lakeshore, he allowed himself to play in the sand. This

evoked a number of childhood fantasies, and he believed that it helped to alleviate his troubled state of mind. These experiences stimulated Jung to consider the potential therapeutic value of play as a means of accessing the unconscious and promoting the normal healing tendencies of the ego.

In 1911, H. G. Wells published his first book, *Floor Games* (1911/1976), which described how he played on the floor with his two sons. Wells believed in stimulating the creative imagination of his children through constructive play. In his book, he admonished the toy manufacturers of his time for not developing better products for children. He was dissatisfied with types of available miniature figurines that he believed either cost too much or were too militaristic.

Margaret Lowenfeld, a child psychiatrist, read *Floor Games,* and this influenced her to create her own version of therapeutic play. She collected many miniature figurines, buildings, and greenery, as well as other toys, and stored them in what she called the "Wonder Box." In the same room, she also had a large tray of sand and a tray of water. One day a child unknowingly constructed the first sand tray by combining the objects of the Wonder Box with a tray of sand. Later workers observing such play behaviors called these constructions "worlds."

Another child psychiatrist, Dora Kalff, was greatly impressed by Lowenfeld's presentation of the sand tray technique at various international conferences and went on to study the procedure with her. A Jungian analyst, she consulted with Jung himself on her adaption of the sand tray technique. Although Kalff is generally credited with introducing the sand tray technique to the mental health community, the earlier influence of Jung, Wells, and Lowenfeld must be acknowledged.

My own discovery of the therapeutic value of sand play in the treatment of dissociative conditions occurred serendipitously. I was unaware of the work of Kalff or her predecessors and never had heard of the sand tray technique. One day, a highly regressed and dissociated hospitalized patient showed me a sand tray that she had constructed from the materials available in the ward psychiatrist's office. This patient had been virtually mute and unable to communicate verbally throughout her admission. I was immediately struck by the variety and intensity of affect and the overall expressivity displayed in her sand tray creation. Sensing that this might be a way to reach this patient, I decided to experiment further with this technique. The remainder of this chapter focuses on describing the case history of this patient and the role that the sand tray has played in her treatment.

Case Study

The patient was a 41-year-old married white female born in a large midwestern city. Her given history is that her parents were members of a transgenerational satanic cult into which she was initiated at birth.

At this point, it is difficult to speak with certainty as to how to understand such allegations from patients. The child abuse and dissociative disorders fields are torn with controversy over whether such reports are historical, metaphorical-allegorical, or inaccurate. There is dispute as to whether one or more of the available hypotheses can offer an inclusive explanation, or whether each case report involves a unique and confusing combination of contributants. The interested reader may wish to consult recent clinical research (Young et al. 1991), expressions of opinion (Ganaway 1989; Lanning 1991; Putnam 1991), and a book on the subject (Sakheim and Devine 1992). In any case, it is the experience of most clinicians that such material, whatever its origin, does not respond reliably to any intervention other than its being treated as serious clinical material requiring respectful exploration, abreaction, and working-through traumatic memories. The latter stance was taken with the patient.

She reported being violently and sadistically abused on a daily basis throughout her childhood. When she began attending school, she reports that she concurrently was placed in a satanic cult education program in which she reportedly was drugged and forced to learn about the cult symbols, rituals, and practices. All Christmas holidays or special occasions had their satanic cult counterpart. For example, she would have two birthday celebrations, two Christmas holidays, and so on, one at home and one in the cult.

Her school records showed that she was absent more days than most pupils throughout elementary school. Her academic performance was erratic. She reported being humiliated by the other children at school on a regular basis because of her bizarre behavior. For example, she would be given an enema at lunchtime as a punishment to cleanse her from evil and told to hold it when she returned to school. Ultimately, she would lose sphincter control and soil her clothes. She would be teased by her schoolmates and sent home by the teacher. At home she would be punished again for soiling her clothes and being sent home from school.

During her high school years, the patient alleges she was apprenticed as a high priestess in her original cult group. She was trained by her mother to make "administrative decisions" about issues related to sacrifices and ceremonies. In addition, she states that she formed her own teenage peer cult group, recruiting members from a black motorcycle gang. This group met regularly but never interacted with her transgenerational group. This gang's activities typically were modified rituals borrowed from the patient's earlier indoctrination, and included drug taking, bizarre sex, and the sacrifice of small animals and occasionally a small child.

After graduating from high school, she enrolled in a teacher's college. She dropped out after completing 2½ years because she could not meet her course obligations. During this period, she abandoned her peer cult affiliations but remained active in her own transgenerational cult group. Over the next 10 years, she held 10 different jobs, most of which involved caring for nursery school children. She was fired on several occasions because of suspected child abuse. Eventually, she completed her college degree and became employed as an elementary school teacher.

She married a Vietnam veteran who was neither affiliated with a cult nor aware of her history of such activities. Their premarital relations were asexual. Her husband became aware that she was abusing alcohol. He encouraged her to leave her teaching job to enter treatment in a local alcohol treatment center. The patient was eventually diagnosed as having a complex dissociative disorder. She was found to have many fragments (Braun 1986) in addition to several well-developed personality states. Such cases have been described by Braun (1986) as polyfragmented multiple personality and by Kluft (1988) as highly complex MPD. In my experience, this type of dissociative disorder appears to be related to a given history of chronic ritualized abuse.

When initially admitted to the hospital, the patient was in an extremely regressed and dissociated state. She was uncommunicative, fearful, easily agitated, and appeared to relive terrifying past experiences spontaneously. At times she was very childlike; she carried around a baby doll that she alternately nurtured and abused. At other times she appeared to be reenacting sexual experiences. She would masturbate in public, expose herself, and engage in seductive behaviors.

Treatment, of course, involved efforts toward behavioral containment and redirection from disruptive activities. In terms of individual psychotherapy, the development of trust was the first treatment issue to be addressed. Because the patient switched rapidly through a large number of nonverbal personality fragments, standard verbal communication was almost impossible at times. Her switches were so frequent that at times she was unable to complete a sentence either in writing or in speech. To overcome this problem, I would sit and talk with her in a quiet, soothing, hypnotic manner, attempting to create an atmosphere of empathy and safety.

The next step in therapy was to establish some type of nonverbal communication channel with the patient. I established ideomotor signals for "yes," "no," and "stop." This permitted some interaction with the patient and some insight into her inner world. Nonetheless, her defenses were so fortified and her switching so chaotic that it was difficult to get much useful information.

She had been hospitalized for almost 2 months when she discovered a sand tray and shelves of figurines in the waiting room of the office of one of the psychiatrists. She brought me to this office, pointed to the sand tray, and said, "Me do?" Permission was obtained, and the patient spent the next 3 hours doing her first sand tray. I gave her no instructions and left her to work on her own.

The most striking aspect of this first sand tray was the overwhelming sense of chaos that it depicted. Its chaos was paralleled in her writing and artwork. It was a mirror of her own perception of her own internal psychological structure. There were more than 300 pieces and figurines in the sand tray. Representations of violence and sexual abuse were interspersed with religious figures or objects, a poignant commentary on her reported history and its impact on her.

Although other staff members and I were deeply moved by the trauma depicted in this sand tray, the patient herself had no immediate overt emotional response to what she had represented. However, when I attempted to process the sand tray with her the following day, she experienced a flood of sensory images and affective responses. Although she had no verbal explanation for or conscious knowledge of what was depicted on the sand tray, when she saw it, her pelvis started to writhe, she turned her head, covered her eyes, and began screaming, "No! No! No! Not true!" This reaction was more congruent with the affective intensity displayed in the sand tray than with her weak verbal disclaimer.

These observations led me to try to find out more about the use of the sand tray and to explore its potential applications for the diagnosis and treatment of dissociative conditions. In my initial efforts, no set procedures or instructions were used with the patient. She was allowed to do what she wanted with no guidance or imposed structure. On completing the sand tray, she would show me what she had created. I would use ideomotor signals to question her.

After 3 to 4 weeks, the sand trays began to get more organized. Specific incidents of abuse were depicted. Inquiries made via ideomotor signals allowed the identification of specific personality fragments and the clarification of many reported incidents. This helped the patient to understand her own internal structure and its adaptive function. The patient seemed compulsively driven to make sand trays whenever I was present, and to "take down" the depictions before I left. The patient felt safe to build sand worlds and reveal herself only during those times; she feared exposing her inner world to others. Gradually, it became clear that three distinct yet parallel sections recurrently appeared in all of her sand trays. They were divided by lines drawn in the sand in the following manner:

1. The section farthest to the right contained miniature figurines representing the patient's thoughts and feelings in the here and now.
2. The middle section was the largest and was replete with scenes of sadistic torture, both sexual and physical, representing her involvement with her transgenerational satanic cult.
3. The left section portrayed the wide variety of bizarre physical and sexual abuses she had experienced in her home environment.

I began to understand that I could access the patient's daily condition by examining the first section. This included indications of the patient's reactions to treatment and the nature and extent of her current homicidal and suicidal ideation. The middle section allowed me to understand the highly organized and complex nature of the training and activities of her satanic cult. For example, she depicted a scene in this section in which she represented herself as being forced by cult members to insert a crucifix into her vagina in order to induce premature labor. The left section provided information about the precult training she had received at home as a child, and the nature of the ongoing abuses that occurred in between cult meetings (e.g., pornography, snuff films, prostitution, drug involvement). During the first 10 months of treatment, the patient vacillated between accepting and denying the validity of the history depicted in her sand trays. She became better able to understand and accept her past when she was eventually able to write and finally to speak about these experiences. This was accomplished between months 12 and 18 of intensive hospital treatment.

After 2 years of treatment, the patient was able to offer thoughtful reflections upon her experience with the sand tray. She wrote,

> The sand was set up in small sections, and each section contained a different kind of abuse or form of torture. I rarely would complete a whole section at one time. . . . The building became too painful, and we would switch and add to or complete another section. . . . Items were tested and fragments inside would tell me when they were ready to have the information come out. . . . It was my life in the

sand. A life we could not talk about and that was not perfect. They would tell what we could not.

This account demonstrates the utility of the sand tray in accessing previously dissociated apparent memories. Past abuses that once could not be remembered consciously and expressed verbally could be depicted in the sand. It is instructive to reflect that this was one way of protecting a patient—someone who has been forced to promise her tormentors that she would never talk of what had happened to her—in a safe and more controlled manner. The pictures in the sand changed over the course of therapy as issues were resolved in treatment.

Over time, other patients on the unit began to request time to "play" with the sand tray, possibly because of the special attention and interest that was given to the first patient. This afforded me an opportunity to try variations on the initial technique in order to find out what was most effective in the treatment process. However, this case clearly illustrates some of the possible applications of this technique. At least in some cases, it can allow the therapist access to a patient's inner world when traditional methods of inquiry fail to yield this type of data. We can only hope that, as other therapists begin to use this potentially valuable technique, its applications for the assessment and treatment of patients with dissociative disorder will become better understood and more widely appreciated.

References

Braun BG: Towards a theory of multiple personality and other dissociative phenomena. Psychiatr Clin North Am 7:171–193, 1984

Braun BG: Issues in the psychotherapy of multiple personality disorder, in Treatment of Multiple Personality Disorder. Edited by Braun BG. Washington, DC, American Psychiatric Press, 1986, pp 1–28

Braun BG, Sachs RG: The development of multiple personality disorder: predisposing, precipitating, and perpetuating factors, in Childhood Antecedents of Multiple Personality Disorder. Edited by Kluft RP. Washington, DC, American Psychiatric Press, 1985, pp 37–64

Ganaway GK: Historical truth versus narrative truth: clarifying the role of exogenous trauma in the etiology of multiple personality disorder and its variants. Dissociation 2:205–220, 1989

Hilgard E: Divided Consciousness: Multiple Controls in Human Thought and Action. New York, Wiley, 1977

Kluft RP: Introduction: multiple personality disorder in the 1980s, in Childhood Antecedents of Multiple Personality Disorder. Edited by Kluft RP. Washington, DC, American Psychiatric Press, 1985, pp viii–xiv

Kluft RP: First-rank symptoms as a diagnostic clue to multiple personality disorder. Am J Psychiatry 144:293–298, 1987

Kluft RP: The phenomenology and treatment of extremely complex multiple personality disorder. Dissociation 1(4):47–58, 1988

Lanning KV: Commentary: ritual abuse: a law enforcement view or perspective. Child Abuse Negl 15:171–174, 1991

Putnam FW: Commentary: the satanic ritual abuse controversy. Child Abuse Negl 15:175–179, 1991

Sakheim DK, Devine SE (eds): Out of Darkness: Exploring Satanism and Ritual Abuse. New York, Lexington, 1992

Schacter D: Implicit memory: history and current status. J Exp Psychol 13:501–508, 1987

Spiegel H, Spiegel D: Trance and Treatment. New York, Basic Books, 1978

Wells HG: Floor Games (1911). New York, Arno Press, 1976

Young WC, Sachs RG, Braun BG, et al: Patients reporting ritual abuse in childhood: a clinical syndrome. Child Abuse Negl 15:181–190, 1991

Section IV

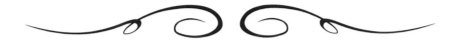

Contemporary Issues and Concerns in the Study of Multiple Personality Disorder

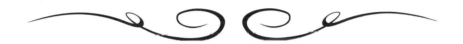

Chapter 16

Multiple Personality Consultation in the Public Psychiatric Sector

Philip M. Coons, M.D.

I first met Connie Wilbur, M.D, in late 1973, when she spoke on multiple personality disorder (MPD) to the Indiana Psychiatric Society. At the time, I was a second-year psychiatric resident struggling to understand my first MPD patient. Before 1973, my only exposure to MPD had been hearing a case presentation at the Purdue University Student Health Center during a senior medical student elective. I had been assured that MPD was a rare disorder and that I probably would not see more than one case during my career. No member of the faculty of the Department of Psychiatry at Indiana University School of Medicine was aware of ever having seen a case of MPD. However, several of my supervisors were very helpful and supportive of my efforts to explore the phenomenon and to seek consultation elsewhere. Dr. Wilbur was gracious enough to spend time with me during a noontime luncheon when she was in Indianapolis, so I proceeded to "pick her brain." What I remember best about Connie's advice was the admonition "listen to the patient." She maintained that the answers to my questions would be provided by the patient in due time. My task was to provide a safe environment, develop trust, and foster inquisitiveness.

I found the book *Sybil* (Schreiber 1973) extremely helpful in my work with my first MPD patient. There were few resources to which I could turn. Over the next 2 years, my search of the professional literature in the dusty stacks of several university and research libraries in Indiana and Illinois unearthed only 150 references on MPD. Many of these were in very obscure sources, and only 11 were from the years 1950–1957. I found contributions by Myers (1903), Prince (1905), Taylor and Martin (1944), Thigpen and Cleckley (1957), Sutcliffe and Jones (1962), Ludwig and colleagues (1972), and Ellenberger (1970) especially helpful at that time. My explorations were not easy. In 1973, MPD was not even listed in the *Index Medicus*. Unbeknownst to me at the time, Myron Boor, a psychologist, was doing a similar search of the literature. We eventually met and collaborated on the first comprehensive bibliography of MPD (Boor and Coons 1983). Since 1970, the professional literature on MPD has exploded with hundreds of new articles, book chapters, and books (collected in bibliographies by Boor and Coons 1983; Coons 1986–1990; Damgaard et al. 1985) and the publication of *Dissociation,* a specialized journal.

In 1977, Connie Wilbur and Ralph Allison participated in the first panel on MPD ever held at an annual meeting of the American Psychiatric Association. Since 1978, a continuing medical education course on MPD has been (with the exception of 1980) an annual occurrence. I feel fortunate to have been included on the faculty of most of these courses. Workshops on a national level have also been given by the American Society for Clinical Hypnosis, the American Orthopsychiatric Association, the Society for Clinical and Experimental Hypnosis, and the International Society for the Study of Multiple Personality/Dissociation.

In Indiana I have spearheaded efforts to educate both professional and lay audiences about MPD. I have given a number of Psychiatry Grand Rounds presentations at Indiana University School of Medicine and have spoken to professional and lay audiences at local hospitals, outpatient clinics, churches, and child protective services. I had been codirector of the Indianapolis Study Group for many years and have made numerous radio and television appearances in central Indiana to educate the lay public. Finally, I have been active in educating the Indiana medical community through a continuing medical education article (Coons 1986a).

In 1984 I opened a Dissociative Disorders Clinic in the Psychiatry Department at Indiana University School of Medicine. I have functioned as its director and have provided both consultation and supervision of treatment of MPD to psychiatric residents and other mental health professionals in both inpatient and outpatient settings. Since the Dissociative Disorders Clinic opened, 285 patients have been evaluated, and 107 were diagnosed with MPD.

Over the years I have evolved a characteristic style of interviewing and consulting with patients suspected of having MPD (Coons 1986b). If the patient is being seen in consultation for another clinician, that clinician is invited to participate in the evaluation session(s) to become more familiar with both the diagnostic process and the treatment of MPD. Two to three 50-minute sessions are often necessary to elicit a full psychiatric history, including present and past psychiatric difficulties, medical history, review of systems, family history, social history, and mental status examination. The referring clinician often can provide a good description of overt dissociation if it has occurred and been witnessed. At the end of the first session the patient is administered the Dissociative Experiences Scale (DES) (Bernstein and Putnam 1986), a checklist for symptoms of dissociation and posttraumatic stress disorder, and the Minnesota Multiphasic Personality Inventory (MMPI; Hathaway and McKinley 1970). A neurological examination electroencephalogram (EEG) and other psychological and medical tests may be administered if necessary. Collateral interviews are scheduled with parents, spouses, and others to confirm or disconfirm a history of prior dissociation and child abuse (Coons 1980, 1984). By the end of the second session I have usually gathered enough material to make me fairly confident of a diagnosis, and the patient has become comfortable enough with me so that I can elicit alter states if they exist.

My technique for eliciting alter states often varies on a patient-by-patient basis. In 20%–25% of patients my work is easy, because spontaneous dissociation into an alter occurs sometime during the course of the evaluation. In an equal number of patients I am able to talk to an alter by merely calling that alter's name with the primary personality's permission or inquiring whether "anyone else" wants to talk to me. In approximately 50% of the cases, such accessing does not occur easily, so I tell the patient to close his or her eyes, relax, and "go back into the head" as he or she did when younger in an attempt to avoid pain, fear, or knowledge of child abuse, while I call forth an alter. This technique takes advantage of the patient's tendency to dissociate. If this technique fails (as in less than 5%–10% of MPD cases), I perform a formal hypnotic induction to search for alter states (Kluft 1982).

To make a diagnosis of MPD, in addition to the patient's fulfilling DSM-III-R diagnostic criteria (American Psychiatric Association 1987), I require both the presence of a history of amnesia (Coons 1984) and the observation of actual dissociation or switching of personalities. I have been fooled at least once by a patient who proved to have factitious MPD. As a result, I learned that it is important to observe the patient over more than a relatively short period of time to search for inconsistencies in history and presentation. I take care to observe the patient for signs of the overdramatization seen in factitious cases and malingerers (Coons 1984; Orne et al. 1984).

A portion of the third or final session is spent sharing the results of my findings and recommendations with the patient and the consulting clinician. In situations where the therapeutic rapport is tenuous, I am careful to share only as much as I think the patient can handle. Many patients experience the most circumspect explanation of their circumstances as overwhelming. Some patients have been known to flee therapy because of their fear of loss of control. Unless the therapist already has ample information about MPD, he or she is given a packet of five or six articles on the diagnosis and treatment of MPD (e.g., Boor and Coons 1983; Damgaard et al. 1985; Kluft 1985a, 1985b, 1987). Finally, the clinician is invited to join the Indianapolis Study Group, which meets monthly to discuss the treatment of MPD. A number of consultees, mainly psychiatric residents, have elected to continue in supervision with me while they treat their patients with long-term psychodynamic psychotherapy and hypnosis. Clinicians who do not know hypnosis and wish to use it are advised to obtain experience in its use through various continuing education courses or training programs offered around the country (American Society for Clinical Hypnosis, Society for Clinical and Experimental Hypnosis, and accredited training programs in psychiatry and psychology).

Examples of Case Consultations

What follows are illustrations, drawn from my experiences as a consultant, of a number of common problems encountered in the diagnosis and treatment of MPD. For the sake of clarity, a short discussion follows each case vignette. (For further discussion on consultation and transference and countertransference in the treatment of MPD, see Chu 1988a, 1988b; Fine 1989; Greaves 1988; Kluft 1988a, 1988b, 1990; see also Chapter 4.)

Diagnosis

Case Study 1—False-Positive Misdiagnosis

The patient was a 26-year-old male referred for hospitalization with the diagnosis of "multiple personality." He gave a history of violent agitated behavior during blackouts. He indicated that these blackouts occurred when "Oscar" bothered him. The patient maintained that Oscar was initially an imaginary playmate who had "turned bad" when he was 16 years of age. Collateral history sources revealed that the patient had lied extensively and had participated in much antisocial behavior during his life. Further examination revealed that although Oscar could talk through the patient, Oscar did not emerge spontaneously and could not be elicited, even with the aid of hypnosis. Eventually it was discovered that the patient was seeking disability and that he had used the ruse of Oscar whenever he needed to evade responsibility.

The diagnosis in this case was malingering. Interestingly, the referring clinician was greatly disappointed that the patient did not have MPD, because she had never seen such a case.

Case Study 2—False-Negative Misdiagnosis

The patient was a 25-year-old woman who had been hospitalized 6 times in 6 years. Her symptoms included sudden mood swings and suicidal urges, angry and/or inappropriate behavior for which she was amnesic, different handwriting styles, use of different names, inner voices, self-starvation, self-mutilation, and sexual frigidity. Her history revealed suspected child abuse by her schizophrenic mother. Despite her history, which was strongly suggestive of MPD, her manifestation of many signs considered indicators of MPD, and reports from the nursing staff of dissociative behavior, her therapist discounted this information and made the diagnosis of schizoaffective disorder. The patient languished, essentially untreated and unimproved, for 2½ months until she was transferred to another clinician, who made the correct diagnosis of MPD and instituted appropriate therapy.

This case represents a not-uncommon problem among psychiatric professionals: disbelief in MPD. Although the reasons for this particular clinician's disbelief are unknown, Goodwin (1985) and Benedek (1984) indicate that the following mechanisms may be operative: identification with the aggressor, revulsion at the child abuse, or anxiety about involvement in a difficult clinical situation that might make the clinician angry or sexually stimulated. Still another factor in clinicians' disbelief is having been exposed to training that dogmatically asserts that all tales of sexual seduction are fantasy and/or the mistaken belief that MPD is rare (Coons 1980).

Case Study 3—False-Negative Misdiagnosis

A 19-year-old woman was referred for hospitalization. She had been hospitalized four times before in another hospital for "psychotic episodes" that consisted of 2- to 4-hour periods of crying, screaming, visual hallucination, and head-banging. She was amnesic for some of these episodes, which did not seem to respond to phenothiazines. The episodes that she could remember she described as feeling as if she were having a "bad dream" or reliving the past. She had a long history of childhood physical and sexual abuse. In addition, she had "inner voices," amnesia for childhood events, frequent severe headaches, and conversion paralysis. In this case, hypnotic inquiry proved necessary and revealed evidence of alter states, which were subsequently observed spontaneously emerging on the ward.

Another extremely common problem encountered with MPD is misdiagnosis. In this case the flashbacks of past abuse had been interpreted mistakenly as evidence of psychosis.

Case Study 4

A 38-year-old woman was referred by her therapist for assessment of possible dissociative disorder. Symptoms included amnesia episodes since childhood, childhood physical and sexual abuse, self-mutilation, and a vague feeling of being split into different "little girl" parts. Hypnosis confirmed the existence of MPD. Continued contact revealed significant alcohol abuse in one of her adult personalities, so treatment with Antabuse was instituted as she continued in treatment for her MPD.

This case represents an example of the majority (about 75%) of my consultative work with MPD patients and their therapists. A clinician asks for consultation to help diagnose possible MPD, the diagnosis is made, treatment is instituted, and the patient proceeds slowly and fairly uneventfully toward integration.

Treatment

Case Study 5

A 29-year-old woman with MPD was referred for treatment by her therapist, who wished to terminate the treatment abruptly. The therapist had treated the patient for depression and suicidal thinking for 5 years and had only recently become aware of the MPD. The patient had become overly involved with both her therapist and her minister. Both had engaged in much hugging and hand-holding, both inside and outside their professional contacts with her. The therapeutic relationship was abruptly terminated after the patient staged a fake abduction and rape in her attempt to extract more sympathy from her therapist. This patient eventually found another therapist who was able to set firm limits and resist her infantile demands. Consultation with the minister enabled him to set firm limits also.

Case Study 6

In a similar situation, a clinician engaged in hugging and hand-holding with a 30-year-old MPD patient who, as a child, had been sexually abused by her father. On a number of occasions she was invited into her therapist's home. Although the clinician had been warned that his overfamiliar behavior was inappropriate, it continued.

Despite enjoying this boundary-violating behavior in some alters, these unwarranted intimacies provoked strong negative responses in other alters. These alters eventually became so enraged that (in these alters) the patient threatened her therapist's life. At this point he considered termination of therapy.

Overinvolvement with patients is an ever-present danger. It is particularly hazardous with MPD patients, who are extremely needy because of their experiences with chronic child abuse and neglect. If the clinician gives in to and indulges the patient's inappropriate demands for attention, regression rather than benefit is a likely outcome. Demands for attention may escalate, eventually exhaust the clinician, and ultimately lead to the abrupt termination of therapy, as occurred in these two later cases.

In several other instances, patients have revealed to me that the overfamiliarity in therapy had actually progressed to sexual contact. In no case was this therapeutically beneficial; in one case a malpractice action was brought against the clinician. For the patient, such unwarranted behavior represents a continuation of the abuse that began in childhood, still another victimization at the hands of a purported caretaker. The retraumatization during therapist-patient sexual contact usually leads to premature termination of therapy, which is interrupted until a replacement therapist can be found. Clinicians wishing more information on sexual contact between therapists and MPD patients should consult Kluft (1989, 1990).

Case Study 7

A 40-year-old professional woman with MPD was hospitalized for an acute intercurrent depression that resolved rapidly. However, both she and her therapist became so fascinated with the exploration of her dissociative illness that discharge was delayed for months. In her attempt to become one of the most fascinating patients on record, she scoured the professional literature on MPD; she even considered writing a book and making television appearances. As a result of consultation, the patient's attempts to obtain disability were short-circuited, and she eventually returned to work. Outpatient therapy became bogged down, however, because both the patient and the therapist continued their fascination with MPD and had difficulty prioritizing legitimate psychotherapeutic goals.

Kluft (1988a) indicates that the initial fascination with MPD is a normative experience for novice MPD therapists. However, we concur that continued fascination combined with a disability-seeking, narcissistically invested patient can be an invitation to therapeutic disaster. The inexperienced and minimally skilled mental health professional may find him- or herself simply overwhelmed, as in the following examples.

Case Study 8

A 25-year-old professional call girl with MPD had experienced both physical and sexual abuse in childhood. She evolved an eroticized and sexually provocative alter who alternated with her frightened, reserved, and inhibited host or original personality. Her boyfriend (and procurer) attended therapy sessions with her. Unfortunately, his agenda was to attempt to maintain the status quo.

The patient's therapist was so inexperienced and limited in his therapeutic repertoire that despite consultation, he was unable to set limits and exclude the boyfriend from therapy. Therapy was terminated by the patient's move to another city, and it was never resumed.

Case Study 9

A 20-year-old indigent single mother of an infant was diagnosed as having MPD during a psychiatric hospitalization. She was referred to a public psychiatric clinic in her local community for follow-up care on discharge. Her inexperienced therapist threatened that if she continued to dissociate, her child would be taken away from her on the grounds of child abuse. She dropped out of therapy and moved to a different community where she continued to dissociate, but declined to seek further treatment.

The question of inexperienced clinicians is a thorny one. I have consulted with a variety of clinicians with a wide range of experience, including psychiatrists, psychiatric residents, psychologists, psychology interns, social workers, nurse clinicians, and occupational therapists, who have made excellent MPD therapists. The successful clinicians, regardless of their age or experience, appeared to have a number of characteristics in common. These included a solid grounding in psychodynamic psychotherapy, an ability to listen and empathize, a willingness to explore and learn about MPD and its therapy, a willingness to challenge old misconceptions about child abuse, a capacity to tolerate frustration, and an ability to set firm limits.

In certain circumstances, the consultant becomes involved in a situation for which no resolution is immediately apparent.

Case Study 10

A 40-year-old male with MPD was found not guilty by reason of insanity for kidnapping, assault, and intent to murder. He was confined to a state hospital for treatment. Although he became apparently integrated for a short period of time, the integration was not lasting. Continued treatment became almost impossible for a number of reasons. There was a lack of administrative support for the therapeutic endeavor. Frequent changes in the structure of the institution led to frequent changes of therapists; some of these therapists knew nothing about MPD and were unwilling to learn. A series of potent phenothiazine medications were administered in the course of fruitless attempts to treat the MPD as a psychotic delusional system. Finally, the powerful lobbying efforts of politicians and community activists prevented this man's release back into the community, even though he no longer presented a danger.

This final case represents a situation in which it is almost impossible to render adequate care for the patient. The efforts to provide appropriate therapy encountered elements of disbelief, mistreatment, and downright prejudice. Thankfully, an increasingly small number of patients with MPD are encountering such deleterious experiences.

Conclusions

If I leave the interested reader and clinician with one caveat about MPD, I would like to demystify the disorder and say that it is not a "special" disorder, nor are people who have MPD "special patients." Neither are they freaks who deserve to be held in awe. The problems encountered in treating MPD are no more unusual or complicated than the problems encountered in treating borderline personality disorder. Therapy may be arduous, but it is also very gratifying. There is no substitute for sound psychotherapeutic technique, especially one with firm limits and boundaries combined with a listening empathetic ear. If a clinician has these attributes, the acquisition of the few remaining skills needed to treat MPD should be easy. We should all be grateful to the wisdom of Connie Wilbur's example and for her insistent advice about the importance of listening to the patient.

References

American Psychiatric Association: Diagnostic and Statistical Manual of Mental Disorders, 3rd Edition, Revised. Washington, DC, American Psychiatric Association, 1987

Benedek EP: The silent scream: countertransference reactions to victims. American Journal of Social Psychiatry 4:49–52, 1984

Bernstein E, Putnam F: Development, reliability, and validity of a dissociation scale. J Nerv Ment Dis 174:727–735, 1986

Boor M, Coons PM: A comprehensive bibliography of literature pertaining to multiple personality. Psychol Rep 53:295–310, 1983

Chu JA: Some aspects of resistance in the treatment of multiple personality disorder. Dissociation 1(2):34–38, 1988a

Chu JA: Ten traps for therapists in the treatment of trauma survivors. Dissociation 1(4):24–32, 1988b

Coons PM: Multiple personality: diagnostic considerations. J Clin Psychiatry 41:330–336, 1980

Coons PM: The differential diagnosis of multiple personality disorder: a comprehensive review. Psychiatr Clin North Am 7:51–57, 1984

Coons PM: Dissociative disorders: diagnosis and treatment. Indiana Med 79:411–415, 1986a

Coons PM: Treatment progress in 20 patients with multiple personality disorder. J Nerv Ment Dis 174:715–721, 1986b

Coons PM: Abstracts of recent articles. Newsletter of the International Society for the Study of Multiple Personality and Dissociation 4–8, 1986–1990

Damgaard J, Benschoten S, Fagan J: An updated bibliography of literature pertaining to multiple personality. Psychol Rep 57:131–137, 1985

Ellenberger EF: The Discovery of the Unconscious: The History and Evolution of Dynamic Psychiatry. New York, Basic Books, 1970

Fine CG: Treatment errors and iatrogenesis across therapeutic modalities in MPD and allied dissociative disorders. Dissociation 2:77–82, 1989

Goodwin J: Credibility problems in multiple personality disorder and abused children, in Childhood Antecedents of Multiple Personality Disorder. Edited by Kluft RP. Washington, DC, American Psychiatric Press, 1985, pp 1–19

Greaves GB: Common errors in the treatment of multiple personality disorder. Dissociation 1(1):61–66, 1988

Hathaway SR, McKinley JC: Minnesota Multiphasic Personality Inventory, Revised. Minneapolis, MN, University of Minnesota, 1970

Kluft RP: Varieties of hypnotic interventions in the treatment of multiple personality. Am J Clin Hypn 24:230–240, 1982

Kluft RP: Making the Diagnosis of Multiple Personality Disorder (MPD) (Directions in Psychiatry, Vol 5, Lesson 23). Edited by Flach FF. New York, Hatherleigh, 1985a, pp 1–11

Kluft RP: The Treatment of Multiple Personality Disorder (MPD): Current Concepts (Directions in Psychiatry, Vol 5, Lesson 24). Edited by Flach FF. New York, Hatherleigh, 1985b, pp 1–11

Kluft RP: An update on multiple personality disorder. Hosp Community Psychiatry 38:363–373, 1987

Kluft RP: On giving consultations to therapists treating multiple personality disorder: fifteen years' experience, I: diagnosis and treatment. Dissociation 1(3):23–29, 1988a

Kluft RP: On giving consultations to therapists treating multiple personality disorder: fifteen years' experience, II: the "surround" of treatment, forensics, hypnosis, patient-initiated requests. Dissociation 1(3):30–35, 1988b

Kluft RP: Treating the patient who has been exploited by a previous therapist. Psychiatr Clin North Am 12:483–500, 1989

Kluft RP: Incest and subsequent revictimization: the case of therapist-patient sexual exploitation, with a description of the sitting duck syndrome, in Incest-Related Syndromes of Adult Psychopathology. Edited by Kluft RP. Washington, DC, American Psychiatric Press, 1990, pp 263–287

Ludwig AM, Bransma JM, Wilbur CB, et al: The objective study of a multiple personality, or, are four heads better than one? Arch Gen Psychiatry 26:298–310, 1972

Myers FWH: Human Personality and Its Survival of Bodily Death, Vol 1. New York, Longmans, Green, 1903

Orne MT, Dinges DF, Orne EC: On the differential diagnosis of multiple personality in the forensic context. Int J Clin Exp Hypn 32:118–169, 1984

Prince M: Dissociation of a Personality. New York, Longmans, Green, 1905

Schreiber FR: Sybil. Chicago, IL, Regnery, 1973

Sutcliffe JP, Jones J: Personal identity, multiple personality, and hypnosis. Int J Clin Exp Hypn 10:231–269, 1962

Taylor WS, Martin MF: Multiple personality. Journal of Abnormal and Social Psychology 29:281–300, 1944

Thigpen CH, Cleckley HM: The Three Faces of Eve. New York, McGraw-Hill, 1957

Chapter 17

Eating Disorders in Survivors of Multimodal Childhood Abuse

Jean M. Goodwin, M.D., M.P.H.
Reina Attias, Ph.D.

M any classic clinical descriptions of multiple personality disorder (MPD) and incest victimization syndromes contain accounts of disordered eating behaviors. The extreme multimodal childhood abuse that is almost invariably present in these patients may involve abnormal eating experiences, including starvation, force-feeding, forced ingestion of nonfood substances, and emotional abuse around eating or weight, in addition to oral rape and forced fellatio (Dietz and Bienfang 1985).

Cornelia B. Wilbur's 11-year treatment of "Sybil" dealt with several types of disordered eating. Dr. Wilbur traced the origins of these symptoms to specific characteristics of Sybil's childhood abuse. Neither "eating disorder" nor "anorexia" is mentioned in the index of *Sybil* (Schreiber 1974). However, close reading indicates that this patient was 22 years of age and weighed 79 pounds when she met Dr. Wilbur. At a height of 5 feet 5 inches, her ideal body weight would have been 123 pounds. At 65% of her ideal body weight, she falls well within the DSM-III-R (American Psychiatric Association 1987) guidelines defining anorexia nervosa (Thorn and Cahill 1974). The text leaves it unclear whether the depressed host personality ate too little, simply fasted, or found some other way to achieve this weight. At least three other alters—one child alter, and two who enjoyed eating—complained that Sybil was not feeding the body. The body images of the 16 alters in Sybil's system ranged from "plump" to "chunky" to "willowy" to "small" to "pale and thin." They ranged in age from toddler to middle-aged. Two male alters complained about looking like a girl; they wanted male genitals and bodies. Although repetitive vomiting is not described in this account, Sybil did complain of difficulties swallowing. Another somatic symptom, massive diarrhea, probably also interfered with her ability to gain weight. Conflicts about eating and conflicts about body image became more intense as treatment progressed and alters became more coconscious.

As Sybil recovered memories of her childhood, it became more understandable why eating and swallowing were so difficult. Because of daily physical and sexual abuse in childhood, she was often too angry, frightened, humiliated, or depressed to feel like eating. In addition, her mother insisted on absolute control of Sybil's body. She imposed force-feeding and forced defecation on her daughter through the use of enemas and laxatives. Sybil's diarrhea may have been a somatosensory memory of those episodes. Her difficulty swallowing related not only to the force-feedings but also to being gagged by having rags stuffed into her mouth and being hit in the throat. One time she was struck so violently that her larynx was fractured. By refusing to eat, Sybil avoided memories of the abusive feeding and elimination practices and of the assaults on her mouth and throat. Her very low weight also avoided the secondary sexual characteristics that might have panicked child and male alters as well as those alters phobic of sexuality because of sexual abuse (Bruch 1973).

Other therapists working with patients with multiple personality and related dissociative states have documented other eating disorder behaviors: binge eating, induced vomiting, fear of food, and laxative abuse (Bliss 1986; Kluft 1985). Torem (1986) treated two patients with bulimia nervosa whose altered states of consciousness during episodes of bingeing and purging were the clue to the fact that these behaviors were part of a dissociative disorder. One of these bulimic patients gorged when in an ego state that had been starved by the mother. The patient's purging, on the other hand, was the adaptive effort of an ego state that had been forced to eat rotten food and vomitus. In this case, each limb of the bulimia represented both sensations related to a dissociated memory of abuse and behaviors that constituted realistic but displaced efforts to defend against parental assaults.

Early clinical accounts of eating disorders and of incest victimization syndromes occasionally describe patients with both conditions. Bruch (1973) described a 14-year-old girl with abdominal pain, anorexia, vomiting, aphonia, anger, and sexual preoccupations who revealed genital fondling by her father. Crisp (1984) described a 16-year-old girl with both anorexia and bulimia whose symptoms had begun subsequent to her widowed father's first frank sexual advances. She also became alcoholic. Eating disorders have been described acutely in other survivors of childhood sexual abuse (Bagley 1984; Conte and Schuerman 1988; Jorne 1979; Peters 1976). Annie Katan (1973) treated an adult woman who presented with agitation, anxiety, and depression. This patient had been genitally fondled by her father from about age 2; at age 5, she had fellated an unknown adult male who approached her at school. After the episode of fellatio, she had problems involving gagging, vomiting, and an inability to swallow, and she could eat only a few special foods.

The current view of both anorexia and bulimia is that they are complex disorders that probably include many subgroups. Some patients have coexisting major affective symptoms; some have borderline personality disorder (BPD); some cases develop after a traumatic event, such as a rape or attempted rape (Abraham and Beaumont 1982; Damlouji and Ferguson 1985; Herzog and Copeland 1985; Swift et al. 1986). For many patients with eating disorders, this is part of a more extensive syndrome of psychological suffering. Amongst the patients described in the first 19th-century English accounts of anorexia nervosa, one refused to speak, and was enuretic and encopretic; another had intense headaches and shivering (Silverman

1988). Bruch (1973) estimated that 10% of anorexic patients have an atypical "hysterical" pattern that includes a later age at onset, conversion symptoms, sexual preoccupation, and dysphoria about weight loss. Among patients with bulimia, the lifetime rates of additional psychiatric disorders are high, not only for mood disorders but also for substance use and anxiety disorders (Hudson et al. 1987; Swift et al. 1986). Studies of family patterns of these patients are just becoming available (Johnson and Flach 1985).

Preliminary data suggest that survivors of childhood abuse may be more likely to assort into that subgroup of patients whose eating disorders are accompanied by other severe symptoms. One study (Goodwin et al. 1988) described 10 adult incest survivors whose severe symptoms had led to multiple psychiatric hospitalizations. All had been physically and emotionally mistreated and sexually abused. Seven had eating disorders, all involving purging with anorexia, normal weight, or obesity; four had been hospitalized because of their eating disorders. Five of the seven connected their purging with prior fellatio experiences. Two additional survivors had episodes of either fasting or vomiting that had not been previously diagnosed as eating disorders. Associated symptoms, present in more than half of these survivors, included dissociative symptoms, BPD, legal involvements (particularly loss of child custody), alcohol and substance abuse, rape victimization, spousal abuse victimization, multiple suicide attempts, major affective disorder, and somatic complaints.

Some statistical studies of incest survivors and of patients with eating disorders have begun to quantify this area of overlap. Sedney and Brooks (1984) surveyed a nonclinical population of college women for both childhood sexual experiences and symptoms. They found higher percentages of both weight loss and being overweight in those subjects with a history of intrafamilial or extrafamilial childhood sexual abuse. However, these differences were not statistically significant. Finn and colleagues (1986) also failed to find significant associations. However, Runtz and Briere (1986), in a similar study of 278 undergraduate women, found that eating problems were more likely to be found in the group with prior sexual abuse. The sexually abused group admitted to problems with both overeating and undereating more frequently than the nonabused group. However, only the undereating item reached significance. Other questionnaire items that were significantly different between abused and nonabused women included school problems, conflict with authority, early sexual behaviors, dissociation, somatization, anxiety, and depression (Briere and Runtz 1988).

Oppenheimer and colleagues (1985) reported that 31% of patients with anorexia nervosa and 42% of patients with bulimia described experiences of childhood sexual abuse. Pyle and colleagues (1988) report an identical percentage, 42% ($n = 24$), in 58 patients with bulimia nervosa. In addition, 74% ($n = 43$) reported enduring prior physical abuse and 94% ($n = 55$) psychological abuse. In this sample, 30% ($n = 17$) reported self-mutilation. Powers and colleagues (1988) found a higher percentage of childhood sexual abuse in patients with morbid obesity (37% [$n = 10$] of 27) than in bulimia nervosa (29% [$n = 12$] of 31) or anorexia nervosa (27% [$n = 4$] of 15). Other estimates of the frequency of childhood sexual abuse in patients with eating disorders range from 29% to 82% (Root and Fallon 1988; Sloan and Leighner 1986). However, it is unclear whether these percentages are higher than expected, because 44% of women in the general population (Russell 1983) have experienced rape or attempted rape before age 18. Also, because we are postulating child abuse as only one of many possible etiologies for eating disorders, comparison of raw frequencies of prior abuse is not the definitive test of the hypothesis. More detailed qualitative data are needed describing both the nature of the childhood sexual abuse and other abuse and the development of the eating disorder.

If further studies support the finding of a childhood sexual subgroup among patients with eating disorders, this would fit with other findings:

1. High hypnotizability in bulimic and anorexic patients (Bliss 1986; Torem 1986);
2. The presence of dissociative symptoms in as many as 75% of bulimic patients (Abraham and Beaumont 1982); and
3. Minnesota Multiphasic Personality Inventory (MMPI; Hathaway and McKinley 1970) and other test similarities between incest survivors and anorexic patients (Scott and Thoner 1986).

Sexual dysfunction is yet another symptom associated with traumatic child abuse (Goodwin 1987). In a study of 27 males with bulimia and anorexia (Herzog et al. 1984), 26% ($n = 7$) were homosexual, and almost all had problems with sexuality and sexual behavior. Because males are less pressured toward abnormal eating by societal preoccupations (Steiner-Adair 1986), all-male samples may include higher percentages of patients whose eating disorder reflects childhood trauma.

A Theoretical Framework for Exploring Connections Between Child Abuse and Eating Problems

In a previous article (Goodwin et al. 1988), it was proposed that some self-abusive behaviors in adulthood represent a continuation of childhood abuse, with the survivor now incorporating the role of the parent-perpetrator. Thus, the child who has been thrown into walls later throws himself into them or walks into them "accidentally." "Stripes," originally the result of lashings, are reenacted as the thin cuts of the delicate self-mutilator. Sexual abuse becomes promiscuity, often with sadistic partners. In this model, starvation of the child, labeled earlier as failure to thrive, would become self-starvation; force-feeding could be reenacted as gorging; and compulsive laxative use could take the place of parental overcontrol of elimination.

However, case studies already cited indicate the situation is even more complex. Reenactments are only one way in which fragments of dissociated memories of childhood abuse resurface. Braun (1988a, 1988b) has proposed a model describing four separate aspects of memory that can be dissociated or retrieved: behavior, affect, sensation, and knowledge. Braun uses the mnemonic BASK to represent these four aspects. Within this model, enactments—gorging, self-starvation—are only one mode in which traumatic memories can resurface. Feeling states are another. Another mode is the sudden experiencing of sensations—such as the difficulty in swallowing experienced by Sybil—which only later are recognized as memory fragments.

Another way in which eating behaviors function in the life of an abuse survivor is to defend against the initial assaults or the memories of them. Thus, Torem's (1986) patient ate greedily because in the displaced time of her memory she was being starved; she purged to rid her system of poison. Sybil avoided disruptive flashbacks by staying away from kitchens and food and the act of swallowing.

Still another way in which eating disorders can emerge in these survivors is as a secondary effect of the posttraumatic and dissociative disorders that are the primary sequelae of the abuse. The chronic anxiety, depression, hostility, and guilt that characterize posttraumatic stress disorder (PTSD) are not conducive to normal enjoyment of food. When dissociation has split the body image into multiple fragmentary identities, the tasks of identifying and achieving an ideal weight become hopelessly complicated. This is the case with MPD patients. With alters eating different menus at various times of day, often unbeknownst to each other, good nutritional control becomes the exception rather than the rule. Once leaving the body becomes the preferred defense against abuse and flashbacks, the normal triggers of hunger and satiety are left behind.

Multiple Eating Disorders in a Patient With MPD

In the following complex case, multiple forms of disordered eating illustrate all three categories of impingements from prior child abuse.

Case Study 1. Anita is a 33-year-old single obese chronic mental patient whose multiplicity was diagnosed only when she was 32. At 19, she was hospitalized for anorexia nervosa. At present she weighs 220 pounds and has had multiple emergency room visits for vomiting and dehydration. At one point Anita explained her vomiting: "We're sick. Someone's been beating us up." A persecutor alter was reenacting (via self-mutilation) the genital mutilation that her grandfather had practiced, leaving her with pain, nausea, and vomiting. The vomiting was complicated by fasting related to several fragmented affective aspects of the memory. Nine-year-old Maggie was too angry to eat. Three-year-old Caroline was too sad: "She only cries; she doesn't drink." Betty was too anxious, and her hyperventilation made the nausea worse. Helen fasted "to get closer to God." A "psychotic" alter saw food "as bugs." One alter was specialized to do all the vomiting for the system; she smelled the stench of the outhouse in which she had been locked at age 3 by the grandfather as punishment for refusing his sexual advances.

This symptom complex, in addition to being a container endlessly repeating various dissociated fragments of the memory, could also be used as a powerful resistance to remembering. Often, when reconstruction was proceeding rapidly, Anita would call to cancel a treatment session, saying "They've made me too nauseated to go in today." At other times, the vomiting alter rescued the system from potentially lethal overdoses and illegal drugs (grandfather, too, had given Anita substances to sedate her).

Anita's disordered eating is entwined with every aspect of her dissociative disorder. Among her 20 alters are infants, animals, demons, and spirits whose "nutritional requirements" vary as greatly as do their body images.

Eating Disorders in Incest Survivors With Mixed Posttraumatic and Dissociative Symptoms

Whereas in patients with MPD one finds multiple eating disorders as a response to multiple types of child abuse, in less disturbed incest survivors, it is more possible to focus on single eating dysfunctions and single types of child abuse.

Disordered Eating as Memory Equivalent
Case Study 2.   Ann is a 27-year-old woman who entered psychotherapy to explore emerging memories of incest with her father. Her diagnostic exploration revealed beatings by both parents from an early age; sexual abuse, including genital touching and fellatio between ages 7 and 12; emotional abuse, including overcontrol of eating and excretion; and exploitation of her capacity to work. She was making meals and caring for younger siblings from age 7.

Although her cognitive memories of the incest seemed clear and complete, she usually showed very little feeling about the abuse. Feelings tended to surface for her around 4 P.M., when she would experience anxiety and dysphoria and stuff herself with food. Further exploration of this experience revealed that it contained cognitive and behavioral aspects of her childhood experience, as well as some of her feeling states. She realized that stuffing herself with food was how she comforted herself after the fellatio with her father, which generally had taken place about 4 P.M.

We have seen other instances in which abnormal eating behavior represented a fragment of a dissociated memory. One patient remained unaware of her incest pregnancy until delivery, then rerepressed the entire experience after the baby died. During the years when she was amnesic—both for the incest and the traumatic delivery—she remained severely obese and vomited secretly every morning. She had also concealed her morning sickness during pregnancy. During this period when she was unable to access knowledge and memory, her overeating, vomiting, shame, and obesity represented behavioral, affective, and sensory fragments of the lost memory.

Some incest survivors who have been diagnosed as bulimic describe certain foods as triggering intense nausea, dysphoria, and the feeling that they are choking. Often they can control their bulimia by avoiding foods such as milk, tapioca pudding, rice pudding, mayonnaise, and egg whites. Some of these survivors state clearly that these foods reevoke the somatic sensations that they felt when the abuser ejaculated into the mouth.

Disordered Eating as Defense Against Memory

Once we understand that eating behaviors and associated sensations can contain dissociated memories and trigger flashbacks, it becomes more understandable how eating in all of its aspects, as with sexuality and all of its aspects, can become the focus of multiple secondary posttraumatic symptoms as the patient attempts to use numbing mechanisms to avoid remembered pain. In addition, body weight is a powerful tool for changing body image. Thus some survivors are able to become grossly obese to escape any identification with the childlike body image that would trigger flashbacks to the abuse. Other survivors become thin, maintaining a prepubertal or quasi-masculine low body weight, to avoid fears of rape or impregnation that might erupt, together with memories of the abuse, if their body image were that of a young adult woman.

Continuation of Case Study 2.   Ann's weight remained normal until her marriage. She found that she was able to enjoy sex with her husband, but she experienced vivid visual flashbacks of her father after intercourse. As her weight climbed, the flashbacks decreased in number. Although her current weight of more than 200 pounds is seriously interfering with her health, she is afraid that if she complied with medical recommendations to lose weight, she would no longer be able to have sex with her husband.

Case Study 3.   Barbara entered treatment at age 25 because of extreme dysphoria and the intrusion of disorganized memory fragments whenever she saw her father. In psychotherapy she was able to reconstruct extreme incestuous abuse from her father between ages 3 and 11. This included fellatio and forced vaginal intercourse. There was physical abuse (including strangulation) and emotional abuse around eating. Barbara's weight fluctuated. At one point she became thin and obtained work as an artist's model. She became increasingly panicked at the attention men gave her and began to mutilate herself.

Case Study 4.   Christine is a 22-year-old woman who had been victimized by physical and sexual abuse from her father, her mother, two uncles, and a cousin, between ages 4 and 17. From age 8 until age 17, she had regular vaginal intercourse with her father. Although she has never been diagnosed as having an eating disorder, she says of herself, "I never eat and I never have periods." She maintains her weight between 80 and 90 pounds. She says that she was terrified of pregnancy from the time the oral sexual intercourse progressed to vaginal intercourse at age 8. She did not menstruate until age 16 and still has only 1 or 2 menstrual periods each year.

Case Study 5.   Darlene is a 26-year-old woman who has been diagnosed as having bulimia nervosa. She was sexually abused by her father and her brother from ages 2 to 16. She describes her purging as follows: "It's like cleaning out your system. If I can get the semen out of my system, I feel better. Sometimes I eat and think about the guys who raped me. Afterward it's like I pretend I'm purging all over them."

For the patient in Case Study 5, the eating disorder functioned both as a healing ritual and a revenge fantasy. In the other case studies, a shift in self-image is important in the defensive strategy. For these survivors of multimodal childhood abuse who do not have access to the alters available in MPD, different weight and body images seem to offer ways to change state in order to avoid the unpleasant cognitive or affective aspects of dissociated memories. For example, the two patients who became obese not only distanced themselves from the child body image that inhabited their flashbacks but also decreased courting advances and sexual triggers from men. The first patient describes her obesity as a comprehensively numbing state. She feels that all sensations and some affects, especially anger, are muted by her encasing layers of fat. This parallels recent physiologic studies finding depressions in both sympathetic and parasympathetic activity associated with increasing body fat (Peterson et al. 1988). Where a weight state has become an important mechanism for numbing, it becomes as conflicted as other such mechanisms, such as substance abuse or anorgasmia. The patient needs it but hates needing it.

Understanding the meanings of weight and eating as they relate to dissociated memories of abuse and defenses against them can help the therapist understand the intense preoccupation with weight and eating with which some incest survivors are obsessed. For a survivor desperately attempting to avoid flashback images of his or her body, it can be helpful to substitute more abstract elements of body image, such as weight or clothing size, for the dangerous visual images that would otherwise be used to represent the self mentally. These patients may become preoccupied with attaining a certain body weight or wearing a certain outfit because their real aim is to attain a particular ego state. A therapist who grasps this aspect may be able to help the obese patient reduce to a compromise weight that allows some further exploration of sexuality without producing so many sexual triggers that he or she becomes frightened and more symptomatic. The female anorexic patient, too, may be able to gain to a compromise weight that is physically safer but still allows her long periods of amenorrhea.

Conclusions

Nurturance comes from the Latin word for "suckling," so it is perhaps not surprising that survivors of inadequate or distorted nurturance have difficulty feeding and swallowing. The concept of "orality" is based on this analogy but may be too abstract and metaphorical to capture the concrete eating disabilities we are describing here. Nor is it surprising that those who feel powerless and betrayed turn to eating as a last bastion of autonomy and self-expression. Centuries of fakirs, saints, and "hunger artists" have taught us to expect this, too (Bell 1985; Bruch 1973; Mogul 1980).

Reviews of the literature and case studies suggest that childhood abuse survivors might present a qualitatively different picture from some other subgroups of patients with eating disorders. Some possible distinguishing characteristics are later age at onset, greater conflict about eating, greater variety of disordered eating practices, presence of altered states of consciousness, and the presence of associated severe symptoms. These include BPD, other family violence problems, alcohol and substance abuse, self-mutilation and suicidality, flashbacks, depression, and somatization, including conversion disorders.

We recommend that the therapist remain alert to the possibility that abnormal eating behaviors represent fragments of dissociated memories or ways to defend against those memories, or that they occur as epiphenomena related to posttraumatic or dissociative sequelae of child abuse.

Previous investigators have described distorted body images in some patients with eating disorders. Our experience indicates that this disturbance may be even more profound than previously thought, extending to absent body image or multiple body images

(L. Bienz, F. Irigoyen, unpublished data, October 1985). Such disturbance may be an inevitable consequence of overusing dissociative exits from the body. "Who would not leave a burning house?" asked one of our patients. Another described being oblivious to both her ongoing anorexia and her previous sadistic child abuse until she caught sight of her reflection in a subway window. "That looks like someone who just got out of a concentration camp," she thought, and then recognized the reflection as her own. The preoccupation with weight seen in some patients may be like the preoccupation with clothes shown by H. G. Wells's *Invisible Man* (1897/1987); he was not trying to cover up a wounded or deformed body image, but one that was not there at all. Further study of this disrupted population may help us learn more about the construction of body and self-image during normal child development. The developmental linkages between autobiographical memory and self-image may turn out to be so numerous and intricate that we will learn to look for gaps in memory whenever we find disturbances in self-image, and vice versa (Nelson 1988; Touyz et al. 1984).

References

Abraham S, Beaumont PJV: Varieties of psychosexual experience and patients with anorexia nervosa. International Journal of Eating Disorders 1:10–19, 1982

American Psychiatric Association: Diagnostic and Statistical Manual, 3rd Edition, Revised. Washington, DC, American Psychiatric Association, 1987

Bagley C: Mental health and the in-the-family sexual abuse of children and adolescents. Canada's Mental Health 32:17–23, 1984

Bell RM: Holy Anorexia. Chicago, IL, University of Chicago Press, 1985

Bliss EL: Multiple Personality, Allied Disorders, and Hypnosis. New York, Oxford University Press, 1986

Braun BG: The BASK (behavior, affect, sensation, knowledge) model of dissociation. Dissociation 1(1):4–23, 1988a

Braun BG: The BASK model of dissociation: clinical applications. Dissociation 1(2):16–23, 1988b

Briere J, Runtz M: Symptomatology associated with childhood sexual victimization in a nonclinical adult sample. Child Abuse Negl 12:51–59, 1988

Bruch H: Eating Disorders: Obesity, Anorexia and the Person Within. New York, Basic Books, 1973

Conte J, Schuerman JR: Factors associated with increased impact of child sexual abuse. Child Abuse Negl 11:201–211, 1988

Crisp AH: The psychopathology of anorexia nervosa: getting the "heat" out of the system, in Eating and Its Disorders. Edited by Stunkard AL, Stellar E. New York, Raven, 1984

Damlouji NF, Ferguson JM: Three cases of posttraumatic anorexia nervosa. Am J Psychiatry 142:362–363, 1985

Dietz WH, Bienfang D: Obesity, family violence and medicine, in Unhappy Families: Clinical and Research Perspectives on Family Violence. Edited by Newberger EH, Bourne R. Littleton, MA, PSG, 1985

Finn S, Hartman M, Leon G, et al: Eating disorders and sexual abuse: lack of confirmation for a clinical hypothesis. International Journal of Eating Disorders 5:1051–1060, 1986

Goodwin J: Developmental impacts of incest, in Handbook of Child Psychiatry, Vol V. Edited by Noshpitz I, Berlin J, Call R, et al. New York, Basic Books, 1987

Goodwin J, Cheeves K, Connell V: Defining a syndrome of severe symptoms in survivors of extreme incestuous abuse. Dissociation 1(4):11–16, 1988

Hathaway SR, McKinley JC: Minnesota Multiphasic Personality Inventory, Revised. Minneapolis, MN, University of Minnesota, 1970

Herzog DB, Copeland PM: Eating disorders. N Engl J Med 313(5):295–303, 1985

Herzog DB, Norman DK, Gordon C, et al: Sexual conflict and eating disorders in 27 males. Am J Psychiatry 141:989–990, 1984

Hudson JI, Pope HG, Yurgelun-Todd D, et al: A controlled study of lifetime prevalence of affective and other psychiatric disorders in bulimic outpatients. Am J Psychiatry 144:1283–1287, 1987

Johnson C, Flach A: Family characteristics of 105 patients with bulimia. Am J Psychiatry 142:1321–1324, 1985

Jorne PS: Treating sexually abused children. Child Abuse Negl 3:285–290, 1979

Katan A: Children who were raped. Psychoanal Study Child 28:208–224, 1973

Kluft R: The natural history of multiple personality disorder, in Childhood Antecedents of Multiple Personality Disorder. Edited by Kluft RP. Washington DC, American Psychiatric Press, 1985

Mogul SL: Asceticism in adolescence and anorexia nervosa. Psychoanal Study Child 35:155–175, 1980

Nelson K: The ontogeny of memory for real events, in Remembering Reconsidered: Ecological and Traditional Approaches to the Study of Memory. Edited by Neisser U, Winograd E. New York, Cambridge University Press, 1988

Oppenheimer R, Howells K, Palmer L, et al: Adverse sexual experience in childhood and clinical eating disorders: a preliminary description. J Psychol 19(213):357–361, 1985

Peters JJ: Children who are victims of sexual assault and the psychology of offenders. Am J Psychother 30:398–421, 1976

Peterson HR, Rothchild M, Weinberg CR, et al: Body fat and the activity of the autonomic nervous system. N Engl J Med 318:1077–1083, 1988

Powers PS, Coovert DL, Brightwell DR: Sexual abuse history in three eating disorders. Paper presented at the Annual Meeting of the American Psychiatric Association, Montreal, May 1988

Pyle RL, Perse T, Mitchell JE, et al: Abuse in women with bulimia nervosa. Paper presented at the Annual Meeting of the American Psychiatric Association, Montreal, May 1988

Root MP, Fallon P: The incidence of victimization experiences in a bulimic sample. Journal of Interpersonal Violence 3:161–173, 1988

Runtz M, Briere J: Adolescent "acting-out" and childhood history of sexual abuse. Journal of Interpersonal Violence 1(3):326–334, 1986

Russell DEH: The incidence and prevalence of intrafamilial and extrafamilial sexual abuse of female children. Child Abuse Negl 7:133–146, 1983

Schreiber FR: Sybil. New York, Warner Books, 1974

Scott R, Thoner G: Ego deficits in anorexia nervosa patients and incest victims: an MMPI comparative analysis. Psychol Rep 58:829–846, 1986

Sedney MA, Brooks B: Factors associated with a history of childhood sexual experiences in a nonclinical female population. Journal of the American Academy of Child Psychiatry 23:215–218, 1984

Silverman JA: Anorexia Nervosa in 1888. Lancet 1:928–930, 1988

Sloan G, Leighner P: Is there a relationship between sexual abuse or incest and eating disorders? Can J Psychiatry 31:656–660, 1986

Steiner-Adair C: The body politic: normal female adolescent development and the development of eating disorders. J Am Acad Psychoanal 14(1):95–114, 1986

Swift WJ, Andrews D, Barlage NE: The relationship between affective disorder and eating disorders: a review of literature. Am J Psychiatry 143(3):290–299, 1986

Thorn GW, Cahill GF: Gain in weight; obesity, in Harrison's Principles of Internal Medicine. Edited by Wintrobe M, Thorne G, Adams R, et al. New York, McGraw-Hill, 1974

Torem MS: Dissociative states presenting as an eating disorder. Am J Clin Hypn 29:137–142, 1986

Touyz SW, Beaumont PJV, Collins JK, et al: Body space perception and its disturbance in anorexia nervosa. Br J Psychiatry 144:167–171, 1984

Chapter 18

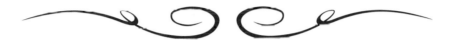

Eating Disorders in Patients With Multiple Personality Disorder

Moshe S. Torem, M.D.

T he diagnosis of multiple personality disorder (MPD) poses a con-
siderable challenge, even for experienced clinicians. This is because
MPD is a clandestine disorder (Kluft 1985); it is hidden from the
clinician as well as the patient (Coons 1984; Kluft 1985, 1987). It is
also a great masquerader. The presenting symptoms of MPD are so
variable that patients with MPD are frequently misdiagnosed (Coons
1988; Kluft 1987). A typical MPD patient acquires three to four alternate diagnoses and has been in the mental health care system for 6
to 8 years before being accurately diagnosed (Putnam et al. 1986).

It is not uncommon for MPD patients to seek treatment for a variety of psychophysiological symptoms (Coons 1988). Bliss (1980) reported on the occurrence of gastrointestinal symptoms in 14 MPD
patients he studied.

Eating disorder symptoms may be among the presenting symptoms. In a previous discussion (Torem 1984), I presented a number
of cases in which anorexia nervosa was the presenting clinical
picture of an underlying case of MPD. Later, I reported (Torem

1986) that patients with eating disorders may also experience dissociative states. Putnam and his colleagues (1986) reported a 35% incidence of nausea and vomiting ($n = 35$) in their series of 100 MPD patients. Putnam and colleagues (1986) found anorexic symptoms in 25% of the cases ($n = 25$) they studied and bulimia symptoms in 15% ($n = 15$).

However, my conversations with colleagues in the field suggest that pathological eating behavior in MPD patients may be more common than previously thought (Torem 1987). It seemed worthwhile to study this connection, both to improve the treatment of patients with apparent eating disorders who might have unrecognized concomitant dissociative disorders, and to determine whether eating disorder symptoms might be a clue to initiate inquiry for the presence of MPD.

Methods

I designed a questionnaire to study both the frequency of pathological eating behaviors and the coexisting eating disorder symptoms in the histories of patients currently being treated for MPD. The questionnaire included questions regarding the following:

1. Basic demographic data;
2. Previous diagnoses of eating disorders;
3. Previous treatments in an eating disorders program;
4. Response to such treatment;
5. Whether the treatment was in an outpatient or inpatient eating disorders program;
6. Whether specifically defined eating disorder symptoms were still in existence at the time of the study;
7. Whether the known pathological eating behavior was the result of an underlying dissociative mechanism;
8. Whether the pathological eating behavior was associated with the influence of one or more than one ego state or alter;
9. Whether the host personality had conscious awareness of the pathological eating behavior; and

10. Whether the eating problem had improved since treatment started to address the issue of multiplicity, as compared to previous treatments that had not addressed this issue.

The questionnaire also included questions to explore the underlying dynamics of pathological eating behavior such as self-punishment, reenactment of trauma, flashbacks, or conflicts around sexuality and gender identity. Another question explored the history of forced fellatio in those patients who had a history of sexual abuse. The questionnaires were sent to clinicians who had been trained in the diagnosis and treatment of MPD and who were experienced in working with such patients. These clinicians were from Ohio and neighboring states.

Seventy-eight clinicians were sent the survey. Of those, only 34 (44%) clinicians responded. However, three responses did not include useful information and were discarded. The completed surveys of 31 clinicians (40%) provided data on 84 MPD patients.

Results

Demographics

Of the 84 patients, 80 (95%) were female and 4 (5%) were male. Most of the patients (51%) were in the range of 31 to 40 years of age; 33% were between 21 and 30; 12% were 41 to 50 years of age. Only 2% were younger than 20, and 2% were over 51. Thirty-nine percent of the patients were single, 29% were married, and 21% were divorced. A total of 53% of the patients were employed, 30% were unemployed, and 2% were disabled.

History of Patterns of Pathological Eating Behavior

Seventy-seven patients (92%) had a known history of pathological eating behavior. For 6 patients (7%), there was no known history of pathological eating behavior. For 1 patient, no historical information addressed the presence or absence of such symptoms.

Table 18–1 illustrates the various pathological eating behavior symptoms in the 77 patients positive for such symptoms.

In summary, 231 eating disorder symptoms were reported by 77 patients, for an average of about 3 per patient.

Thirty-seven patients (44%) had had a previous diagnosis of an eating disorder, while 43 (51%) did not. Among the 37 patients who had received prior diagnoses of eating disorders, 16 (43%) had been diagnosed with bulimia, 14 (38%) had been diagnosed with anorexia nervosa, and 10 (27%) carried the diagnosis of atypical eating disorder.

Of a total of 84 patients, 24 (29%) had been treated previously for an eating disorder. Of these, 16 patients (67%) had been treated in an outpatient eating disorders program, and 14 patients (58%) had been treated in an inpatient eating disorders program. At the time of this study, 59 patients (70%) had active eating disorder symptoms. Of these 59 patients 39 (66%) had symptoms of binge eating, 19 (32%) had symptoms of self-induced vomiting, 30 (51%) had symptoms of self-starvation or excessive dieting, and 5 (8%) had symptoms of laxative abuse.

Pathological Eating Behavior and Dissociation

Seventy-two patients (86% of all reported and 94% of those with eating disorder symptoms) were judged to have their pathological eating behavior as a presentation of an underlying dissociative mechanism. Of these 72 patients, in 27 (38%) the bingeing and purg-

Table 18–1. Eating disorder symptoms in 77 subjects with a history of pathological eating behavior

Eating disorder symptom	Number	Percentage
Bingeing	64	83
Excessive dieting	49	64
Self-induced vomiting	39	51
Extreme weight fluctuations	35	45
Laxative abuse	21	27
Excessive exercising	19	25
Ipecac abuse	4	5

ing was done by one personality or ego state; in 25 (35%) the binge-ing and purging was done by more than one personality or ego state; in 28 (39%) the host personality had conscious awareness of the bingeing and purging behaviors; and in 15 (21%) the host per-sonality had amnesia to the bingeing and purging behaviors.

Influence of Treatment on Eating Disorder Symptoms

Because these patients were diagnosed as having MPD and treated accordingly, it is instructive to note the impact of their treatment on their eating disorder symptoms (Table 18–2).

It seems apparent that in many cases, treatment directed at MPD leads to improvement in such symptoms, but that in the majority of cases no such conclusion can be drawn. It remains unclear whether this is related to the type or the duration of the treatment. Our data do not allow us to know whether some MPD patients' eating dis-orders are epiphenomena of their MPD, whereas others are autono-mous conditions that will require a different therapeutic approach.

Underlying Dynamics of Eating Behaviors
The clinicians treating 68 of the patients with eating disorder symp-toms believed that they had discerned the underlying dynamics of these symptoms (Table 18–3).

Table 18–2. Influence of treatment on eating disorder symptoms among 84 subjects

Eating disorder symptom	Number	Percentage
Eating problem has improved since the beginning of treatment	35	42
Eating problem has become worse since the beginning of treatment	7	8
Eating problem has not changed since the beginning of treatment	24	29
Unknown	18	21
Total	84	100

History of Forced Fellatio

The majority of patients who have MPD have a history of being sexually abused in childhood (Putnam et al. 1986). In this study, 48 patients (58%) were reported to have a history of having endured forced fellatio.

Discussion

It is rather astounding that 92% of the MPD patients studied in this project had a known history of pathological eating behavior and that 44% had a history of previously being diagnosed with an eating disorder. Furthermore, 24 patients (29%) had a history of previous treatment for an eating disorder, in the course of which the diagnosis of their MPD was missed. At the time of the study, 59 patients (70%) were still having symptoms of an eating disorder.

Table 18–3. Underlying dynamics of eating behavior among subjects with known eating behavior dynamics ($n = 68$)

Specific dynamics	Number	Percentage
Eating behavior is a manifestation of self-punishment	40	59
Eating behavior is a manifestation of a regressed childhood ego state or alter	39	57
Eating behavior is a manifestation of a posttraumatic flashback	21	31
Eating behavior is a manifestation of conflicts around sexuality and one's gender identity	21	31
Eating behavior is a manifestation of internal battle among alters and ego states because of a delusion of separateness	21	31
Eating behavior is a manifestation of boredom	1	1
Eating behavior is a manifestation of other causes (anxiety, restlessness, etc.)	2	2

It is clear that it is necessary to increase the awareness of the staff of eating disorders programs regarding dissociative disorders. It will be helpful if they can recognize the possibility that some patients with eating disorders may have an underlying dissociative mechanism (e.g., Torem 1986) and that some may even have diagnosable MPD (Kluft 1985; Torem 1984).

That eating disorders are conditions with multiple interrelated causes and consequences, and that their etiology is not uniform, is not a new concept. It already has been discussed by Powers and Fernandez (1984). In the ideal scenario, the competent clinician will be successful in ascertaining the etiology of the patient's eating disorder symptoms, and this knowledge will inform and guide the patient's treatment. For example, some patients with eating disorders have an underlying major affective disorder. These patients may respond well to treatment with antidepressant medications and mood stabilizers. Severe family conflicts and enmeshment may be at the core of other patients' problems, and these patients may respond well to family therapy (Minuchin et al. 1978). Goodwin and Attias (Chapter 17) described a special subgroup of patients with eating disorders in whom the underlying etiology was related to a history of multimodal childhood abuse. In another publication, Goodwin and her colleagues (1988) described eating disorder pathology in survivors of severe incestuous abuse.

Still other patients with eating disorders may have MPD at the root of their difficulties (Bliss 1986; Torem 1988, 1990). These patients must be treated with psychotherapy that addresses the internal dynamics of their multiplicity and posttraumatic stress disorder (PTSD). In fact, in a previous report (Torem and Curdue 1988), it was pointed out that some cases of PTSD initially may present with the symptoms of an eating disorder. Ego-state therapy (Torem 1989) was also found effective in the treatment of dissociative eating disorders.

An interesting aspect of the current study was the issue of patients' responses to treatment. Thirty-five patients (42%) showed an improvement in their pathological eating behavior. These patients were diagnosed as having MPD, and the treatment was directed at their underlying multiplicity. However, 24 patients (29%) showed no significant change in their pathological eating behavior; and in 7 patients (8%), the pathological eating behavior got worse. As we look at the total number of these patients, we find out that it is higher than 59. An explanation for this is that some patients at one time showed an improvement in some symptoms of their pathological eating behavior, and at other times some of these symptoms got worse.

Eating and swallowing may represent acts of internalization through incorporation, introjection, and finally identification with the external object or idea. Some ideas and dynamics may be portrayed in connection with eating. Our language has innumerable metaphorical expressions regarding eating, and its implied meanings (e.g., "I couldn't swallow it"; "I was unable to stomach that stuff"; "He was so disgusting, he made me puke"; "She was starving for love and attention"). Although in some MPD patients eating may express an attempt to reenact childhood traumata, in others it may be a matter of an attempt at self-love and self-nurturing in the face of neglect, loneliness, and emptiness. In still others, it may result from efforts of an alter personality created to protect the patient by making him or her heavier (even obese) and therefore sexually unattractive. Self-induced vomiting may symbolically represent self-hate or an attempt to expel a hateful, unwanted, introjected object.

Another curious finding is the fact that 48 patients (57%) had a history of being sexually abused by forced fellatio. This may mean that pathological eating behavior may symbolically express some of the unresolved conflict and traumata surrounding such experiences. I have studied more intensively a number of patients with the symptom of self-induced vomiting who had experienced forced fellatio. In one of these cases, the patient as a child was forced to swallow the semen of the abuser, who ejaculated in her mouth. She developed a fear of becoming pregnant and forced herself to vomit following that incident. In her case, the self-induced vomiting was the result of a child alter reenacting the trauma as an attempt to master it, doing so in order to prevent a pregnancy. In another case, self-induced vomiting represented the patient's unconscious reenactment of the trauma with an attempt to master it, and at the same time to symbolically reject and expel the abuser who literally forced himself into the patient's body.

It is difficult to compare the findings of this study with the observations in the general literature on MPD. Few have addressed these considerations, which are fairly new. For example, a 1984 article by Coons does not list the eating disorders as possible differential diagnoses for MPD. In a later article, Coons (1988) does mention that some patients with MPD do have eating disorder symptoms. Bliss (1980) studied 14 cases of patients with MPD. He reported that 91% of them had complaints of stomach upsets, 73% of them complained of having severe nausea, 91% had complaints of abdominal pain, and 73% complained of severe constipation. However, Bliss does not mention anything about the existence of pathological eating behavior. Putnam and his colleagues (1986) published the results of a study in which they reviewed the variability of the clinical presentation of 100 MPD patients. They reported that 35% of their studied cases had complained of nausea and vomiting, 25% of anorexia, and 15% of bulimia.

How can we reconcile the discrepancy between the findings in this study and those in previous reports? Perhaps one way to understand is that patients who engage in binge eating and a variety of purging behaviors are rather secretive, and they will not report spontaneously on these behaviors unless questioned directly or actually observed by their clinicians (Herzog 1982). Another possible explanation is the fact that this study focused *specifically* on pathological eating behavior and eating disorder symptoms. It studied patients' eating behavior in much greater detail. The other studies included symptoms of nausea, upset stomach, vomiting, anorexia, and bulimia (among many other symptoms) but were designed more to look at the general clinical picture of patients with MPD. Clinicians without a special interest in eating disorder symptoms may not have considered asking about them in connection with MPD.

What are the implications of the results of this study? Kluft (1987) emphasizes that MPD often has a polysymptomatic presentation suggestive of one or more commonplace conditions, and false-negative diagnoses are quite common. One type of condition that may be suspected while MPD itself remains covert is the eating disorders. It is essential that all patients with eating disorders be screened for underlying or concomitant dissociative disorders. MPD patients with eating disorders may be treated in a specialized eating disorders program (even an inpatient program) while no attention is given to the underlying MPD. Such patients may be perceived as treatment failures in traditional behavior modification or drug therapy approaches. For many of these patients, the underlying MPD must be diagnosed and treatment directed at the underlying dynamics of the patient's dissociation and multiplicity to effect an improvement in their pathological eating behavior (Torem 1987, 1990).

References

Bliss EL: Multiple personalities. Arch Gen Psychiatry 39:1388–1397, 1980

Bliss EL: Multiple Personality, Allied Disorder, and Hypnosis. New York, Oxford University Press, 1986

Coons PM: The differential diagnosis of multiple personality disorder. Psychiatr Clin North Am 7:51–67, 1984

Coons PM: Psychophysiologic aspects of multiple personality disorder. Dissociation 1(1):49–53, 1988

Goodwin JM, Cheeves K, Connell V: Defining a syndrome of severe symptoms in survivors of severe incestuous abuse. Dissociation 1(4):11–16, 1988

Herzog FB: Bulimia: the secretive syndrome. Psychosomatics 23:481–487, 1982

Kluft RP: The natural history of multiple personality disorder, in Childhood Antecedents of Multiple Personality. Edited by Kluft RP. Washington, DC, American Psychiatric Press, 1985, pp 197–238

Kluft RP: An update on multiple personality disorder. Hosp Community Psychiatry 38:363–373, 1987

Minuchin PS, Rosman BL, Baker L (eds): Psychosomatic Families: Anorexia Nervosa in Context. Cambridge, MA, Harvard University Press, 1978

Powers PS, Fernandez RC: Current Treatment of Anorexia Nervosa and Bulimia. Basel, Switzerland, Karger, 1984

Putnam FW, Guroff JJ, Silberman EK, et al: The clinical phenomenology of multiple personality disorder: review of 100 recent cases. J Clin Psychiatry 47:285–293, 1986

Torem MS: Anorexia nervosa and multiple dissociated ego states. Paper presented at the First International Conference on Multiple Personality/Dissociative States, Chicago, IL, September 1984

Torem MS: Dissociative states presenting as an eating disorder. Am J Clin Hypn 29:137–142, 1986

Torem MS: Eating disorders in MPD patients. Paper presented at the Fourth International Conference on Multiple Personality/Dissociative States, Chicago, IL, November 1987

Torem MS: A modified ego-strengthening technique as a crisis intervention for the MPD patient. Trauma and Recovery 1(2):7–12, 1988

Torem MS: Ego-state hypnotherapy for dissociative eating disorders. Hypnos 16(2):52–63, 1989

Torem MS: Covert multiple personality underlying eating disorders. Am J Psychother 44:357–368, 1990

Torem MS: Eating disorders, in Clinical Hypnosis With Children. Edited by Wester W, O'Grady D. New York, Brunner/Mazel, 1991, pp 230–256

Torem MS, Curdue K: PTSD presenting as an eating disorder. Stress Medicine 4:139–142, 1988

Chapter 19

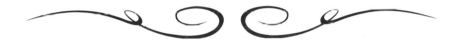

A History of Multiple Personality Disorder

George B. Greaves, Ph.D.

In 1791, Eberhardt Gmelin, a contemporary of Franz Anton Mesmer, reported a case of what he called *umgetaushte Persönlichkeit* (exchanged personality). The case was described in detail in Ellenberger's (1970) classic history of psychodynamic psychiatry *The Discovery of the Unconscious.* It involved a 20-year-old German woman from Stuttgart. The incident occurred in 1789, the year the U.S. Constitution was ratified and the year the French Revolution began. During the uprising, French aristocrats fled across the border into Stuttgart to escape massacre.

To everyone's surprise, a young woman of Stuttgart began to speak perfect French and to behave like a highborn French lady. She now spoke German with a French accent. As the "French Woman," she remembered everything she said and did. As the German woman, she knew nothing of the "French Woman." Gmelin somehow discovered that he had the ability to make her shift easily from one personality to another by a wave of his hand. Gmelin's 87-page report of this astonishing young woman was published in his 1791 *Materialen fur die Anthropologie.*

355

It would be strange, indeed, were we to surmise that in humankind's vast history, what we now know as multiple personality disorder (MPD) should not have existed prior to 1789, springing suddenly as Athena from the brow of Zeus. But from an epistemological viewpoint, no knowledge can properly be said to exist before it is conceptualized; and from an empirical perspective, no objective entity exists until it is rendered independently verifiable. For an alternative to this stance, see Ellenberger (1970) and Kluft (1991), both of whom, in essence, understand multiple personality as the secularization of what were widely prevalent possession syndromes.

What Gmelin described has been given many names. "Exchanged personality," when observed by French scientists seeing similar patients, was called *double conscience* and came to be described by English-speaking scientists as "dual consciousness," "alternating personality," "multiple personality," and "split personality." By the mid-1980s, it was being called "multiple personality disorder," which, in 1987, became its official designation in DSM-III-R (American Psychiatric Association 1987).

The still-elusive and ever-changing name of this disorder is an issue of major importance in the history of what will be called for the time "Gmelin's syndrome." The specific implications of this issue will be discussed later in this chapter.

Although we know little of the long-term impact of Gmelin's case, we know much about the detail and impact of the Mary Reynolds case, published 25 years later. The curious circumstances involving Mary Reynolds first came to light in 1815 and were first published in 1816 in *Medical Repository* in New York, by Dr. S. L. Mitchell.

The main facts are these: Ms. Reynolds was born in 1785 in Birmingham, England. Her family emigrated to Meadville, Pennsylvania, in the Western Allegheny region. She was the second oldest of 8 children; 20 years separated the births of the oldest and youngest. She was described as having been brought up in a strongly religious atmosphere. As a child, she seemed melancholy, shy, and given to solitary religious devotions and meditations.

[Nevertheless] she was considered normal until she was about eighteen . . . when she began to have occasional "fits," which were evidently hysterical. One of these attacks, when she was about nineteen years old, left her blind and deaf for five or six weeks. Some three months later, she slept eighteen or twenty hours and awoke seeming to know scarcely anything that she had learned. She soon became familiar with her surroundings, however, and within a few weeks learned reading, calculating, and writing, though her penmanship was crude compared to what it had been. Now she was buoyant, witty, fond of company and a lover of nature. . . . After five weeks of this new life, she slept again, and awoke as her "normal" self, with no memory of what she had experienced since her recent lapse. (Greaves 1980)

Such a précis gives little justice to the wealth of detail presented in historical multiple personality cases, nor to the importance accorded them. Indeed, the Mary Reynolds case was written about many times throughout the 19th century in ever-greater detail, including an autobiography by Ms. Reynolds herself. The published case literature on 19th- and early 20th-century multiple personality would occupy several volumes if published as a single edited work.

I have been known to speak at length on the events that led to multiple personality being regarded as an uncommon but by no means rare condition in the 19th century—and certainly an occurrence worthy of great study—while being regarded as an anomaly and annoyance throughout much of the 20th century. Such lectures can be reduced to a single statement: French-speaking psychiatry dominated the English-speaking world during the 19th century; German-speaking psychiatry has dominated much of the 20th.

A hundred years ago, French psychiatry and neurology were intensively focused on 1) hypnosis and hypnotic phenomena; 2) puzzling divisions of consciousness with amnesia; and 3) the quasi-neurologic anomalies of hysteria, led by Jean Martin Charcot and later by Pierre Janet. On the American shore stood William James and Morton Prince, both intensively interested in divided states of consciousness. It was a marriage made in heaven: the Salpêtrière, France's famous hospital, in the flower of its influence, was communicating through its professors with Harvard University, during its own greatest period of psychological and philosophical discovery (Ellenberger 1970).

The consummate event in the first period of the history of interest in Gmelin's syndrome occurred in 1906. Pierre Janet, the author of a famous book on dissociation, was invited to speak at the Harvard Medical School. He spoke on Felida X, the most extensively documented case of multiple personality known to French physicians at the time, and he compared her with Mary Reynolds. In the meantime, William James had already published on Ansel Bourne (1890), Morton Prince (1906) had gone to press with the Christine Beauchamp case, and all three scholars knew the Mary Reynolds case well. This was the first known transatlantic meeting on the subject of multiple personality.

1907–1943

The period from the first description of Gmelin's syndrome in 1791 to the first transatlantic meeting of scholars at Harvard in 1906 covers a period of 115 years—years rich in such reports.

Interest in Gmelin's syndrome certainly did not die in 1906 following Janet's Harvard lecture; in fact, it increased. Prince published more examples of the syndrome. He founded the still-published *Journal of Abnormal Psychology*—partially as a vehicle for further describing such cases as might be found by himself and others—and *Dissociation of a Personality* created a fervor of interest in the field. As late as the 1960s and 1970s, the Beauchamp case was cited in almost all major psychiatric and abnormal psychology texts as the prototypical example of multiple personality.

Looking back with the inevitable wisdom of hindsight, this has proved to be unfortunate, both in terms of adding to the deficiencies of textbook education of mental health professionals and in contributing to the difficulties that they have encountered with certain kinds of patients. It implies no disrespect for Prince and his enormous contributions to observe that in retrospect, and by contemporary standards, the perception of the case of Ms. Beauchamp as paradigmatic is misleading in many regards. Those now specializing in the field of treating Gmelin's syndrome are still struggling to deal with certain aspects of the Beauchamp case study, which in many ways leaves itself open to the interpretation that multiple personality is a hypnotically mediated iatrogenic phenomenon. Iatrogenesis is the subject of four papers and a discussant's lengthy summary in an issue of *Dissociation* (Coons 1989; Fine 1989; Greaves 1989; Kluft 1989; Torem 1989). In sum, the consensus of contemporary experts is that many phenomena of MPD can be induced on a transient basis with relative facility, but there is no evidence that true and stable clinical MPD can be created iatrogenically.

There is no reason to believe that the existence of Gmelin's syndrome has ever declined in frequency, given what we now know of its origins; we have no reason either to believe that its prevalence has increased. We do know that reports have increased geometrically since 1980.

The crucial importance of how an observable (empirical) entity is described and how it is classified is one of Aristotle's ultimate contributions to science. How our use of language influences how we think and act (i.e., how the use of language affects outcomes) is the great contribution of the 20th-century school of British analytical philosophy.

Earlier I mentioned the problem of what Gmelin's syndrome should be called. Consider the brief quote from Bleuler's psychiatric text:

> It is not alone in hysteria that one finds an arrangement of personalities one succeeding the other. Through similar mechanisms schizophrenia produces different personalities existing side by side. As a matter of fact there is no need delving into those rare though most demonstrable hysterical cases, we can produce the very same through hypnosis. (Bleuler 1924, p. 138)

Eugene Bleuler, the author of the above passage, thereby included at least some instances of Gmelin's syndrome in his global diagnosis of schizophrenia. Those remaining cases, which he deemed hysterical, he relegated (at least by implication) to the realm of hypnotic artifacts.

In today's world, psychiatrists and clinical psychologists abound;

textbooks and scientific papers are published by the thousands each year. From this perspective, it is difficult to imagine how the writings of a handful of turn-of-the-century European psychiatrists should have an impact on the field for decades to come.

However, a century ago there were few psychiatrists; and although comparatively few writings appeared, they often were of extremely high caliber and widely read. How do we account for their continuing influence, despite their inaccuracies? Social psychologists have come to know this phenomenon as "inoculation theory" and have studied it intensively. Roughly speaking, this means that whoever relates information first—"whoever gets there the firstest with the mostest"—is in a highly advantaged position. This is because the first storyteller is the one who sets the stage around which all else, at least initially, revolves. Applied inoculation theory may be described as follows.

An eminently successful tort attorney explained the principle to me in his own words:

> When a civil damages suit is brewing, even if your client has obviously done the damage, you always look for a way of finding a legitimate way of filing a suit of complaint against the aggrieved party before they have a chance to file. You always want to be in the plaintiff's position in a damages suit, if there is any way to get there. You want to be first to explain to the jury what the issues in the case are and their legal origin. You want to be in the position of the first to accuse of wrongdoing. You want to set the tone of the case. And this process can go on and on for hours and days. No matter how worthy the aggrieved's complaint, their suit is reduced to a countersuit. They have the burden not only of proving their grievance, but also of overcoming all the testimony and points of law made against them, even before they have had a chance to utter a single word in court. (Henderson, personal communication, July 1988)

This is not meant to imply that Bleuler had any intent of using "inoculation" as a way of conscripting Gmelin's syndrome into his fold of ideas. It merely serves to demonstrate how powerful the phenomenon is, and how it can be used deliberately to one's advantage.

Profound upheavals in Europe during the second period I have selected to describe brought a stream of brilliantly educated, German-speaking psychiatrists to the comparatively safe havens of English-speaking nations. Although many, if not most, were Jewish men and women escaping from the terrible events in Germany and German-occupied and German-influenced nations, their intellectual heritage and orientation reflected German psychiatry's values and tenets. They wrote diligently of what they knew; they had their previous and current writings translated into English; and they exerted an enormous influence on a world much insulated from high European scholarship, and with them many brought the rich traditions of Freud, Bleuler, and Kraepelin.

The relatively peaceful English-speaking nations, struggling to understand the insanity of the world, readily embraced these explanations of madness (even if they did not fully understand them) and published them widely. That is why, through this inoculation of ideas, English-speaking countries have come to be dominated by the peculiarities of Germanic psychiatric ideas.

By 1943, Gmelin's syndrome had been pronounced extinct by an eminent immigrant author. In a world filled with woe, in which countless millions of "civilized people" were being killed willy-nilly in a seemingly senseless conflagration, who cared whether some civilian in Stuttgart suddenly spoke French and did not remember it?

What the world needed was aggregate data in order to treat its psychiatric casualties in a planet gone insane. That it got: from Kraeplin, Bleuler, and Freud.

1944–1979

In 1944, only months after MPD had been declared "extinct," Taylor and Martin (1944) published a celebrated review paper in the journal founded by Morton Prince, which is now called *The Journal of Abnormal Psychology*. For 30 years this landmark paper, which surveyed all the world's cases known to its authors, was the most quoted reference in the history of the illness. Its tabular and columnar presentation of extremely difficult cases; its use of unfamiliar terms such as "coconsciousness," which can be either "one way or two way"; its uninterrupted, chronological series of cases; and its listing of the number of personalities are all precursors to Richard Kluft's method of presentation of much of his serial data. Ironically, the principal historical use of Taylor and Martin's review as a citation has been to prove both that multiple personality exists and that it is rare.

For 13 years after the publication of this pivotal paper—blackout time—no classical case of Gmelin's syndrome was published in extensive form. Then, in 1957, Corbett Thigpen and Hervey Cleckley published *The Three Faces of Eve*. Few realize that Thigpen and Cleckley's scientific studies of Chris Costner Sizemore, including electroencephalogram data, psychological testing, and so forth, were first published in 1954 in Morton Prince's journal.

Upon discovering Chris's inescapably explicit multiplicity, the Augusta, Georgia, psychiatrists sought sources on how to treat her and were led to Morton Prince's puzzling case of Christine Beauchamp, from which they received little direction.

Cleckley's gift was that of a great descriptive writer. He noticed small things and could weave them into a pattern of great discernment into which "everything fit." His *Mask of Sanity* (1964) remains a classic work in the description and diagnosis of "psychopaths."

Cleckley's pen is everywhere in *Eve*. It is an evenhanded description of what he and Corbett Thigpen experienced. There is no hype, no misplaced optimism, no treatment plan, no promises. *Eve* the book reads as the faithful monitoring of two psychiatrists, senior and junior, who haven't the slightest idea how to treat the patient and who dismiss her at the end, when she is somewhat stabilized, wishing her well and knowing that she still experiences amnesia.

The Academy Award–winning movie is quite different in many ways from the book it was based on, but the portrayal by Joanne Woodward of the "switching" of personalities is so clinically accurate, so typical of explicit cases of MPD, that the effect is chilling.

The whole world cannot be collectively fooled by any fraud or propaganda. *The Three Faces of Eve* rang true. Common sense dictates that whatever rituals comfort adults in their mourning, forcing a young child to kiss the body of her dead grandmother on the lips would leave a lasting, albeit not positive, impression on the child's mind. Common knowledge would also lead us to suspect that parents who would be so insensitive as to enforce such an act, despite the young child's screaming, could be insensitive to the child in other ways.

The symptoms of flagrant multiple personality were brilliantly described by Thigpen and Cleckley. They were less successful in outlining issues of etiology and treatment, although the strange illness seemed to be linked with childhood trauma and was minimally responsive to their therapeutic efforts.

In 1971, a remarkable paper appeared seemingly out of nowhere, authored by Margareta Bowers and six other contributors, entitled "Therapy of Multiple Personality." This article is noteworthy for several reasons. First of all, with little explanation, it outlines a canon of rules for treating multiple personality, most of which almost every expert in the field follows scrupulously to this day. Second, the paper is rarely cited. Third, almost no scholar in the field seems to give this paper much weight. Fourth, it appeared to be based on experience with patients with Gmelin's syndrome at a time in which such unpublished aggregate treatment accumulated experience with these allegedly rare patients was totally unheard of. A fifth peculiarity of this work is that it was published in the *International Journal of Clinical and Experimental Hypnosis,* rather than in Prince's still-surviving journal. The sixth oddity is that the data base from which the paper obviously derives is missing and is not even alluded to in passing.

The summation of the paper by Bowers and her colleagues, brilliant as it was, is that were a clinician to see a rare case of Gmelin's syndrome, he or she should treat it thus and so. In 1971, even in its accuracy, the paper fell stillborn from the press. Fourteen years had passed since the Eve case; the paper, in its time, was considered irrelevant. If submitted today, editors of major journals would be clamoring for it, insisting on publishing the data base. The Bowers paper would be lengthy and detailed and would produce a progeny of follow-up papers. Instead, it fell through the cracks, like so many advances published before their time.

While *The Three Faces of Eve* was still in press, Cornelia Wilbur was struggling to understand and treat a young woman from Nebraska who had most remarkable symptoms. The therapy required 16 years and has become the most important clinical case of multiple personality in the twentieth century, *Sybil*.

The case of *Sybil* (Schreiber 1973) has become a landmark for many reasons, of which I will mention two. For one thing, *Sybil* was written, based on notes of historical transactions between Dr. Wilbur and her patient, by a third person, a professor of English and a professional writer. This lent a whole new dimension to traditional case studies. Instead of first- and second-person accounts of interpersonal transactions—you, me, and we—we are introduced for the first time to the linguistic objectivity of third-person accounts. A skilled observer and organizer of ideas, immune to the intense transference and countertransference emotions inherent in the relationship between doctor and patient, Flora Rheta Schreiber was able to describe the complex of interactions and the participants in a unique way. What resulted is a rare view into a patient's uninterpreted symptoms, a psychiatrist's frustrations, and the teasing-out of what is going on between the two. Flora Rheta Schreiber became the Boswell to Wilbur's (and Sybil's) Dr. Johnson.

The second landmark value of the Sybil case is that of the tenacity of Dr. Wilbur in validating what her patient had told her. She interviewed Sybil's parents, she took Sybil to the home of her childhood, she spoke with Sybil's doctor and reviewed his records: everything fit. In short, this single case study is a classic in the study of the sequelae of child abuse. Dr. Wilbur received much criticism from her peers for publishing such an intimate and provocative case in the public press, though she had been denied publication in psychiatric journals (Wilbur 1989).

Allison and Kluft

Meanwhile, Ralph Allison, a Stanford-trained psychiatrist in California, had been seeing large numbers of patients with Gmelin's syndrome, and was being severely criticized by colleagues for making the diagnosis (Allison and Schwarz 1980). Nevertheless, he published and lectured on what he saw, his publications being often relegated to obscure journals.

Richard Kluft, a Harvard-trained physician moving toward a career in psychoanalysis, watched his practice almost wither and die when he started diagnosing and talking to his colleagues about Gmelin's syndrome. Like Drs. Wilbur and Allison, Dr. Kluft was also refused publication of his findings in mainstream psychiatric journals.

I also came into the picture during this time. Trained as a scholar in philosophy and psychology specializing in the mind-body problem, analytic philosophy, personality theory, and clinical psychology, I could not understand how I could come upon a florid case of multiple personality during my first year of clinical practice, be referred a second case 3 years later by a general surgeon, meet Cornelia Wilbur and David Caul a few months later and learn that they were identifying these patients in great numbers, be referred yet another such patient 3 years later, and reconcile these data with the notion that multiple personality is rare or nonexistent.

The numbers did not fit; the clinical presentation of the patients did. For a year of lengthy Fridays, I combed the stacks of my university library, searching for any detail I could learn about multiple personality. Out of this research came a lengthy and explosive review article on the subject.

1980–1984

The gathering storm culminated in five independent landmark publications in 1980, the watershed year of clinicians' unwavering interest in Gmelin's syndrome.

The first of these was the description of multiple personality as a separate diagnostic entity in the new DSM-III (American Psychiatric Association 1980), divorcing it from both hysteria and schizophrenia, to which it had been tied.

The second cannon to fire was the book by Ralph Allison and Ted Schwarz, *Minds in Many Pieces* (1980), for which one can basically create a précis as follows: "I don't care who you guys think you are; I'm a Stanford-trained psychiatrist; I see this case as Gmelin's syndrome, I've got to treat this patient for what I see as being wrong. If you want data, go to meetings, read my papers, and read my book."

The third important publication of the year was Milton Rosenbaum's (1980) realization that, based on Bleuler's text, Gmelin's syndrome may have been inadvertently tied to the diagnosis of schizophrenia in the minds of psychiatrists. If so, those reading Rosenbaum's paper thought, patients with Gmelin's syndrome may be being precisely mistreated. Gmelin's syndrome requires psychotherapy and hypnotherapy; schizophrenia requires neuroleptic pharmacology.

My extensive review (Greaves 1980) and analysis of the known world's literature on the subject was published in October 1980 as the lead article in *The Journal of Nervous and Mental Disease,* including tracts and summaries of the Allison and Schwarz book, which had become available as my paper was in press. This paper, which stressed that Gmelin's syndrome was wholly plausible, understandable, and probably not rare, soon replaced Taylor and Martin (1944) as the standard reference in the field.

Finally, in December 1980, Eugene Bliss first advanced his now-famous hypothesis that subjects of Gmelin's syndrome had what he has repeatedly characterized as an "autohypnotic illness." He reported 14 examples from his recent clinical experience. In Bliss's formulation of the problem, therapists do not induce Gmelin's syndrome; patients do.

Suddenly, a whole new ball team had come to town.

Myron Boor (1982), upon reading my paper, further explored one of his many contentions: that the presumed rarity of multiple personality was a self-fulfilling prophecy. Boor located 29 additional cases in the recent literature that I had overlooked, and the *Journal of Nervous and Mental Disease* put another paper on Gmelin's syndrome in press during 1982. Between the two papers, the two of us were able to demonstrate that half again as many cases of multiple personality were known in the 1970s alone as had been reported in the preceding century and a half.

The effect of the 1980–1982 papers can be compared to offensive linemen opening a hole in the defensive line for a swift halfback to run through. In a sense this analogy is completely false, for in 1980–1982 there was neither a true team nor a sense of the game being played. As a figure in this history, I did not even know there were any halfbacks available to run the ball. That had changed dramatically by 1984. However, even in 1980, there was an amazing sense of camaraderie among those few professionals who had encountered the strange phenomenon of Gmelin's syndrome and had become aware of one another's work. They were drawn to one another, as if all had had a close encounter of the third kind.

By 1984, there was so much interest in Gmelin's syndrome in the psychiatric world that four journals devoted entire special issues to the subject: *Psychiatric Annals, Psychiatric Clinics of North America, The International Journal of Clinical and Experimental Hypnosis,* and *The American Journal of Clinical Hypnosis* (the latter dated 1983, but in fact distributed in 1984). Papers were flying everywhere, at dizzying speeds—not just any papers, but some excellent ones. It was as if a dam had broken, unable to resist the gravity and force of the flood of waters behind it.

The Case of Billy Milligan

1981 saw the publication of Daniel Keyes's *The Minds of Billy Milligan* (1981). It was the second of the Sybil-type case reports. Written by a professional writer, also a professor of English, *Milligan,* like *Sybil,* benefited from the advantages of a third-person account. Keyes, unlike a psychotherapist, was free to interview anybody and everybody about any matter at any time, limited only by the willingness of other potential resource persons to talk to him. Because of Keyes's dogged scholarship, the Billy Milligan case is the best-documented and most contextualized case study of multiple personality ever written.

To give a précis of the Milligan account: Young adult females living on and around the campus of Ohio State University reported being raped. The impression among the public developed that there existed a demented "campus rapist" who preyed on young coeds. A furor ensued. A suspect was picked up; the forensic psychologist who interviewed him suspected that he had MPD. A famous and ultraconservative psychiatrist offered the facilities of his hospital to study the patient. He consulted with Cornelia Wilbur and David Caul, who concurred that the patient had flagrant multiple personality. The psychiatrist exhaustively documented the patient's condition to the judge in the case. Ultimately, the patient was found "not guilty" of his crimes "by reason of insanity." Acquittal means innocence of criminal intent but does not mean freedom. Milligan, the adjudicated, instead was remanded into treatment with Dr. Caul, the medical director of a state hospital. He did well under Dr. Caul's care. However, he was accused of committing unsubstantiated crimes while out on passes. His treatment with Dr. Caul was interrupted, and Milligan was sent to several locked facilities for criminally insane inmates.

The Founding of the ISSMP&D

In the first 18 months following the publication of my 1980 "Mary Reynolds" paper, I received requests for more than 5,000 copies of my work from more than 55 countries. Such events are exceedingly unusual in scientific publishing. Clearly, the paper spoke to concerns of thousands of clinicians.

During the summer of 1982, I began forming a "steering committee" to guide me in understanding the impact of these ideas and to bring together others of a similar mind. By November 1982, this group consisted of myself, David Caul, Emmanuel Berman (Israel), John Burns, Jane Yates, Jackie Damgaard, Helen Coale, and Jeffrey Brandsma.

A computer was purchased to handle the still-burgeoning mail within my office. Mailing lists were compiled from my correspondence and from Ralph Allison's list of those to whom he had sent his brief-lived newsletter *Memos on Multiplicity*. The Atlanta study group was born, meeting on a weekly basis. *The ISSMP Newsletter* began to be published on a quarterly basis, containing all the latest news in the field, and the idea was born to form an organization of and for clinicians who had encountered and had expressed an interest in Gmelin's syndrome. Dues in the prospective organization were to be $12.00 per year to cover the cost of mailings, and those who joined in the first year could become charter members.

The response was unbelievably vigorous and the new paperwork awesome. It soon became evident that there existed a vast, almost secret underground of loosely networked clinicians who were intensively studying Gmelin's syndrome and had compiled highly esoteric, unpublished knowledge about it.

In March 1983, I was fortunate to make contact with Chris Sizemore ("Eve") in Atlanta, while she was on a speaking tour. Mrs. Sizemore had become a major advocate for the mental health field and had a large constituency. Upon explaining my plans for organizing the field, she readily agreed to support the effort and agreed to become a part of the steering committee (Sizemore 1989). This was followed by a trip to New York that April to meet with Richard Kluft, Bennett Braun, Frank Putnam, Roberta Sachs, and Jane Dubrow. All but Ms. Dubrow were faculty members at what was by then an annual American Psychiatric Association training workshop on Gmelin's syndrome, first presented in 1978, with Ralph Allison as the director and with David Caul and Cornelia Wilbur among the faculty.

By the end of that long, dream-filled meeting, where we discussed where we would like to see the field headed, all the practitioners present agreed to join the Steering Committee of the fledgling International Society for the Study of Multiple Personality. An implicit agreement was made to assist one another in completing individual projects that seemed impossible to achieve within the time frames discussed. Braun would organize international meetings; Kluft would further the interest of scholarship; Putnam would serve as the organizer of scientific research; I would continue to organize the field as a specialized discipline; and Sachs would serve at any point position, as needed. This division of labors continued to exist along the original lines conceived for several years. As for Ms. Dubrow, she and Dr. Braun later married.

1985–Present

Every impossible dream discussed at that table at Mama Leone's Restaurant on the evening of April 30, 1983, has been realized in abundance. The fledgling Society, renamed the International Society for the Study of Multiple Personality and Dissociation, grew from 11 members in the autumn of 1982 to more than 2,750 members by the end of November 1992. Frank Putnam has written a landmark book in the field, integrating 356 general resources with his own clinical work (1989). Colin Ross (1989) published another general text of importance. The Seventh Annual International Conference on Multiple Personality/Dissociation met in Chicago in 1989. The DSM-III-R was published, and it removed the label of "rare" from MPD.

Books and articles on the subject proliferated during this period—some of enormous importance (e.g., Braun 1986; Kluft 1985; Putnam 1989), the greater and the lesser all carefully collected, catalogued, and annotated in *The ISSMP&D Newsletter* by Philip Coons and Richard Loewenstein, updating earlier comprehensive collections of the literature by Boor and Coons (1983) and Damgaard and colleagues (1985). This consolidated collection of titles, available from the ISSMP&D, is decidedly more comprehensive than that available from computerized abstracting services.

Hospital programs for the treatment of MPD patients have sprung up nationwide in Chicago, Atlanta, Akron, Denver, Birmingham, Dallas-Fort Worth, and Philadelphia. *The ISSMP&D Newsletter,* edited by Braun, and published by the Ridgeview Institute, has a constantly expanding readership. *Dissociation,* the official journal of the ISSMP&D, edited by Kluft and published by Ridgeview Institute, attracted more than 3,100 subscribers during its first 48 months of existence.

This period was one of consolidation in the organization, study, and treatment of multiple personality and dissociative states. Given the vehicle of a professional confederation—by which is meant a voluntary union of factions, united for a common purpose, willing to follow agreed-upon principles of procedure—more publications and presentations on multiple personality-related topics has occurred during this brief period than in any previous period of history. Outstanding among them has been Richard Kluft's series of papers and lectures that, in tandem with his earlier works, will inevitably become a permanent legacy in the history of psychiatry.

The Future

It is now more than a century since the publication of William James's great psychological masterwork of 1890 that, among other things, articulated in detail the phenomena of altered and divided states of consciousness, including multiple personality. During this century, interest in multiple personality has come full circle, from a period of intense focal interest, to a period of extreme neglect, to a period of focal interest once again. As in 1890, there is renewed scholarly and clinical interest in hypnosis, dissociation, and the work of Janet and certain other 19th-century French physicians.

The good news is that as the pendulum of interest in Gmelin's syndrome has swung back to the forefront of psychiatry; the syndrome is much better understood by more people than ever before; an enormous and detailed literature has appeared in the course of a single decade; and all of this is underpinned by a highly successful, steadily growing professional society. To paraphrase Richard Loewenstein's (1989) comments at the First Eastern Regional Conference on MPD and Dissociation:

> Never in the history of psychiatry have we ever come to know so well the specific etiology of a major mental illness, its natural course, its treatment. . . . nor has there ever been such a grass roots movement to research and understand such a disorder.

The bad news is that there are few therapists trained up to the task of treating these patients (Greaves 1980, 1988), that many clinicians have developed irrational reactions both to these patients and to the colleagues who treat them (Allison and Schwarz 1980; Dell 1989; Goodwin 1985; Greaves 1988), that there are still some serious gaps in the literature, that considerable "educational lag" exists in psychiatry in the form of pervasive "myths" about the illness (Dell 1989), and that "conceptual anomalies" continue to exist in the field that need to be addressed and resolved (Greaves 1989).

For the remainder of this chapter, I will focus on what I regard as one of the vexing central problems in the history of Gmelin's syndrome, alias "multiple personality," "split personality," "MPD," and so on. The following I regard as one of the understressed areas in the literature, which tends to keep MPD studies "unintegrated" with the mainstream of psychiatric thinking and intersects with some of the other issues I have discussed. This is the area of "conceptual anomalies."

The Syndrome in Search of a Name

The etymological variations of the term "multiple personality" are fascinating in that they describe a condition in which individuals typically call themselves by numerous names and experience themselves in vastly different ways. However, it is somewhat unsettling that the scientific community, like the patients it studies, has encountered a psychiatric entity for more than 200 years that cannot pin it down with a suitable name.

The term "Gmelin's syndrome," although enjoying the advantage of neutrality, does not describe currently known conditions as they have been encountered, which are typically far more complex than Gmelin's example.

"Multiple personality," as this group of conditions has been known throughout the present century, suffers as a construct in that the term is an oxymoron (i.e., paired words containing contradictory concepts; Greaves 1989). The term "personality" refers to the collective range of behavior an individual exhibits over time; hence, one logically cannot exhibit more than one collective range of behavior, let alone many. Despite how an MPD patient might experience and therefore describe her or his state of being, different people of varying ages and sizes and sexes with different minds and souls do not, in fact, inhabit the same body.

My focus here is on two related points. First of all, it is admittedly difficult for psychiatrists or anyone else trained in systematic thinking to "believe" in a logically impossible construct. It is quite true, conceptually, that "multiple personality" per se cannot exist. But it does not follow thereby that there might not exist a corresponding empirical syndrome that is conceptually ill-conceived and consequently misnamed. Second, although all master psychotherapists learn their patients' patois and symbol systems as a medium of communication, the ability to communicate in the patient's language is in no way an endorsement of the patient's ideas or behavior.

To address the second point first, the master's principle above is effective only when a strong boundary exists between patient and therapist and is established and maintained by the therapist, which allows for the patient's struggle to communicate his or her experiences and personal truth. This is the basis for the interpretive process in psychotherapy; the therapist cannot interpret what he or she has not yet learned to understand in the patient's idiosyncratic language-symbol-conceptual system.

Many professional therapists never become masters because they have never learned to hear; they only tell rigidly. But there is the corollary error: some therapists learn their patients' language-symbol-conceptual system so well that they forget their own, disregard their ego-boundaries, and become so drawn into their patients' internal object world that they assimilate huge masses of their patients' "object" world as their own. When this blurring of ego boundaries and intradyadic object relations occurs, the stage is set for the most amazing misadventures in psychotherapy (Greaves 1988).

How this language aspect fits into treatment run awry is that an alarming number of therapists working with Gmelin's syndrome patients actually believe they are working with different people. Once they lose sight of a patient's intrinsic wholeness (an error that often occurs as soon as the diagnosis is made), treatment may become chaotic unless the therapist correctly reconceptualizes the nature of the problem he or she is dealing with.

The dissociative disorders field has repeatedly addressed the problem of both describing and naming Gmelin's syndrome. It is due to many individual (probably unconscious) insights into the language problem of multiple personality that we owe the term "multiple personality disorder", by which all contemporary writers refer to Gmelin's syndrome. It is easier to smuggle an extra word into a descriptive term than to change the term entirely. By encouraging the use of the term "disorder," it is my impression that those who took up the use of the term and the committee that wrote the Dissociative Disorders section of DSM-III-R were trying to mitigate the problem by creating a term which meant "a disorder with the traditional properties of multiple personality." This intervention has worked rather well for those familiar with the field, who have seized upon the use of "MPD" as a neutral term, much as I have employed the use of "Gmelin's syndrome" here.

One problem with this deft move is that the words "personality" and "disorder" become paired in the new construction. The authors of DSM-III-R never have intended to include multiple personality among the personality disorders, a group of disorders involving longstanding maladaptive behavior patterns and traditionally regarded as rather refractory to treatment.

The unfortunate outcome of the MPD language construct is that many newcomers to the contemporary literature believe that the authors themselves construe MPD as a type of personality disorder. This notion is reinforced when, as a peer reviewer of case records, I see "multiple personality" listed as an Axis II diagnosis. When other case reviewers subsequently observe how difficult these patients can be to treat, they are twice convinced that MPD is a character disorder, excusing altogether any consideration that it may be flaws in both the therapist and the therapy that is the primary cause of the treatment difficulty.

Kluft has taken note of this language problem, and in a lengthy discussion in *Dissociation* (1988), he began to speak of multiple personality as a "disaggregate self state disorder" (Kluft 1988b, p. 51). Although the selected term is exquisitely true of MPD patients, its opposite is not true of normal personality. Normal personality is a functionally integrated unit of many components, not an aggregate of components. Historically, this point has been brilliantly argued in Immanuel Kant's reply to David Hume's "bundle theory" of the self in Kant's masterpiece, *Critique of Pure Reason*.

Calling a Spade a Spade

"Multiple personality" is what analytic philosophers like to call a "silly concept." I have reviewed briefly several struggles with the term and some attempts to repair it. However, once one works with many patients with Gmelin's syndrome, it becomes clear that one is struggling with two conceptual problems, not one. It is not only impossible to conceive of several "persons" occupying one body (or "one person occupying several bodies," as one often hears the subjective experience formulated by patients); it is also impossible to regard Gmelin's syndrome as a neurosis.

When a 38-year-old patient "switches" in one's office, believes earnestly that she is a 13-year-old boy at her uncle's house in St. Louis and that the year is 1965, and then spontaneously reenacts an anal rape (which is why, in trance logic, "she" believes she is a "boy"), hallucinating the therapist as the uncle, the patient is disoriented as to person, place, time, and situation on mental status. That is what "psychosis" is known to mean in the examination of psychiatric patients: a gross breakdown in reality and orientation, whether transient, episodic, or chronic, based on the clinician's understanding of the patient's history. Furthermore, many of these patients hallucinate, experience lengthy periods of profound agnosia (i.e., an inability to recognize familiar people, objects, and places), and are otherwise so grossly disoriented in all spheres that they require complete supervision. These same patients are not only refractory to the use of antipsychotic medications, but most grow increasingly psychotic with their use.

Based on these recurring experiences, one is led to conceive of MPD as a "transient, episodic, recurrent dissociative psychosis of traumatic origin." The problem with this definition is that it does not distinguish well between MPD and posttraumatic stress disorder (PTSD), nor does it distinguish the central feature of MPD: that it is a disorder of identity.

The Essence of MPD

MPD patients uniquely experience "multiple identity disorder." Most believe themselves to be different people, caught up in different times, with enormous gaps of memory and discontinuity of attitude and experience, depending on where they believe themselves to be at the moment. They are "disordered" because they cannot perform consistently in any given social role. From moment to moment they may be lovers, infants, attackers, helpers, teachers, parents, and so on, in a disturbingly inappropriate way. Viewed from the standpoint of role theory, MPD patients periodically exhibit cacophonous role behavior. Viewed from the standpoint of object relations theory, MPD patients periodically experience chaos in their internal object relations, which leads to the acute deterioration of their role performances. Why this is so has been extensively but not exhaustively explored as sequelae to actual trauma.

MPD and Schizophrenia

It may be argued that researchers in MPD may simply be describing schizophrenia in more delineated and precise terms than ever before. There is some merit to this claim, because it has been shown above that (at least in terms of nomenclature) there has been a historical overlap of quite some significance between these disorders, following Bleuler (1911/1980). Furthermore, were this to be true, it would be a happy event for psychiatry.

Fortunately or unfortunately, this surmise is not accurate. Let us consider just a few of the variables that distinguish MPD from schizophrenia. MPD is highly responsive to psychotherapy; schizophrenia is not. MPD is negatively responsive to the use of neuroleptics; schizophrenia is highly responsive. MPD patients, as a group, are highly susceptible to hypnosis; schizophrenic patients are comparatively nonresponsive—in fact, poorly responsive. Acute psychotic episodes in MPD patients tend to be transitory, lasting a few moments to a few hours; such episodes in schizophrenic patients tend to persist for days. MPD patients, while disoriented as to person, place, time, and the role and identity of others, do not tend to exhibit ongoing schizophrenic mentation processes. Nowhere in the extensive literature on schizophrenia is there any consistent mention of such patients assuming diverse identities, nor is it a diagnostic criterion of the disorder, whereas multiple identity formations is the hallmark of MPD. The list of differences could go on and is probably worthy of another extensive comparison at this point in time.

Conclusions Based on the Current Literature and Lore

Multiple personality is a major mental illness, known to be widely distributed in the populations of the United States and Canada. It takes the form of recurrent episode psychoses, in which overtly normal individuals suddenly, overtly, and earnestly believe they are different people. It rarely takes the form of so-called past life experiences. It is highly correlated with reports of extreme, historical traumatic events in which the patient has had to rely on an emergency anxiety defense—dissociation—in order to survive the traumatic experience(s) psychologically. Such experiences usually begin during early childhood and tend to have been repeated a number of times over the course of many years, often under the drive of repetition compulsion and in the context of a nonhealing family.

The disorder is manifested in adulthood by drastic and unexplainable alterations in role performance, usually accompanied by symptoms of profound amnesia, which is explained away by the subject on confrontation through expert and often convincing confabulation.

The treatment of choice is intensive psychotherapy, the focus of which is consistent with what Kluft (1988a) has called "strategic integrationism" or "tactical integrationalism," facilitated with hypnosis, combined with the judicious use of ancillary chemotherapy, mainly the prescribing of anxiolytics and occasionally antidepressants (Barkin et al. 1986).

To summarize and supplement the salient points above, multiple personality, in its classical form is:

1. A major mental disorder;
2. By no means rare;
3. Characterized by recurrent psychotic episodes in which the subject experiences him- or herself as being completely different and separate persons;
4. During these periods of dissociated, disjunctive identity, which may occur with great frequency or infrequency, the patient may

experience him- or herself as existing in completely different time settings;

5. Such alterations in subjective identity experiences are readily observable by others, to a greater or lesser degree, based on the subject's skill at hiding his or her condition;

6. No other psychiatric syndrome shares the essential feature ("hallmark sign") of multiple personality—that of a consistently established *multiple identity process;*

7. The disorder is of apparent traumatic origin, though not necessarily of brutal origin;

8. The syndrome is propagated by many or most patients through unconscious and excessive use of primitive anxiety defenses, including splitting, autohypnotic dissociation with amnesia, denial, projection, regression, and projective identification;

9. Primary higher-order ego defenses are most often of the obsessive-compulsive type; and

10. The syndrome seems to be best treated by psychotherapists familiar with both the treatment of maladaptive preoedipal psychic defense structures and the pathognomy of hypnotic disorders.

If ever a fertile hunting ground existed for the followers of the rich self psychology theories of Heinz Kohut (1971; Wolf 1989), it is in the field of MPD. A decade of intensive writing on MPD has occurred with nary a flutter from psychoanalysts oriented toward self psychology. The absence of the long tradition of self theory from the current MPD writings is both a loss of opportunity to MPD scholars and to the traditional scholars of self theory. One would expect this lapse of common knowledge to be integrated during the next decade.

References

Allison RB, Schwarz T: Minds in Many Pieces. New York, Rawson, Wade, 1980

American Psychiatric Association: Diagnostic and Statistical Manual of Mental Disorders, 3rd Edition. Washington, DC, American Psychiatric Association, 1980

American Psychiatric Association: Diagnostic and Statistical Manual of Mental Disorders, 3rd Edition, Revised. Washington, DC, American Psychiatric Association, 1987

Barkin R, Braun B, Kluft R: The dilemma of drug treatment for multiple personality disorder patients, in The Treatment of Multiple Personality Disorder. Edited by Braun BG. Washington, DC, American Psychiatric Press, 1986, pp 107–132

Bleuler E: Textbook of Psychiatry. Translated by Brill AA. New York, Macmillan, 1924

Bliss E: Multiple personalities: a report of 14 cases with implications for schizophrenia and hysteria. Arch Gen Psychiatry 37:1388–1397, 1980

Boor M: The multiple personality epidemic: additional cases and inferences regarding diagnosis, ctiology, dynamics and treatment. J Nerv Ment Dis 170:302–304, 1982

Boor M, Coons P: A comprehensive bibliography of literature pertaining to multiple personality. Psychol Rep 53:295–310, 1983

Bowers M, Brecher-Marer S, Newton BW, et al: Therapy of multiple personality. Int J Clin Exp Hypn 22:216–233, 1971

Braun BG (ed): Special issue on multiple personality disorder. Am J Clin Hypn 26, 1983

Braun BG (ed): Symposium on multiple personality. Psychiatr Clin North Am 7(1), 1984

Braun BG (ed): Treatment of Multiple Personality Disorder. Washington, DC, American Psychiatric Press, 1986

Cleckley H: The Mask of Sanity, 4th Edition. St. Louis, IL, CV Mosby, 1964

Coons P: Iatrogenic factors in the misdiagnosis of multiple personality disorder. Dissociation 2:70–76, 1989

Damgaard J, Benschoten SV, Fagan J: An updated bibliography of literature pertaining to multiple personality disorder. Psychol Rep 57:131–137, 1985

Dell P: Professional skepticism about MPD. Paper presented at First Eastern Regional Conference on Multiple Personality and Dissociation, Alexandria, VA, June 24, 1989

Ellenberger H: The Discovery of the Unconscious: The History and Evolution of Dynamic Psychiatry. New York, Basic Books, 1970

Fine C: Treatment errors and iatrogenesis across therapeutic modalities in MPD and allied dissociative disorders. Dissociation 2:77–82, 1989

Gmelin E: Materialen für die Anthropologie. Tübingen, Germany, Cotta, 1791. Quoted in Ellenberger H: The Discovery of the Unconscious: The History and Evolution of Dynamic Psychiatry. New York, Basic Books, 1970, p 127

Goodwin J: Credibility problems in multiple personality patients and abused children, in Childhood Antecedents of Multiple Personality Disorder. Edited by Kluft RP. Washington, DC, American Psychiatric Press, 1985, pp 1–19

Greaves G: Multiple personality 165 years after Mary Reynolds. J Nerv Ment Dis 168:577–596, 1980

Greaves G: Common errors in the treatment of multiple personality disorder. Dissociation 1(1):61–66, 1988

Greaves G: Observations on the claim of iatrogenesis in the promulgation of multiple personality disorder: a discussion. Dissociation 2:99–104, 1989

James W: Principles of Psychology (3 vols). Cambridge, MA, Harvard University Press, 1890 (reprinted 1981)

Keyes D: The Minds of Billy Milligan. New York, Random House, 1981

Kluft RP (ed): Special issue on multiple personality disorder. Psychiatric Annals 14(1), 1984

Kluft RP (ed): Childhood Antecedents of Multiple Personality Disorder. Washington, DC, American Psychiatric Press, 1985

Kluft R: Editorial: Today's therapeutic pluralism. Dissociation 1(4):1–2, 1988a

Kluft R: The phenomenology and treatment of extremely complex multiple personality disorder. Dissociation 1(4):47–58, 1988b

Kluft R: The iatrogenic creation of new alter. Dissociation 2:83–89, 1989

Kluft RP: Multiple personality disorder, in American Psychiatric Press Annual Review of Psychiatry, Vol 10. Edited by Tasman A, Goldfinger S. Washington, DC, American Psychiatric Press, 1991, pp 161–188

Kohut H: The Analysis of the Self. New York, International Universities Press, 1971

Loewenstein R: Dissociative spectrum and phenomenology of MPD. Paper presented at First Eastern Conference on Multiple Personality and Dissociation, Alexandria, VA, June 24, 1989

Mitchell SL: A double consciousness, or a duality of persons in the same individual. Medical Repository 3:185–186, 1816

Prince M: The Dissociation of a Personality. New York, Longmans, Green, 1906

Putnam F: Diagnosis and Treatment of Multiple Personality Disorder. New York, Guilford, 1989

Rosenbaum M: The role of the term schizophrenia in the decline of the diagnosis of multiple personality. Arch Gen Psychiatry 37:1383–1385, 1980

Ross C: Multiple Personality Disorder: Diagnosis, Clinical Features and Treatment. New York, Wiley, 1989

Schreiber F: Sybil. Chicago, IL, Regnery, 1973

Sizemore CC: A Mind of My Own. New York, Morrow, 1989

Taylor W, Martin M: Multiple personality. Journal of Abnormal and Social Psychology 39:281–300, 1944

Thigpen C, Cleckley H: A case of multiple personality. Journal of Abnormal and Social Psychology 49:135–151, 1954

Thigpen C, Cleckley H: The Three Faces of Eve. New York, McGraw-Hill, 1957

Torem M: Iatrogenic factors in the perpetuation of splitting and multiplicity. Dissociation 2:92–99, 1989

Wilbur C: The making of "Sybil." Address delivered at First Easter Regional Conference on Multiple Personality and Dissociation, June 22, 1989

Wolf B: Heinz Kohut's self psychology: a conceptual analysis. Psychotherapy: Theory, Research, and Practice 26(4):545–554, 1989

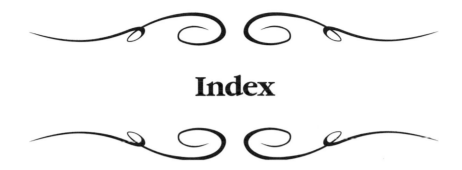

Index

Page numbers printed in **boldface** *type refer to tables.*